2022

ADVANCES IN PSYCHIATRY AND BEHAVIORAL HEALTH

EDITOR-IN-CHIEF
Deepak Prabhakar

SECTION EDITORS
Aryandokht Fotros
Carly Johnco
Lauren M. Osborne
Claudia L. Reardon
Eric A. Storch
Andres G. Viana

ELSEVIER

Editor: Megan Ashdown
Developmental Editor: Hannah Almira Lopez

Editorial Office:
Elsevier, Inc.
1600 John F. Kennedy Blvd,
Suite 1800
Philadelphia, PA 19103-2899

International Standard Serial Number: 2667-3835
International Standard Book Number: 13: 978-0-323-92015-5

CONTRIBUTORS

ESTHER AKINYEMI, MD
Clinical Assistant Professor, Department of Behavioral Health, Henry Ford Health, Detroit, Michigan, USA

CINDY MILLER ARON, LCSW, CGP, FAGPA
Senior Director of Clinical Services, Ascend, Consultation in Health Care, LLC, Chicago, Illinois, USA

SUNIL BHAR, PhD
Professor of Clinical Psychology, Department of Psychological Sciences, School of Health Sciences, Swinburne University of Technology, Australia

JENNIFER L. BRYAN, PhD
Houston VA HSR&D Center for Innovations in Quality, Effectiveness and Safety, Michael E. DeBakey VA Medical Center, VA South Central Mental Illness Research, Education and Clinical Center, Menninger Department of Psychiatry and Behavioral Sciences, Baylor College of Medicine, Houston, Texas, USA

PATRICIA CARLSON
Service Chief, TMS Program, Department of Psychiatry, Sheppard Pratt Health Systems, Towson, Maryland, USA

SANDRA L. CEPEDA, MS
Predoctoral Trainee, Department of Psychology, University of Miami, Coral Gables, Florida, USA

JESSAMINE T-H. CHEN, MPsych (Clin), PhD
Professor, Postdoctoral Fellow, School of Psychological Sciences, Centre for Emotional Health, Centre for Ageing, Cognition and Wellbeing, Macquarie University, Sydney, New South Wales, Australia

JONATHAN S. COMER, PhD
Professor, Florida International University, Center for Children and Families, Miami, Florida, USA

JOHANN M. D'SOUZA, MA
Department of Psychiatry and Behavioral Sciences, Baylor College of Medicine, Department of Psychology, Texas Institute for Measurement, Evaluation, and Statistics, University of Houston, Houston, Texas, USA

TANYA DAVISON, DPsych (Clinical)
Director, Research Discovery, Silver Chain, Australia

MIA J. DRURY, BA
Mclean Hospital, Belmont, Massachusetts, USA

JILL EHRENREICH-MAY, PhD
Professor, Department of Psychology, University of Miami, Coral Gables, Florida, USA

JOEY KA-YEE ESSOE, PhD
Center for OCD, Anxiety, and Related Disorders for Children, Division of Child and Adolescent Psychiatry, Department of Psychiatry and Behavioral Sciences, Johns Hopkins School of Medicine, Baltimore, Maryland, USA

HARRIS EYRE, MBBS, PhD
Neuroscience-Inspired Policy Initiative, OECD, PRODEO Institute and Meadows Mental Health Policy Institute, Deakin University Institute for Mental and Physical Health and Clinical Translation, Global Brain Health Institute at University of California, San Francisco, San Francisco, California, USA; Department of Psychiatry, Baylor College of Medicine, Department of Psychiatry, The University of Texas Health Science Center at Houston, Houston, Texas, USA

ARIANNA FERRETTI, BS
Department of Neuroscience, Brown University, Providence, Rhode Island, USA

RAPHAELA SHEA FONTANA, DO
Department of Psychiatry and Behavioral Medicine, Prisma Health – Upstate, Clinical Assistant Professor, University of South Carolina School of Medicine, Greenville, South Carolina, USA

BRENT P. FORESTER, MD, MSc
Mclean Hospital, Belmont, Massachusetts, USA; Harvard Medical School, Boston, Massachusetts, USA

ARYANDOKHT FOTROS, MD, MSc
Department of Psychiatry and Human Behavior, Brown University, Providence, Rhode Island, USA

GABRIELLE F. FREITAG, MS
Doctoral Student, Florida International University, Center for Children and Families, Miami, Florida, USA

JENNIFER FREYTAG, PhD
Houston VA HSR&D Center for Innovations in Quality, Effectiveness and Safety, Michael E. DeBakey VA Medical Center, VA South Central Mental Illness Research, Education and Clinical Center, Houston, Texas, USA

KATHERINE A. GIFFORD, PsyD
Assistant Professor, Vanderbilt Sports Concussion Center, Department of Neurology, Vanderbilt University Medical Center, Nashville, Tennessee, USA

PAUL GORCZYNSKI, PhD, HCPC, CPsychol, AFBPsS
Senior Lecturer, University of Greenwich, School of Human Sciences, Park Row, London, United Kingdom

ANDREA L.B. GOTTLIEB, PhD
Director of Dialectical Behavior Therapy Program, Sheppard Pratt, Baltimore, Maryland, USA

CHRISTINE E. GOULD, PhD
Geriatric Research Education and Clinical Center (GRECC), Veterans Affairs Palo Alto Health Care System, Palo Alto, California, USA; Department of Psychiatry and Behavioral Sciences, Stanford University School of Medicine, Stanford, California, USA

HANNAH L. GRASSIE, BA
Predoctoral Trainee, Department of Psychology, University of Miami, Coral Gables, Florida, USA

ALYSSA G. HERTZ, MS
Department of Psychiatry and Behavioral Sciences, Baylor College of Medicine, Houston, Texas, USA; Philadelphia College of Osteopathic Medicine, Philadelphia, Pennsylvania, USA

NEHA SHROFF HUDEPOHL, MD
Clinical Associate Professor, Department of Psychiatry, University of South Carolina School of Medicine Greenville/Prisma Health, Greenville, South Carolina, USA

HEMALATHA JAYARAM, DPsych (Clinical)
Senior Clinical Psychologist and Academic, Peter James Centre, Aged Persons Mental Health Services, Eastern Health, Australia

AARON SLONE JECKELL, MD
Voluntary Professor, Vanderbilt Sports Concussion Center, Department of Psychiatry and Behavioral Health, Vanderbilt University School of Medicine, Nashville, Tennessee, USA

RAHUL KHANNA, MBBS, FRANZCP
Director, Innovation and Medical Governance, Phoenix Australia, University of Melbourne, Melbourne, Australia

CHRISTOPHER L. KLINGER, LCSW-C
Dialectical Behavior Therapy Program, Sheppard Pratt, Baltimore, Maryland, USA

DEBORAH KODER, PhD
Lecturer and Clinical Supervisor, Department of Psychological Sciences, School of Health Sciences, Swinburne University of Technology, Australia

NICOLE LEISTIKOW, MD
Assistant Professor, Department of Psychiatry, University of Maryland School of Medicine, Baltimore, Maryland, USA

JAN A. LINDSAY, PhD
Houston VA HSR&D Center for Innovations in Quality, Effectiveness and Safety, Michael E. DeBakey VA Medical Center, VA South Central Mental Illness Research, Education and Clinical Center, Menninger Department of Psychiatry and Behavioral Sciences, Baylor College of Medicine, Houston, Texas, USA

LISA MacLEAN, MD
Chief Clinical Wellness Officer, Henry Ford Health System, Detroit, Michigan, USA

DIANA MATOVIC, PhD
Professor, Postdoctoral Fellow, School of Psychological Sciences, Centre for Emotional Health, Centre for Ageing, Cognition and Wellbeing, Macquarie University, Sydney, New South Wales, Australia

CAITLYN E. MAYE, BS
Department of Psychiatry and Behavioral Sciences, Baylor College of Medicine, Houston, Texas, USA

JOSEPH F. MCGUIRE, PhD
Center for OCD, Anxiety, and Related Disorders for Children, Division of Child and Adolescent Psychiatry, Department of Psychiatry and Behavioral Sciences, Johns Hopkins School of Medicine, Baltimore, Maryland, USA

LYDIA J. MCKEITHAN, MD
Vanderbilt Sports Concussion Center, Vanderbilt University School of Medicine, Nashville, Tennessee, USA

KAITLIN R. McMANUS, BA
Mclean Hospital, Belmont, Massachusetts, USA

MEAGHAN O'DONNELL, PhD
Professor, Phoenix Australia, University of Melbourne, Melbourne, Australia

ROSAIN OZONSI, BS
Mclean Hospital, Belmont, Massachusetts, USA

NANCY A. PACHANA, PhD, FAPS, FASSA
Professor, School of Psychology, The University of Queensland, Brisbane, Queensland, Australia

TIMOTHY RYAN PARKER, MD
Department of Psychiatry and Behavioral Medicine, Prisma Health - Upstate, Psychiatry Resident, Prisma Health - Upstate Psychiatry Residency Program, Greenville, South Carolina, USA

AINSLEY K. PATRICK, BS
Center for OCD, Anxiety, and Related Disorders for Children, Division of Child and Adolescent Psychiatry, Department of Psychiatry and Behavioral Sciences, Johns Hopkins School of Medicine, Baltimore, Maryland, USA

REGAN PATRICK, PhD
Mclean Hospital, Belmont, Massachusetts, USA; Harvard Medical School, Boston, Massachusetts, USA

CAITLIN M. PINCIOTTI, PhD
Rogers Behavioral Health System

ALEXANDER J. POZNANSKI, MD
Psychiatry Resident, Department of Behavioral Health, Henry Ford Health, Detroit, Michigan, USA

AVANI PRABHAKAR, MD
Section of Palliative Medicine, Division of General Internal Medicine, Assistant Professor, Department of Medicine, Johns Hopkins School of Medicine, Baltimore, Maryland, USA

DEEPAK PRABHAKAR, MD, MPH
Chief of Medical Staff, Sheppard Pratt, Associate Professor (Ad), Department of Psychiatry, University of Maryland School of Medicine, Baltimore, Maryland, USA

ZHEALA QAYYUM, MD, MMSc
Training Director, Child and Adolescent Psychiatry Fellowship Program, Department of Psychiatry and Behavioral Sciences, Boston Children's Hospital, Harvard Medical School, Boston, Massachusetts, USA

KESLEY A. RAMSEY, PhD
Center for OCD, Anxiety, and Related Disorders for Children, Division of Child and Adolescent Psychiatry, Department of Psychiatry and Behavioral Sciences, Johns Hopkins School of Medicine, Baltimore, Maryland, USA

CLAUDIA L. REARDON, MD
Department of Psychiatry, Professor, University of Wisconsin-Madison School of Medicine and Public Health, Madison, Wisconsin, USA

MONICA RETTENMIER, MD
Service Chief, Electroconvulsive Therapy, Department of Psychiatry, Sheppard Pratt Health Systems, Towson, Maryland, USA

KATLYN REYNOLDS, BS
Center for OCD, Anxiety, and Related Disorders for Children, Division of Child and Adolescent Psychiatry, Department of Psychiatry and Behavioral

Sciences, Johns Hopkins School of Medicine, Department of Mental Health, Bloomberg School of Public Health, Johns Hopkins University, Baltimore, Maryland, USA

NICOLE ROBINSON, PhD
Research Fellow, Department of Electrical and Computer Systems Engineering, Turner Institute for Brain and Mental Health, School of Psychological Sciences, Monash University, Melbourne, Australia

KASSIDY ROGERS-HEALION, BS
Department of Biology, Tufts University

DANIELA SAMPAIO, MD
Psychiatry Residency Program, University of Maryland, Sheppard Pratt, Baltimore, Maryland, USA

ABIGAEL SCHMIDT, BS
Center for OCD, Anxiety, and Related Disorders for Children, Division of Child and Adolescent Psychiatry, Department of Psychiatry and Behavioral Sciences, Johns Hopkins School of Medicine, Baltimore, Maryland, USA; Department of Psychology, Towson University, Towson, Maryland, USA

MARGUERITE REID SCHNEIDER, MD, PhD
Fellow in Child and Adolescent Psychiatry, Department of Psychiatry and Behavioral Sciences, Boston Children's Hospital, Harvard Medical School, Boston, Massachusetts, USA

MARK SILVER, MSW
Coordinator of the Wellbeing Clinic for Older Adults, Department of Psychological Sciences, School of Health Sciences, Swinburne University of Technology, Australia

ERIN SMITH
Global Brain Health Institute, University of California, San Francisco, San Francisco, California, USA; Department of Neurology and Neurological Sciences, Stanford University, Palo Alto, California, USA; Neuroscience-Inspired Policy Initiative, Organisation for Economic Co-operation and Development (OECD), Paris, France

KELSEY SMITH, MD
Resident Physician, Prisma Health/University of South Carolina School of Medicine Greenville – Psychiatry Residency Program (Greenville), Greenville, South Carolina, USA

MILENA H. SMITH, MD, PhD
Instructor, Department of Psychiatry and Behavioral Sciences, Johns Hopkins School of Medicine, Baltimore, Maryland, USA

ERIC A. STORCH, PhD
Department of Psychiatry and Behavioral Sciences, Baylor College of Medicine, Houston, Texas, USA

MEG I. STRIEPE, PhD
California Institute of Integral Studies, San Francisco, California, USA

SAMANTHA TAYLOR, MD
Fellow in Child and Adolescent Psychiatry, Department of Psychiatry and Behavioral Sciences, Boston Children's Hospital, Harvard Medical School, Boston, Massachusetts, USA

HILARY N. TOUCHETT, PhD
Houston VA HSR&D Center for Innovations in Quality, Effectiveness and Safety, Michael E. DeBakey VA Medical Center, VA South Central Mental Illness Research, Education and Clinical Center, Houston, Texas, USA

ALLIE N. TOWNSEND, MA
Department of Psychiatry and Behavioral Sciences, Baylor College of Medicine, Houston, Texas, USA; The Chicago School of Professional Psychology, Washington, DC, USA

ANYA E. URCUYO, BA
Doctoral Student, Florida International University, Center for Children and Families, Miami, Florida, USA

MARC S. WEINBERG, MD, PhD
Mclean Hospital, Belmont, Massachusetts, USA; Harvard Medical School, Massachusetts General Hospital, Boston, Massachusetts, USA

ANDREW D. WIESE, PhD
Department of Psychiatry and Behavioral Sciences, Baylor College of Medicine, Houston, Texas

CHUANG-KUO WU, MD, PhD
Professor, Department of Neurology, The Warren Alpert Medical School, Brown University, Director of

Alzheimer's Disease and Memory Disorders Center of Rhode Island Hospital, Providence, Rhode Island, USA

VIVIANA M. WUTHRICH, MPsych.(Clin), PhD
Professor of Clinical Psychology, School of Psychological Sciences, Centre for Emotional Health, Centre for Ageing, Cognition and Wellbeing, Macquarie University, Sydney, New South Wales, Australia

AARON M. YENGO-KAHN, MD
Vanderbilt Sports Concussion Center, Department of Neurological Surgery, Vanderbilt University Medical Center, Nashville, Tennessee, USA

DEVAL ZAVERI, MD
Director of the Women's Mental Health Program, Department of Psychiatry, Sheppard Pratt Health Systems, Towson, Maryland, USA

ADVANCES IN PSYCHIATRY AND BEHAVIORAL HEALTH

CONTENTS

VOLUME 2 • 2022

evaluate their preferences for treating such symptoms. Our findings demonstrated that providers see a wide range of individuals who have experienced concussion. Preferences for the management of SRC-related symptoms vary among providers and are not associated with patient volume, despite confidence being correlated with volume. The wide variability in treatment preferences and lack of confidence among low volume providers reinforces the need for robust studies and evidence-based guidelines for the management of concussion-related neuropsychiatric symptoms.

Neurosciences

Neuropsychiatric Aspect of Posterior Cortical Atrophy

Chuang-Kuo Wu

The clinical diagnosis of posterior cortical atrophy (PCA) has been established for more than 3 decades. Yet, this diagnostic entity only has obtained valuable academic attention in recent years. The cognitive profile of PCA is well documented and underlying pathology is extensively investigated. By contrast, the neuropsychiatric manifestation of PCA is rarely discussed in the medical literature. Based on the longitudinal observational study, this author has noted 3 stages or aspects of neuropsychiatric presentation of PCA through the disease course. More importantly, without effective treatment, neuropsychiatric symptoms play a major role in causing caregiver burden.

Psychedelics for Alzheimer's Disease Palliative Care

Kaitlin R. McManus, Regan Patrick, Meg I. Striepe, Mia J. Drury, Rosain Ozonsi, Brent P. Forester, and Marc S. Weinberg

Psychedelic compounds (psilocybin, lysergic acid diethylamide, ayahuasca) paired with psychotherapy offer great potential for addressing multiple aspects of unmet palliative care needs for aging patients with Alzheimer's disease and their caregivers. In this review, the authors integrate recent findings from psychedelic and psychedelic-assisted therapy clinical research with key domains of Alzheimer's disease palliative care, from neurobehavioral symptom management to social and spiritual aspects of care in patients and their caregivers. In doing so, they provide a framework for approaching use of these exciting compounds in the Alzheimer's disease population, while recognizing some of the practical challenges faced.

The Therapeutic Potential of Restoring Gamma Oscillations in Alzheimer's Disease

Arianna Ferretti, Kassidy Rogers-Healion, and Aryandokht Fotros

A growing body of research supports an important role in the effect of brain waves and their dynamics on cognitive function. Studies have shown there are differences between the brain rhythms of patients with Alzheimer's disease (AD) and healthy individuals, namely reduction of gamma waves. In this article, we will review the current research about the significance of these changes in brain oscillations and a proposed biological mechanism for decreased oscillations in the gamma frequency. Additionally, we discuss the efforts to stimulate neural networks at this frequency to alleviate symptoms and prevent neurodegeneration.

Psychotherapeutics

Advances in Psychotherapy with Internet-Based Cognitive Behavioral Therapy for Anxiety and Obsessive-Compulsive Disorder

Allie N. Townsend, Alyssa G. Hertz, Johann M. D'Souza, and Andrew D. Wiese

Advances in modern technology have contributed to the recent evolution of virtual therapy options for anxiety disorders and obsessive-compulsive disorder (OCD). This article discusses videoconferencing, self-help, and Internet-based cognitive behavioral therapy (ICBT) for anxiety disorders and OCD. Empirical support for ICBT for panic disorder, social anxiety disorder, generalized anxiety disorder, health anxiety, and OCD is reviewed, as are variables associated with treatment outcomes. Globally, ICBT for anxiety disorders and OCD is an efficacious treatment yet lack of patient engagement is a significant barrier. Lastly, clinical implications and future directions are identified to promote research that further improves these technological interventions.

Advances in Psychotherapy for Older Adults Using Video-to-Home Treatment

Jennifer Freytag, Hilary N. Touchett, Jennifer L. Bryan, Jan A. Lindsay, and Christine E. Gould

Providing telemental health services to older adults has become especially important during the COVID-19 pandemic. Video-to-home (VTH) treatment is an effective treatment modality; research shows that older adults are open to using VTH. However, there are unique barriers to using VTH with older adults. Barriers include access to technology, acceptance of technology, and physical and cognitive limitations. Additional concerns include establishing rapport with older patients and the policy and ethical concerns surrounding the use of VTH. Methods of addressing these barriers have been developed, and more research is needed to develop evidence-based VTH practice.

Recent Advances in Psychotherapy with Virtual Reality: Closing the Research-to-Practice Gap

Joey Ka-Yee Essoe, Ainsley K. Patrick, Katlyn Reynolds, Abigael Schmidt, Kesley A. Ramsey, and Joseph F. McGuire

With consumer devices becoming increasingly affordable, virtual reality (VR) bears therapeutic promise for psychiatry and psychotherapy. Nevertheless, there remains a research-to-practice gap as advances in VR technology outpace clinical research: VR therapeutics practical for day-to-day clinical care remain largely unavailable, inaccessible, or unaffordable. This article returns to three foundational promises of VR: enhancing treatments already feasible in the clinic, making feasible treatments impractical in the clinic, and making possible "impossible" treatments in the clinic. These are discussed in terms of current state of research; whether VR therapeutics are available, accessible, and affordable to frontline clinicians; limitations; and areas of growth via practical examples. This is followed by a discussion on clinical research approach to further bridge the research-to-practice gap: first, using in research only VR devices that are practical for frontline clinics, and second, developing VR-therapeutics with scalability and excellence in mind—through optimization and a team-science approach.

Affective Computing in Psychotherapy

Rahul Khanna, Nicole Robinson, Meaghan O'Donnell, Harris Eyre, and Erin Smith

Affective computing, the discipline aimed at enabling computers to interpret, express, and modify emotion, is rapidly maturing. Although not aimed exclusively at health care, the technology holds promise to increase our understanding of psychotherapy, train future generations of clinicians, and directly deliver care alongside human therapists. It may also enhance autonomous therapy systems to deliver care in a stepped-care model. This article reviews the principles of, and recent advances in, affective computing for psychotherapy. It outlines emerging and potential applications and pitfalls, concluding with steps toward ethical development and clinical adoption.

Women's Mental Health

Perimenopause and Mental Health: Implications for the Assessment and Treatment of Women at Midlife

Nicole Leistikow and Milena H. Smith

Perimenopause is a 4- to 9-year window of risk before menopause in which women may experience new onset or worsening of psychiatric symptoms, particularly depression. Therefore, primary care assessment of women at midlife should include routine depression screening. In addition, psychiatric evaluations of midlife women should also screen for symptoms of perimenopause, including hot flashes and night sweats; sleep disturbance; cognitive complaints; sexual, vaginal, and urinary problems; and joint pain, with concerning symptoms receiving further workup or appropriate referral. Treatment of perimenopausal depression should include treatment of contributing perimenopausal symptoms and consideration of agents with efficacy for vasomotor symptoms.

Infertility and Its Association with Depression, Anxiety, and Emotional Distress: A Current Review

Neha Shroff Hudepohl and Kelsey Smith

Infertility is a complex medical phenomenon with the potential for profound impact on mental health. The relationship between infertility and mental health is bidirectional, with interactions in pathophysiology and treatment. Evidence suggests that depression, anxiety, and emotional distress are more prevalent in those undergoing infertility evaluation and assisted reproductive technology, and that the presence of these mental health conditions may have an impact on the outcomes of evaluation and treatment. Evidence-based treatment approaches in the context of infertility are often administered by infertility centers directly. Screening and referral for appropriate treatment can improve outcomes for patients with infertility.

Child and Adolescent

Intensive Treatments for Youth with Obsessive-Compulsive Disorder and Anxiety Disorders

Caitlyn E. Maye, Caitlin M. Pinciotti, and Eric A. Storch

Anxiety disorder and obsessive-compulsive disorder (OCD) in youth are prevalent and debilitating. Without effective treatment, prolonged symptoms can have significant adverse outcomes later in life. Currently, effective treatments for anxiety disorders often use a cognitive behavioral therapy (CBT) approach. Specifically, for youth with OCD, the gold-standard, evidence-based cognitive behavioral treatment is CBT with exposure and response prevention. Although CBT reduces symptoms and improves overall functioning for youth with OCD or anxiety, this treatment is not effective for all youth.

Moving Beyond the Clinic: Leveraging Telehealth Strategies to Address Youth Mental Health Challenges

Gabrielle F. Freitag, Anya E. Urcuyo, and Jonathan S. Comer

Telehealth treatment formats for youth mental health problems use synchronous interactive communication technologies (eg, videoconferencing) to facilitate real-time interactions between patients/families and providers. Recent years have witnessed a sharp uptick in the evaluation, acceptance, and use of telehealth approaches, and the COVID-19 pandemic pushed telehealth into the clinical mainstream. Against this backdrop, we provide an overview of telehealth practice in youth mental health care, focusing on the rationale, history, practice trends, and supporting evidence. We discuss key administrative, ethical, and policy-related considerations and controversies for telehealth providers working with children and families.

Common Treatment Elements of Manualized Evidence-Based Treatments for Youth Anxiety Disorders

Sandra L. Cepeda, Hannah L. Grassie, and Jill Ehrenreich-May

This review aims to provide a descriptive evaluation on the commonalities and differences across 15 evidence-based treatment protocols for childhood anxiety, with emphasis on guiding clinicians in mapping a personalized treatment plan that most fits a given child and family. The reviewed treatment approaches contain overlapping strategies that are common to theoretical frameworks of cognitive behavioral therapy, mindfulness, and acceptance and commitment therapy. This review suggests that most practitioners may select materials from any of the included programs, but are encouraged to provide at minimum techniques of psychoeducation, cognitive flexibility, and exposure-based strategies to youth with anxiety.

Geriatrics

Promotion of Psychological Well-Being in Later Life and Prevention of Late-Life Mental Disorders

Nancy A. Pachana

The prevention of mental health disorders in later life is greatly facilitated by the active promotion of positive mental well-being across the lifespan, but particularly in later life. A lifespan perspective is vital to helping older individuals achieve psychological well-being and includes the individual's history and context as well as proximal (ie, life events) and distal (ie, biological) influences. An individual's cultural context is increasingly recognized as vital in the context of clinical assessment and treatment. Life transitions may negatively impact well-being; interventions to restore wellbeing in such instances should work toward the patient's own life goals. A clear and shared understanding of the individual's history, context, and their own views of their aging can facilitate effective interventions.

Addressing Mental Health in Aged Care Residents: A Review of Evidence-Based Psychological Interventions and Emerging Practices

Sunil Bhar, Deborah Koder, Hemalatha Jayaram, Mark Silver, and Tanya Davison

The prevalence of mental health conditions in residential aged care facilities is substantially higher than in the community. Yet, most research into evidence-based treatments for late life mental health conditions has involved older adults living in the community, rather than aged care residents. This article provides clinicians with an overview of evidence-based psychological interventions and emerging approaches for supporting the mental health of aged care residents, as well as recommendations for how to customize the delivery of such interventions within this environment.

Advances in the Psychological Management of Older Adult Mental Health

Viviana M. Wuthrich, Jessamine T-H. Chen, and Diana Matovic

The most common mental disorders in later life are unipolar mood disorders, anxiety disorders, and substance use disorders. This review outlines the key information needed for the psychological management of common mental disorders in older adults, as well as the challenges pertaining to the recognition and treatment of mental disorders in later life. Some differences in the prevalence of geriatric mental disorders as well as differences in the clinical presentation of mental disorders require minor modification to the assessment and treatment of symptoms. However, there are more similarities than differences in the overall assessment and treatment techniques needed to work with this population.

Education and Clinical Practice

Training and Education Related to Suicide Prevention

Zheala Qayyum, Samantha M. Taylor, and Marguerite Reid Schneider

Suicide is a large and growing public health problem. While mental health providers certainly have a key role to play in suicide prevention, the data support more universal screening for potential suicidality. There is an emergent need to educate all health care professionals broadly to create a health care system that can more universally deliver compassionate preventative care and treatment of suicidal patient. Suicide prevention education must include practical skills for using evidence-based tools for a complete assessment, triage, and treatment planning following a positive screen, and skills for basic brief interventions for those individuals with suicidality not requiring urgent inpatient care, including safety planning and lethal means restriction. The experience of losing a patient to suicide can have a profound effect on providers, especially when it occurs during training. Therefore, it is essential that institutions develop comprehensive programming for responding to a suicide when one takes place.

Neurostimulation and Women's Health

Deval Zaveri, Monica Rettenmier, and Patricia Carlson

We intend to review the available neurostimulation treatments in psychiatry, namely, Electroconvulsive, therapy, Transcranial Magnetic Stimulation, Deep Brain Stimulation, and Vagal Nerve Stimulation. The article briefly outlines the indications, techniques, for each of these treatment modalities, with a focus on women's health, special consideration for women's reproductive mental health when using these treatment approaches.

The Interface Between Psychiatry and Palliative Medicine

Avani Prabhakar and Lisa MacLean

Palliative medicine provides an interdisciplinary approach to meet the needs of the patient and their family at any stage of serious illness regardless of their prognosis or stage of illness and works in collaboration with the primary treating team with the intention of improving quality of life and minimizing suffering for patients and their families throughout the illness journey. This article aims to explore the interface of palliative medicine and psychiatry and the suggestion that consultation-liaison psychiatry is one way to address the specialized needs of the terminally ill patient with psychiatric needs.

Introduction to Dialectical Behavior Therapy for Psychiatrists and Psychiatry Residents

Andrea L.B. Gottlieb, Christopher L. Klinger, and Daniela Sampaio

Comprehensive dialectical behavior therapy (DBT) is effective in treating emotion dysregulation and associated behavioral problems and well supported in psychotherapy literature. Psychiatrists often interact with patients in DBT programs and for whom DBT principles are warranted. DBT is a set of principles, strategies, and skills that can be applied to not only psychotherapy but also psychiatric care of patients with chronic emotion dysregulation. This article provides key points to help with an introduction to comprehensive DBT in order to benefit psychiatrists in their care of such patients.

Recent Advances in Psychopharmacology

Alexander J. Poznanski and Esther Akinyemi

There is a better understanding of mental illness and the potential underlying mechanisms leading to new medications with novel mechanisms of action. The new medications seek to reduce side effects while optimizing efficacy. Attention-deficit hyperactivity disorder, mood disorders, movement disorders, neurocognitive disorders, psychotic disorders, sexual disorders, and sleep disorders have all had newly approved medications in the last 5 years. Some of the new indications are of older medications being explored for other indications. This article describes these medications, the trials supporting them, and relevant clinical information about each medication.

Advances in Psychiatry and Behavioral Health 2 (2022) xxi–xxii
ADVANCES IN PSYCHIATRY AND BEHAVIORAL HEALTH

Preface

Advances: Carrying the Momentum

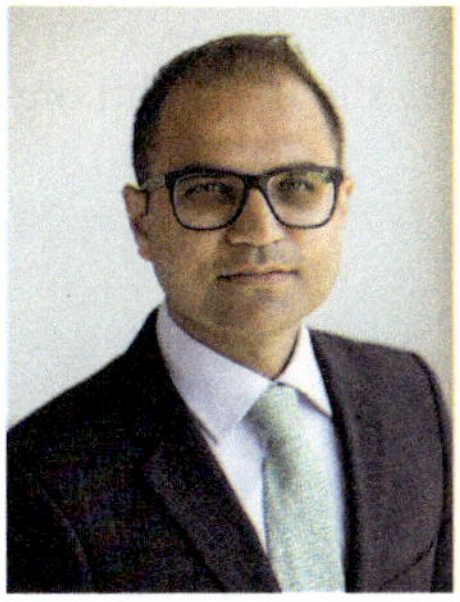

Deepak Prabhakar, MD, MPH,
Editor-in-Chief

It's an absolute privilege to welcome readers to the second issue of *Advances in Psychiatry and Behavioral Health*. What may sound like a hyperbole of gratitude is in fact heartfelt, and why wouldn't it be; ultimately, through the ongoing pandemic and related instability, our team of section editors, Elsevier staff, and contributors have worked diligently to make this issue possible.

The second issue of *Advances in Psychiatry and Behavioral Health* is another step toward facilitating our knowledge and understanding of the progress being made in our field with an emphasis on application in real-world settings. For this issue, we have invited two additional sections. Carly Johnco has edited the inaugural geriatrics section, and Andres G. Viana has edited the section on children and adolescents. Additional content is divided into five sections, all continuing from the first issue: Aryan Fotros has edited the Neurosciences section; Eric Storch has edited the section on advances in Psychotherapy; Lauren Osborne has edited the section on Women's Mental Health; Claudia Reardon has edited a section on Sports Psychiatry; and I have edited the section on Education and Clinical Practice.

Readers will find this issue addressing critical issues in clinical psychiatry. Articles such as impact of bullying on recovery from sports-related concussions, LGBTQ+ mental health in elite sport, the neuropsychiatric aspect of posterior cortical atrophy, and affective computing

https://doi.org/10.1016/j.ypsc.2022.06.006
2667-3827/22/

help broaden our understanding of key concepts for broader application. Similarly, readers are bound to walk away with usable skills and strategies benefiting patients from articles profiled in the sections addressing women's health, child psychiatry, geriatrics, and psychotherapeutics. The section on education and clinical practice addresses important and timely topics such as suicide prevention, neurostimulation in specific populations, and interface of psychiatry and palliative medicine, among others.

It is my hope that readers will find this issue an enriching experience with important takeaways and pearls for clinical application in diverse settings. Work has already begun for the next issue, and what was a message of hope with our first issue has now gradually but surely shifted to the strategy of sustaining the momentum and furthering the mandate of sharing the advances in our field.

Deepak Prabhakar, MD, MPH
Sheppard Pratt
6501 N Charles Street
Baltimore, MD 21204, USA

E-mail address: dprabhakar@sheppardpratt.org

Sports

Advances in Psychiatry and Behavioral Health 2 (2022) 1–7

ADVANCES IN PSYCHIATRY AND BEHAVIORAL HEALTH

Impact of Bullying on Recovery from Sport-Related Concussion

Raphaela Shea Fontana, DO[a,*], Timothy Ryan Parker, MD[b], Aaron Slone Jeckell, MD[c]

[a]Department of Psychiatry and Behavioral Medicine, 10 Patewood Drive, Suite 130, Greenville, SC 29615, USA; [b]Prisma Health – Upstate Psychiatry Residency Program, 701 Grove Road, Greenville, SC 29605, USA; [c]Broward Health Coral Springs, 9600 W Sample Road, Suite 505, Coral Springs, FL 33065, USA

KEYWORDS

• Concussion • Bullying • Pressure • Retirement • Disclosure

KEY POINTS

- Both sport-related concussion (SRC) and bullying in sport (BiS) are ubiquitous occurrences that can significantly impact athletic performance and mental health.
- Athletes may be more vulnerable to biopsychosocial stressors following SRC.
- Features of bullying have been normalized in the athletic domain, which can impact the reporting of symptoms and pressure to return to play (RTP) prematurely and influence early retirement from sport.
- Interventions for coaches, athletes, and other stakeholders should include the optimization of the psychosocial environment during recovery from SRC, open disclosure of symptoms and the mental health resources available to address them, and reinforcement of an antibullying culture.
- The prevalence of bullying during recovery from SRC and its effects merit further study.

INTRODUCTION

Athletes who experience a sport-related concussion (SRC) can develop a myriad of complex physical, emotional, cognitive, and/or behavioral symptoms during their recovery period. Timely recognition of SRC and appropriate management are crucial [1]. Unfortunately, studies indicate that more than half of concussed athletes do not immediately report the presence of concussion-related symptoms [2]. Premature return to play (RTP) after sustaining SRC can lead to negative effects such as a prolonged recovery and increased risk of future concussions or musculoskeletal injury [3]. Research has begun to identify how psychosocial factors may influence an athlete's recovery from SRC, including the rates of symptom reporting and how internal and external pressures play a role in this process. Bullying or harassment has the potential to significantly impact an individual's psychosocial wellbeing. Although empirical evidence on the rates of this phenomenon occurring in sport is extremely limited, the risk of being bullied after SRC may add another layer to the already complicated process of recovery, symptom reporting, and the pressure to RTP prematurely or retire. As a preventable factor, attention should be given to the mitigation of maltreatment of athletes by peers after SRC, and additional efforts should be made to optimize an athlete's psychosocial environment as they recover.

SPORT-RELATED CONCUSSION

There are an estimated 1.6 to 3.8 million SRCs in the United States every year [4]. The prevalence of

*Corresponding author. Prisma Health – Upstate, Department of Psychiatry and Behavioral Medicine, 701 Grove Road, Greenville, SC 29605, USA. *E-mail address:* rsheafontana.do@gmail.com

https://doi.org/10.1016/j.ypsc.2022.03.001
2667-3827/22/

concussion among adolescents in the United States may be as high as 20%, a number that may skew even higher among white males participating in contact sport [5]. A concussion, or mild traumatic brain injury (mTBI), is a common injury caused by an impulse transmitted to the brain that leads to a cascade of neurochemical changes. While the brain requires additional energy as it works to restore neurochemical homeostasis, it is actually in an energy-deficient state. A concussive injury leads to a period of decreased cerebral blood flow, which in turn leads to a deficit in fuel sources of oxygen and glucose. This energy disparity is believed to be the cause of the neuropsychiatric pathology seen in SRC [6]. The impairment seen in SRC is functional rather than structural, and macroscopic tissue injury is typically absent. Recovery takes place in most cases over days to weeks, and approximately 80% of individuals will have recovered within 1 month [1].

Some features that demonstrate an increased risk for sustaining an SRC include sport participation at a young age, a prior history of SRC, previous headache treatment, and a history of attention-deficit/hyperactivity disorder or learning disability [7]. The type of sport can also be a major contributor with high impact contact sports such as American football, rugby, boxing, or hockey conferring the greatest risk of injury [5,7]. Males are more likely to experience SRC, although they also participate in contact sports at a higher rate, and the relationship between SRC risk and sex varies across sports [7,8]. Risk factors for prolonged recovery are equally, if not more, complex, and there is evidence of conflicting data for a number of characteristics [9]. Regardless, research points to the severity of initial symptoms, the development of mood symptoms or headache, and the existence of preexisting mental health issues as being most predictive of a prolonged recovery after SRC [1,9]. Notably, both a personal and family history of mental health disorders can also predict a prolonged recovery [10].

BULLYING IN SPORT

Bullying in sport (BiS) lacks a current consensus definition. As compared with hazing, which has an underlying goal of building team cohesion, the specific goal of bullying is to alienate or exclude a member from the team environment [11]. It can generally be considered any pattern of abuse between peers or teammates with the potential to be dangerous or harmful [12]. Other features include it being reoccurring and intentional with the goal of bringing deliberate harm to the target individual [13]. Newer, or less experienced members of the team, are common targets of bullying in team sport. This can especially be true if a newer member of the team poses a threat to the otherwise established team hierarchy. Bullying can include overt threats or violence, extreme or unwarranted criticism, minimization of accomplishments, verbal or emotional harassment, spreading of rumors, efforts to turn teammates against the victim, or other efforts to exclude the victim from the team community [14,15].

It is estimated that 25% of youths in the general population will experience bullying. Cyberbullying, which can be more insidious, may exist at a rate closer to 50% [16]. BiS has been more difficult to assess, as the role of physical aggression and intimidation in some sports can make detection complicated [17]. Some data support that youths are more likely to experience bullying outside of athletic environments [14,18]. Risk factors for BiS include any feature that distinguishes the victim from peers, the victim being a member of the LGBTQ + community, as well as aspects of the subculture and leadership structure of the team that promote bullying [13,19,20].

Athletes who have been victims of bullying are at a significantly higher risk of developing disorders such as depression, anxiety, and posttraumatic stress disorder [21]. Individuals recovering from SRC have an increased risk of developing mental health disorders as well. Bullying after SRC is important to consider as a possible factor that may influence an athlete's decision to report symptoms. The pressure to perform (either intrinsic/internal or extrinsic/external), competitive level, lack of education about SRC, and stigma are just some of the more studied determinants that have been shown to be involved in reporting patterns [3]. These factors may also impact rates of bullying and harassment-type behaviors. Unfortunately, there is no existing literature examining how bullying may influence a concussed athlete's decision to disclose symptoms, RTP prematurely, or retire. However, based on the high frequency of both SRC and BiS, it is reasonable to surmise that they may coexist and in certain circumstances, BiS may serve as a barrier to help-seeking behaviors after an individual sustains an SRC.

INTERNAL AND EXTERNAL PRESSURES EXPERIENCED AFTER SPORT-RELATED CONCUSSION

SRC, as an "invisible injury," offers a unique set of challenges during recovery. Athletes typically seem "normal" after sustaining this type of injury [22]. It has been established that conditions with invisible symptoms may lead to an increased burden on the individual suffering from them, including negative peer interactions, bullying, low self-esteem, and social isolation [23,24]. SRC recovery can be quite complicated and difficult to understand, and can create a clear distinction between an injured athlete and their peers. As a result, individuals who have experienced SRC may be at an increased risk to experience internal and external social pressures, such as the perceived behavioral norms for symptom reporting and injury recovery.

Many athletes place a significant amount of pressure on themselves already without the added external pressure to succeed. This oftentimes leaves the athlete to push their body in an effort to optimize performance [25]. This is especially true at subprofessional levels whereby the potential for a future career is on the line [26]. SRC can threaten athletic identity, thereby fueling an intrinsic desire to return to sport as soon as possible. Symptom reporting may threaten perceived toughness, playtime, and future role on the team. The Theory of Planned Behavior (TBP) has examined the motivational component behind concussion reporting behaviors among athletes [27]. These behaviors are in part a product of how the athlete thinks others will want them to behave in addition to the importance the athlete places on the opinion of others [27]. Therefore, athletes likely internalize a significant amount of external social pressures or expectations, thus impacting their decision-making process and recovery from injury. These threats of failure or shame can create discomfort within the athlete and play a significant role in symptom disclosure.

External influences (interactions with teammates, coaches, parents, or medical staff) can also influence an athlete's expectation of RTP or retirement after SRC [26]. Athletes have reported a fear of disclosing concussion symptoms due to negative feedback or perception by coaching staff or even teammates [28]. A 2014 survey presented data suggesting that collegiate athletes perceive a decrease in support for reporting concussion symptoms as they advance in sport and gain more exposure to their coaches and the normative reporting behaviors of their sport environment [27]. This study preliminarily suggests that the perception of coaches' attitudes toward concussion reporting by the athletes likely impacts their reporting behaviors [27]. Athletes have also identified experiencing worry about being blamed for losses or ridiculed for poor performance after SRC [29]. Therefore, this may dissuade athletes from disclosing concussion symptoms due to these preconceptions or fear. Participation in athletics, particularly team sport, has empirically demonstrated numerous benefits including improved mood, decreased symptoms of depression, increased feelings of interconnectedness, and improvements in self-esteem [30–32]. Unfortunately, these benefits do not prevent the existence of BiS due to perceived behavioral norms.

Praise of violent collision in sport continues to earn attention from audiences around the world. On the Concussion Alliance's website, they provide a quote by an athlete—"I bet you're fine, you're just a big baby that you can't handle this"—further exemplifying the invalidation received by one's teammate or coach post-SRC [33]. Phrases such as "no pain, no gain" or "pain is weakness leaving the body" can be seen on locker room walls or held as mantras by countless teams. For many years, the television network ESPN had a segment called "Jacked Up" that would highlight the bone-crushing tackles from the past week of National Football League play. Across multiple elite-level sports, athletes have been glorified for returning to play despite experiencing concussion-causing impacts. Athletes who require time off after injury have been portrayed as "weak" or "soft." The culture of extolling big hits and applauding athletes who RTP despite injury has translated to youth sport with disastrous implications. This has likely fostered a perceived norm for many athletes across all levels to diminish the gravitas of SRC symptoms out of fear of blame, alienation, or ostracization—in other words, a form of bullying. Regardless, in response to these intrinsic and extrinsic pressures, many athletes are faced with a difficult decision: return to sport prematurely, disclose symptoms, or retire.

PREMATURE RETURN TO PLAY

The implications of premature RTP after concussion are considerable. The neurochemical cascade and existence of an energy deficit after concussion can lead to increased cellular vulnerability to a second concussive injury [6]. Animal models demonstrate that a second injury during this time has the potential to lead to far more significant neurometabolic changes and axonal injury that may cause long-term deficits [34]. Multiple SRCs in a short period of time have been associated with a prolonged recovery and increased symptom burden [35–38]. As clinicians, coaches, and teammates, it is imperative to prevent secondary injury during this time of vulnerability.

Another concern is the impact that bullying may have on mental health while recovering from SRC. Those experiencing SRC are at an increased risk for developing depression in the immediate period after injury as well as later in life—a risk that increases with the number of concussions experienced [39].

Additionally, those with depression are more likely to experience a prolonged recovery from concussion and experience other postconcussive symptoms [9,40]. A concussion clearly has the potential to create a period of increased vulnerability to biopsychosocial stressors. An athlete may be significantly more vulnerable to any form of bullying during this window of recovery from a concussion, and as bullying is associated with increased rates of suicide, the consequences of this can be tremendous.

Other stressors experienced by injured athletes include missed opportunities, social comparison, unwanted attention, isolation, and pressure to recover [41]. While perhaps not specifically intended to isolate or exclude injured athletes, forms of maltreatment such as coercion, intimidation, or other forms of influence used to pressure athletes to RTP prematurely could be viewed as a form of bullying. Coaches, trainers, teammates, and parents may influence an athlete's recovery by providing (or not providing) educational, emotional, and practical support at different stages of the recovery period [42].

PREMATURE RETIREMENT

In contrast to premature RTP, BiS has the potential to precipitate premature or preemptive retirement from sport. Some of the primary motivations for retirement from sport include injury, age, involuntary exclusion (cut from the team), and voluntary choices related to lifestyle [43]. Retirement from sport is a major transition point with an array of consequences that can be magnified when they occur unexpectedly, such as following SRC or other injuries. A sudden or unexpected transition out of sport can increase the risk of developing mood or other mental health symptoms or disorders [44]. Other results of premature retirement from sport include the loss of the aforementioned benefits of sport as well as loss of the opportunity for education, scholarship, or employment.

Athletes are often encouraged from a young age to invest heavily in their athletic identity, and as a result may experience feelings of loss and helplessness on retirement. An athlete's transition to retirement may be more difficult due to the early age at which they begin and end their competitive careers [45]. Bullying may cause a range of emotional and psychological responses, including anger, shame, and demotivation, which could lead to poor sports performance or premature retirement [46]. Thus, bullying after SRC could potentially expedite an athlete's decision to retire from sport.

RECOMMENDATIONS

There are many steps that can mitigate the risk of BiS after SRC, as well as interventions that may be indicated in the event that it does occur (Box 1). A comprehensive approach to educating athletes, coaches, trainers, and parents, and fostering an empathetic and supportive environment is paramount for appropriately addressing both the common and potential pathologic responses to injury. Interventions should focus not only on medical management but also include psychoeducation to inform stakeholders about the anticipated clinical course and psychological factors that can impact one's recovery.

BOX 1
General clinical recommendations related to bullying in sport (BiS) after sport-related concussion (SRC)

- Immediate recognition of BiS after SRC is crucial
- Identify whether the team or organization has an Emergency Action Plan for mental health or bullying/harassment-related issues
- In cases of BiS, encourage open disclosure of the victim's experiences without suggesting, leading, or influencing their report
- Maintain neutrality and do not denigrate any perpetrator when discussing the situation with the victim of BiS, as overt denigration may make the victim less likely to disclose or open up in session
- Reinforce that SRC and BiS are not the faults of the injured athlete or victim
- Maintain an adult presence in all team functions and settings to mitigate BiS
- Consider contacting the parents of any minor who is experiencing bullying
- Provide appropriate psychoeducation regarding SRC as well as both typical and atypical recovery to the athlete and all involved stakeholders (coaches, athletic trainers, athletic administration, teammates, caregivers, support system, and other members of the health care team)

BOX 2
Detection of bullying after sport-related concussion (SRC)

- Identify whether an injured athlete is isolating more than usual
- Assess whether any nonsanctioned team activities are being held under a high level of secrecy
- Recognize if an injured athlete is experiencing self-imposed isolation or exclusion from team activities
- Identify injury inconsistent with the athlete's sport (eg, bruises on a swimmer's arm)
- Evaluate for the presence of mental health symptoms that are typically attributable to factors other than SRC or concussion recovery, such as psychosis, hypomania/mania, and *preexisting* signs and/or symptoms of depression or anxiety
- Consider whether any symptoms are indicative of a mental health disorder unrelated or only partly related to bullying or concussion

Recognition of BiS following SRC and how this may hinder an athlete's recovery and future participation in sport is an important first step (Box 2). Athletes may present with a number of warning signs that may indicate that BiS is taking place. Consideration should be given to the fact that some of these signs may be indicative of different mental health concerns (other than BiS-related ones) that warrant intervention. To foster a positive environment for future growth and development of athletes, it is imperative that appropriate education and training regarding the occurrence of BiS be provided. This especially pertains to athletes and coaches, so that bullying behavior may be more readily identified and addressed to prevent future bullying and reinforce positive behaviors. Supervision during team activities by coaching staff who have received appropriate education on bullying is paramount to maintaining an antibullying culture in sport [11,15].

RTP following SRC must involve strict adherence to guidelines, and coaches, athletic trainers, and teammates should also work to optimize the psychosocial environment during recovery. Interventions should also target aspects of the coach–athlete relationship. Coaches can play an integral role in creating and reinforcing a team culture that values concussion reporting, as well as open disclosure of symptoms or other struggles. Future research looking at the factors that influence athletes' perceptions of coach support for concussion reporting will be vital to expand on the extrapolated and anecdotal evidence provided in this review [27].

Communication between athletes, coaches, and athletic trainers should remain open to best provide support to the athlete, while also respecting privacy between the athlete and their mental health provider [47]. While the treatment for concussion involves both cognitive and physical rest, athletes should continue to be included in team activities as able and appropriate, while monitoring for signs and symptoms of postconcussion syndrome. Stakeholders must also be informed about the mental health resources available to athletes and how to refer for evaluation and treatment. As we begin to understand the interpersonal factors that play a role in concussion management, we will be able to offer a more individualized treatment approach to athletes while hopefully creating an environment that supports help-seeking behaviors after SRC.

SUMMARY

This article identifies several key components that will hopefully propel future research examining the social intricacies that occur during recovery from SRC. There is a paucity of research examining the degree to which bullying plays a role in an athlete's disclosure of concussion symptoms. Understanding the biopsychosocial factors that may facilitate or hinder symptom reporting behavior post-SRC is not only vital for the development of risk-reducing interventions, but also for an athlete's safety overall. Knowledge of these factors will help create a more robust treatment algorithm postconcussion with the goal of increasing help-seeking behaviors while reducing BiS for athletes in recovery.

CLINICAL CARE POINTS

- After an athlete sustains a sport-related concussion (SRC), look for changes in cognitive, behavioral, and emotional functioning to help guide the next steps in management.
- SRC can predispose athletes to the development or exacerbation of neuropsychiatric pathology. The existence of preinjury neuropsychiatric pathology may

also predispose an athlete to prolonged recovery and increased symptom burden after SRC.

- An athlete with a concussion may experience an increased vulnerability to various biopsychosocial stressors, such as bullying. Therefore, this might impact an athlete's willingness to report symptoms, influence the return to play (RTP) process, or precipitate early retirement from sport.
- Bullying in sport (BiS) can be detrimental to the emotional wellness of an athlete; look for some of the common signs and symptoms that may indicate someone is being bullied such as alienation, ostracization, changes in mood, stolen items from the locker room, or decreased attendance/social isolation in orderto address these concerns immediately.
- To help decrease the occurrence of BiS emphasize the importance of wellness, sportsmanship, and teamwork while avoiding a highly competitive and threatening environment.

DISCLOSURE

The authors have nothing to disclose.

REFERENCES

[1] McCrory P, Meeuwisse W, Dvořák J, et al. Consensus statement on concussion in sport: the 5th international conference on concussion in sport held in Berlin, October 2016. Br J Sports Med. 2017;51(11):838-847. doi:

[2] Asken BM, McCrea MA, Clugston JR, et al. "Playing through it": delayed reporting and removal from athletic activity after concussion predicts prolonged recovery. J Athl Train 2016;51(4):329–35.

[3] O'Connor S, Geaney D, Beidler E. Non-disclosure in Irish collegiate student-athletes: do concussion history, knowledge, pressure to play and gender impact concussion reporting? Phys Sportsmed 2020;48(2):186–93.

[4] Langlois JA, Rutland-Brown W, Wald MM. The epidemiology and impact of traumatic brain injury: a brief overview. J Head Trauma Rehabil 2006;21(5):375–8.

[5] Veliz P, McCabe SE, Eckner JT, et al. Prevalence of Concussion Among US Adolescents and Correlated Factors. JAMA 2017;318(12):1180–2.

[6] Giza CC, Hovda DA. The new neurometabolic cascade of concussion. Neurosurgery 2014;75(Suppl 4):S24–33.

[7] Brett BL, Kuhn AW, Yengo-Kahn AM, et al. Risk Factors Associated With Sustaining a Sport-related Concussion: An Initial Synthesis Study of 12,320 Student-Athletes. Arch Clin Neuropsychol 2018;33(8):984–92.

[8] Lincoln AE, Caswell SV, Almquist JL, et al. Trends in concussion incidence in high school sports: a prospective 11-year study. Am J Sports Med 2011;39(5):958–63.

[9] Iverson GL, Gardner AJ, Terry DP, et al. Predictors of clinical recovery from concussion: a systematic review. Br J Sports Med 2017;51(12):941–8.

[10] Legarreta AD, Brett BL, Solomon GS, et al. The role of family and personal psychiatric history in postconcussion syndrome following sport-related concussion: a story of compounding risk. J Neurosurg Pediatr 2018; 22(3):238–43.

[11] Farrington DP. Understanding and Preventing Bullying. Crime Justice 1993;17:381–458.

[12] Stirling AE. Definition and constituents of maltreatment in sport: establishing a conceptual framework for research practitioners. Br J Sports Med 2009;43(14): 1091–9.

[13] Brackenridge C, Rivers I, Gough B, Llewellyn K, et al. Driving down participation: homophobic bullying as a deterrent to doing sport., . Sport and gender identities masculitinities, femininities, and sexualities. London: Routledge; 2007. p. 120–37.

[14] Steinfeldt JA, Vaughan EL, LaFollette JR, et al. Bullying among adolescent football players: Role of masculinity and moral atmosphere. Psychol Men Masculinity 2012; 13(4):340–53.

[15] Fisher LA, Dzikus L. Bullying in Sport and Performance Psychology. Oxford Research Encyclopedia of Psychology; 2017.

[16] About bullying and cyberbullying. Stomp Out Bullying. Available at: http://www.stompoutbullying.org/. Accessed March 17, 2021.

[17] Coakley J. Sports in society: issues and controversies. 12th edition. New York, NY: McGraw-Hill Education; 2017.

[18] Evans B, Adler A, Macdonald D, et al. Bullying Victimization and Perpetration Among Adolescent Sport Teammates. Pediatr Exerc Sci 2016;28(2):296–303.

[19] Hospital BCs. Bullying prevention in sports. June 28th, 2018. Available at: http://www.beaumont.edu/childrens/specialties/bullying-support-for-children/.

[20] Shannon-McCallum C. Bullying in Recreation and Sport Settings: Exploring Risk Factors, Prevention Efforts, and Intervention Strategies Charlene S. Shannon. J Park Recreation Adm 2013;13:15–33.

[21] Marks SMM, Marcus M. Sexual harrassment and abuse in sports: the role of the team doctor. Br J Sports Med 2012; 46(13):905–8.

[22] Putukian M. How Being Injured Affects Mental Health. In: Brown GT, editor. Mind, body and sport - understanding and supporting student-athlete mental wellness. Indianapolis, Indiana: National Collegiate Athletic Association; 2014. p. 61–4, Chapter 4.

[23] Kundrat AL, Nussbaum JF. The impact of invisible illness on identity and contextual age across the life span. Health Commun 2003;15(3):331–47.

[24] Lempp HK, Hatch SL, Carville SF, et al. Patients' experiences of living with and receiving treatment for fibromyalgia syndrome: a qualitative study. BMC Musculoskelet Disord 2009;10:124.

[25] Connaughton D, Wadey R, Hanton S, et al. The development and maintenance of mental toughness: Perceptions of elite performers. J Sports Sci 2008;26:83–95.

[26] Kerr ZY, Register-Mihalik JK, Kroshus E, et al. Motivations Associated With Nondisclosure of Self-Reported Concussions in Former Collegiate Athletes. Am J Sports Med 2016;44(1):220–5.

[27] Baugh CM, Kroshus E, Daneshvar DH, et al. Perceived coach support and concussion symptom- reporting: difference between freshman and non-freshman college football players. J Law Med Ethics 2014;314–22.

[28] Kerr ZY, Register-Mihalik JK, Marshall SW, et al. Disclosure and non-disclosure of concussion and concussion symptoms in athletes: review and application of the socio-ecological framework. Brain Inj 2014;28(8): 1009–21.

[29] Chrisman SP, Quitiquit C, Rivara FP. Qualitative study of barriers to concussive symptom reporting in high school athletics. J Adolesc Health 2013;52(3):330–5.e3.

[30] Boone EM, Leadbeater BJ. Game on: Diminishing risks for depressive symptoms in early adolescence through positive involvement in team sports. J Res Adolescence 2006;16(1):79–90.

[31] Dunn AL, Trivedi MH, Kampert JB, et al. Exercise treatment for depression: efficacy and dose response. Am J Prev Med 2005;28(1):1–8.

[32] Eime RM, Young JA, Harvey JT, et al. A systematic review of the psychological and social benefits of participation in sport for children and adolescents: informing development of a conceptual model of health through sport. Int J Behav Nutr Phys Act 2013;10:10–98.

[33] The Invisible Injury. Concussion Alliance. Accessed March 20, 2021, Available at: https://www.concussionalliance.org/the-invisible-injury

[34] Prins ML, Hales A, Reger M, et al. Repeat traumatic brain injury in the juvenile rat is associated with increased axonal injury and cognitive impairments. Dev Neurosci 2010;32(5–6):510–8.

[35] Broshek DK, De Marco AP, Freeman JR. A review of post-concussion syndrome and psychological factors associated with concussion. Brain Inj 2015;29(2):228–37.

[36] Manley G, Gardner AJ, Schneider KJ, et al. A systematic review of potential long-term effects of sport-related concussion. Br J Sports Med 2017;51(12):969–77.

[37] Morgan CD, Zuckerman SL, Lee YM, et al. Predictors of postconcussion syndrome after sports- related concussion in young athletes: a matched case-control study. J Neurosurg Pediatr 2015;15(6):589–98.

[38] Zuckerman SL, Yengo-Kahn AM, Buckley TA, et al. Predictors of postconcussion syndrome in collegiate student-athletes. Neurosurg Focus 2016;40(4):E13.

[39] Guskiewicz KM, Marshall SW, Bailes J, et al. Recurrent concussion and risk of depression in retired professional football players. Med Sci Sports Exerc 2007;39(6):903–9.

[40] Solomon GS, Kuhn AW, Zuckerman SL. Depression as a Modifying Factor in Sport-Related Concussion: A Critical Review of the Literature. Phys Sportsmed 2016;44(1): 14–9.

[41] Evans LWR, Hanton S, Mitchell I. Stressors expereinced by injured athletes. J Sports Sci 2012;30(9):917–28.

[42] Podlog LHJ, Schulte S. Psychosocial Factors in Sports Injurt Rehabilitation and Return to Play. Phys Med Rehabil Clin North Am 2014;25(4):915–30.

[43] Lavallee DGJ, Gordon S. The causes of career termination from sport and their relationship to post-retirement adjustment among elite-amateur athletes in Australia. Aust Psychol 1997;32(2):131–5.

[44] Knights S, Sherry E, Ruddock-Hudson M. Investigating elite end-of-athletic-career transition: a systematic review. J Appl Sport Psychol 2016;28(3):291–308.

[45] Lavallee D, Robinson H. In pursuit of an identity: A qualitative exploration of retirement from women's artistic gymnastics. Psychol Sport Exerc 2007;8:119–41.

[46] Vveinhardt JFV. Bullying trends inside sport: when organized sport does not attract but intimidates. Front Psychol 2020;11:2037.

[47] Miller L, Buttell FP. Are NCAA Division I Athletes Prepared for End-of-Athletic-Career Transition? A Literature Review. J Evid Inf Soc Work 2018;15(1):52–70.

Advances in Psychiatry and Behavioral Health 2 (2022) 9–16

ADVANCES IN PSYCHIATRY AND BEHAVIORAL HEALTH

Lesbian, Gay, Bisexual, Trans, and Queer Mental Health in Elite Sport: A Review

Paul Gorczynski, PhD, HCPC, CPsychol, AFBPsS[a,*], Claudia L. Reardon, MD[b], Cindy Miller Aron, LCSW, CGP, FAGPA[c]

[a]University of Greenwich, School of Human Sciences, Park Row, London SE10 9LS, UK; [b]Department of Psychiatry, University of Wisconsin School of Medicine and Public Health, 6001 Research Park Boulevard, Madison, WI 53719, USA; [c]Ascend, Consultation in Health Care, LLC., 737 North Michigan Avenue, 1926, Chicago, IL 60611, USA

KEYWORDS

• Mental health • Mental disorders • Sport • Athletes • LGBT

KEY POINTS

- Elite athletes who identify as LGBTQ+ are at increased risk of experiencing mental health symptoms and disorders.
- Strategies for participatory, collaborative, and multidisciplinary research are needed to better understand the mental health needs of elite LGBTQ+ athletes and how mental health services for these individuals can be improved.
- Policies are needed to address and eliminate discriminatory behaviors and practices that contribute to mental health symptoms and disorders experienced by LGBTQ+ elite athletes.

INTRODUCTION/BACKGROUND

The mental health of elite athletes—those who compete at semielite (eg, highly competitive youth sports, collegiate sports) and world-class elite (eg, Olympics, world championships) levels—has received considerable attention as of late [1,2]. Mental health is a resource that allows athletes to recognize their abilities and potential, cope with various stressors both within and outside of sport, participate in sport productively, and make contributions to their respective athletic and nonathletic communities [3]. Epidemiologic research findings have demonstrated that elite athletes are at risk of experiencing mental health symptoms and disorders [4–6]. Mental health symptoms and disorders can be characterized as having negative effects on a person's cognitions, emotions, behaviors, relationships, and daily functioning. For a diagnosis of a mental health disorder, mental health symptoms must meet specific criteria for duration, severity, and frequency [7]. Such symptoms and disorders can have serious and far-ranging consequences on both the individual athlete as well as the organizations of which they are a part [1,8]. Considerable efforts have been taken by researchers and practitioners to develop better strategies to prevent, treat, and manage mental health symptoms and disorders amongst athletes, as noted by the numerous position statements published on the topic (see Vella, and colleagues for a review) [9]. Despite these extensive efforts, to date very little is known or has been written about the mental health needs of athletes who identify as lesbian, gay, bisexual, trans, and queer (LGBTQ+).

Research from nonathletic populations demonstrates that LGBTQ+ identifying individuals are more

*Corresponding author, *E-mail address:* Paul.Gorczynski@greenwich.ac.uk

https://doi.org/10.1016/j.ypsc.2022.03.002

likely to experience mental health symptoms and disorders compared with populations who are nonminority with respect to their sexual and gender identities [10–12]. For instance, individuals who identify as LGBTQ+ are more likely to experience loneliness, depressive symptoms, anxiety symptoms, substance use, self-harm, and thoughts and attempts of suicide [10,13,14]. LGBTQ+ people are also more likely to experience harassment, discrimination, bullying, and assault [15–17]. With respect to being able to access mental health services, LGBTQ+ people experience challenges. For instance, results from the 2017 National LGBT survey conducted in the UK showed that 72% of individuals who identified as LGBT said it was not an easy process to access mental health services [18]. Many respondents reported long wait times; thoughts of worry, anxiety, or embarrassment about disclosing mental health symptoms or disorders to their health providers; unhelpful or unsupportive health providers; not knowing how or whereby to access mental health services; not knowing who to contact for mental health support; and distances to mental health services that were too far to access. Among the respondents, 54% of individuals disclosed or discussed their sexual orientation with health providers, and of those individuals, 9% stated that their disclosures had a negative effect on their health care experiences. For respondents who identified as trans, 40% stated that they had a negative healthcare experience because of their gender identity. Studies and reviews of LGBTQ+ mental health service use conducted elsewhere in the world have noted similar findings and experiences [12,19–22]. Unfortunately, to date, no studies have evaluated mental health service use among LGBTQ+ athletes.

Mental health providers who work with LGBTQ+ identifying elite athletes are in positions to improve knowledge and pathways to mental health services, address and minimize barriers to mental health services, and enhance mental health service delivery. The purpose of this review is to:

1. Explore the current epidemiologic evidence related to the mental health symptoms and disorders of elite athletes who identify as LGBTQ+; and
2. Understand risk factors for and protective factors against mental health symptoms and disorders for LGBTQ+ identifying elite athletes.

Findings from this review will help structure strategies for collaborative and multidisciplinary research on the mental health needs of LGBTQ+ elite athletes and propose directions for evidence-based practice in mental health service delivery for elite athletes who identify as LGBTQ+.

Methods

For this review, a search strategy of the literature was designed and conducted for the following databases: MEDLINE; CINAHL; APA PsycInfo; and SPORTDiscus. English language literature was searched from inception to December 2021 and focused on the topics of elite athletes who identified as LGBTQ+, mental health symptoms and disorders, and mental health services. A combination of the following keywords was used: "athlete," "sport," "gay," "lesbian," "bisexual," "transgender," "homosexual," "lgbt," "lgbtq," "same sex," "mental health," "mental illness," "mental disorder," and "psychiatric illness." Reference lists of both scientific and gray literature were also reviewed for possible inclusion of additional articles. Where elite athlete-specific or sport-related literature was not available, mental health-related literature from nonelite athletes and the general LGBTQ+ population was used. Findings were grouped broadly into the 2 areas of the purpose statement to provide recommendations for future research and practice.

General information

Epidemiology of mental health symptoms and disorders

Within elite sport, very little is known about the mental health symptoms and disorders of LGBTQ+ identifying athletes, their experiences with accessing or receiving mental health support or treatment, or their journeys through recovery. As noted by Currie and colleagues [23], previous epidemiologic studies of mental health symptoms and disorders in elite sport have underrepresented many significant groups of athletes, including LGBTQ+ identifying individuals. Studies that have been conducted within elite sport do provide some information about the types of mental health symptoms currently experienced by LGBTQ+ athletes, but do not offer evidence with respect to specific disorders, let alone their prevalence or incidence. Most epidemiologic studies that have evaluated the mental health of elite athletes have not collected or published data concerning sexual orientation, or gender identity beyond binary options. For instance, the analysis of the American College Health Association's National College Health Assessment (Fall 2008-Fall 2012 administrations) has provided some information on the general mental health and mental health harms, including substance use, of sexual minority college athletes [24]. Within this assessment, mental health was broadly defined and assessed by 6 questions that asked whether individuals experienced feelings of hopelessness, loneliness, sadness, depression, anxiety, and overwhelming anger.

Furthermore, mental health harms that were examined included intentional self-injury, thoughts of suicide, and suicide attempts. Information was also collected on substance use, which specifically referred to taking illicit and prescription drugs, and binge drinking. Overall, college athletes who identified as sexual minorities were significantly more likely to experience more mental health symptoms and mental health harms than their heterosexual peers. With respect to substance use, individuals who identified as male and part of a sexual minority were significantly more likely to report using illicit drugs than their male-identifying heterosexual comparators, while individuals who identified as female and part of a sexual minority had significantly higher use of illicit and prescription drugs than their female-identifying heterosexual comparators. Other reviews of this health assessment found similar findings [25]. Another study, which examined the mental health literacy of semielite women rugby players in the UK, found that athletes who identified as bisexual were more likely to report lower levels of wellbeing and significantly higher levels of distress when compared with athletes who identified as heterosexual [26]. Although no research has explored the mental health symptoms and disorders of transathletes from an epidemiologic perspective, several researchers and practitioners have noted that transathletes are most likely at an increased risk of mental health symptoms and disorders given reported experiences of nonaccidental violence in sport settings and evidence from nonathletic transpopulations [27,28].

Risk factors for and protective factors against mental health symptoms and disorders

The ecological model provides a basis for mapping and understanding multiple and interacting risk factors for and protective factors against mental health symptoms and disorders [29–31]. Perhaps most importantly, the ecological model allows for an examination of the lives of athletes both within and outside sport. This holistic life perspective views athletes as multidimensional, nonstatic, and constantly acquiring athletic and nonathletic experiences [32,33]. The ecological model, while taking on a holistic life perspective, provides a more complete understanding of the athlete and their mental health needs.

The ecological model can be broken down to examine factors that influence mental health at the intrapersonal, interpersonal, and environmental levels. Reviews published by Reardon and colleagues [1] and Kuettel and Larsen [34] have previously covered such factors for elite athletes. Intrapersonal level factors included physical and psychological characteristics of the individual, such as female sex, previous injuries, surgery, concussions, adverse life events, chronic stress, burnout, perfectionism, poor sleep, career dissatisfaction, competitive failure, forced retirement, and strong athletic identity. Interpersonal level factors included the interactions athletes had with other individuals, including family, friends, teammates, coaches, referees/officials, and fans. These factors included low social support from teammates, coach conflicts, and relationship difficulties with family and friends. Environmental level factors concerned the physical, cultural, and political environments whereby sport was practiced and played. This would also cover travel and movement between locations used for training and competition. Some instances of environmental risk factors included playing individual sports, participating in aesthetic sports, forced retirement, and experiencing nonaccidental violence.

With LGBTQ+ elite athletes, different levels of the ecological model and the intersectionality of multiple factors must be considered with respect to the risk of mental health symptoms and disorders. In addition to the risk factors listed above, careful attention must be given to minority stress [35]. Minority stress refers to stressors that are socially and culturally based, that affect marginalized communities, and that are not typically experienced by individuals outside of those communities [36]. Minority stress can be experienced distally and proximally. Distal minority stressors are external to the minority individual and include aspects of rejection and discrimination, such as hearing discriminatory language [37]. Proximal minority stressors are held internally by the individual and are often based on experiences with distal minority stressors. Proximal minority stressors can include an expectation of experiencing rejection and discrimination, concealment of one's identity for fear of negative repercussions, and possessing self-stigmatizing beliefs and attitudes [35]. The accumulation of both distal and proximal stress experiences can lead an individual to experience mental health symptoms and disorders [35]. Individuals who possess multiple minority statuses may experience minority stress in different ways and to different extents, which may lead to the exacerbation of mental health symptoms [38].

Although it has been recommended that strategies be designed for LGBTQ+ people to enhance or strengthen intrapersonal psychological characteristics, like resilience and coping skills, to address minority stress [39,40], strategies that address heterosexist environments in sport as well as nonaccidental violence are desperately needed [8]. In effect, strategies are needed within the elite sport to enhance inclusivity of diversity to enhance the likelihood of participation in sport for LGBTQ+ people, at any level of competition [28,41–44]. Heterosexism refers to the assumption that all individuals are or should be heterosexual [45]. Such noninclusive beliefs and attitudes are a major barrier to participation in sport for LGBTQ+ people and a major reason why some LGBTQ+ identifying individuals choose to leave sport [46,47]. Heterosexism within sport is often built on very narrow and limiting definitions of masculinity and femininity [47]. Behaviors within sport, like disparaging jokes or homophobic, biphobic, or transphobic slurs, reinforce such binary definitions of gender and perpetuate noninclusive attitudes and behaviors [46–48]. The effects of heterosexism and nonaccidental violence can be traumatic and push an athlete into isolation, which may precipitate and then exacerbate mental health symptoms and disorders, including eating disorders, anxiety symptoms, depressive symptoms, and contemplation of suicide [8]. Such isolation may also impact whether an athlete will seek mental health support [49].

Research from the European Union that has explored the opinions of LGBTI* (lesbian, gay, bisexual, trans, intersex, and *other queer identities) athletes found that 90% of individuals considered homophobia, biphobia, transphobia, and other forms of discrimination to be problematic within sport, with 82% having witnessed or experienced discriminatory language in the previous year [37]. A total of 8% of LGBTI* athletes officially reported incidents of discrimination based on gender or sexuality while a total of 32% of respondents stated they did not know who or which organization to contact in instances of discrimination based on gender and/or sexuality within sport. Facing negative personal experiences of discrimination based on gender and/or sexuality resulted in 5% of LGBTI* individuals quitting sport altogether.

Careful attention needs to be given to environmental level factors, including local and national policies that perpetuate the discrimination of LGBTQ+ individuals wherever athletes may practice or compete. Within elite sport, the 2014 Sochi Olympics may be seen as an example whereby a nation's stance on sexual minorities had an impact on the concentration, performance, and mental health of LGBTQ+ athletes [50]. Before the Games, Russian lawmakers passed a federal bill that prohibited the distribution of information about same-sex relationships to children. The bill was signed into law by Russian President Vladimir Putin shortly after it passed the State Duma. The law was criticized heavily internationally as it prevented LGBTQ+ advocacy.

Discussion

Strategies for participatory, collaborative, and multidisciplinary research

Researchers who wish to explore the mental health needs of LGBTQ+ elite athletes should adopt an inclusive participatory approach that is rooted in the health equity promotion model [51]. The model calls for acknowledging: a) heterogeneity among LGBTQ+ identifying individuals; b) structural and environmental contexts that contribute to mental health symptoms and disorders; and c) health-promoting pathways that take into consideration biological, psychological, behavioral, and social processes. The model further acknowledges the need to address multiple contexts and lived experiences across the lifespan of the individual. With LGBTQ+ elite athletes, this would include attention paid to both athletic and nonathletic contexts across their lifespan, including experiences of childhood through to retirement. Additionally, researchers should adopt good epidemiologic practice to better understand the incidence and prevalence of mental health symptoms and disorders of LGBTQ+ athletes, as well as risk and protective factors associated with their mental health needs. This would include the design of participatory, collaborative, and multidisciplinary research agendas, the collection of demographic data pertaining to sexual and gender identities, and the collection of demographic data that would allow comparative analyses across race, ethnicity, (dis)ability, age, income, class, and geography to better understand diversity and intersectionality within LGBTQ+ populations [10,52,53]. Researchers should follow previously published suggestions on mental health data collection, including the use of validated and reliable questionnaires that are athlete specific [54]. Researchers need to also be mindful of the sorts of experiences LGBTQ+ athletes may have with mental health services. This means structuring studies to better understand the mental health literacy needs of LGBTQ+ athletes, barriers to and enablers of mental health services use, strategies for enhanced mental health practice, and strategies to enhance recovery and return to play. Overall, research rooted in the health equity promotion model would help create inclusive policies, address and prevent heterosexism and nonaccidental violence in sport, and enhance individual practice to diagnose and treat mental health symptoms and disorders.

Evidence-based practice in mental health service delivery

Practitioners need to be aware of research showing that public and self-stigma, low levels of mental health literacy, negative experiences with previous use of mental health services, lack of faith in patient confidentiality, and busy schedules have all been reported to create barriers to seeking treatment of mental health symptoms and disorders for elite athletes [55]. Additionally, many elite athletes are not open about their sexuality, which may compound the difficulty for these individuals to seek appropriate support for mental health symptoms and disorders [55,56]. Practitioners should use strategies to enhance mental health literacy, a key factor in enhancing help-seeking behavior and decreasing public and self-stigma, and design those strategies in a culturally competent manner, one that respects the lived experiences of individuals and their multiple identities [57,58]. Sports teams, leagues, and organizations need to embrace strategies to address heterosexism and the various forms of discrimination against LGBTQ+ athletes. The National Collegiate Athletic Association (NCAA) has investigated and established strategies for best practice in this area, including the creation of LGBTQ inclusive nondiscrimination policies, LGBTQ inclusive codes of conduct, communication material that includes LGBTQ inclusive and nondiscriminatory language, the creation and availability of LGBTQ resources for athletes and coaches, and annual training opportunities for staff and students [59,60]. Practitioners should also follow the further recommendations from the NCAA including raising the visibility of LGBTQ athletes and providing access to mental health services [61]. Strategies to enhance diagnosis and treatment, including both psychotherapy and psychiatric medication, have been extensively reviewed by Chang and colleagues, Reardon and colleagues, and Gouttebarge and colleagues [1,54,62]. Practitioners should establish and maintain a therapeutic alliance with LGBTQ+ identifying athletes, regardless of the specific modality of care. Service providers should initiate any interaction with athletes by asking them their preferred names and pronouns whereby this would enhance inclusivity [63,64]. An inclusive and respectful therapeutic alliance – a collaborative relationship between the athlete and mental health provider, which recognizes and validates an athlete's gender and sexual identity – may act as a key contributor to treatment adherence and overall symptom reduction [63,65,66]. Practitioners should note that athletes may choose to change their preferred names and pronouns, as well as sexual identities, during their course of treatment and recovery. Affirmative therapy takes a positive view of LGBTQ+ identities and relationships and acknowledges the impact of homophobia, biphobia, transphobia, and heterosexism. At times, within psychotherapy, it may be necessary to ask difficult questions that may pertain to an athlete's gender and/or sexual identity. For example, the athlete may wish to acknowledge and address experiences of proximal minority stress or explore areas of their various gender and/or sexual identities. Practitioners should approach these questions and discussions carefully, with sensitivity and respect, rooted in a well-designed and maintained therapeutic alliance.

SUMMARY

Within elite sport, very little is known about the mental health symptoms and disorders of LGBTQ+ identifying athletes, their experiences with accessing or receiving mental health services, or their journeys through recovery. Mental health researchers and providers who work with elite athletes who identify as LGBTQ+ are in positions to improve knowledge and pathways to mental health services, address and minimize barriers to mental health services, and enhance mental health service delivery. Participatory, collaborative, and multidisciplinary research that is rooted in the health equity promotion model may help better understand and address structural and environmental challenges within elite sport while acknowledging the heterogeneity and intersectionality of LGBTQ+ athletes. Inclusive, rigorous research will ultimately help structure mental health services to better address the mental health needs of LGBTQ+ elite athletes.

CLINICS CARE POINTS

- Ensure mental health literacy resources are inclusive of LGBTQ+ people and offer connections to LGBTQ+ supportive services and providers.
- Routinely ask athletes their preferred names and pronouns to enhance inclusivity.
- Familiarity with affirmative therapy whereby LGBTQ+ identities and relationships are acknowledged and respected may facilitate a stronger therapeutic alliance

DISCLOSURE

The authors have nothing to disclose.

REFERENCES

[1] Reardon CL, Hainline B, Miller Aron C, et al. Mental health in elite athletes: International Olympic Committee consensus statement (2019). Br J Sports Med 2019; 53:667–99.

[2] Swann C, Moran A, Piggott D. Defining elite Athletes: issues in the study of expert performance in sport psychology. Psychol Sport Exerc 2015;16:3–14.

[3] World Health Organization. Strengthening mental health promotion (Fact sheet, No 220). Geneva, Switzerland: World Health Organization; 2001.

[4] Gorczynski PF, Coyle M, Gibson K. Depressive symptoms in high-performance athletes and non-athletes: a comparative meta-analysis. Br J Sports Med 2017;51: 1348–54.

[5] Gouttebarge V, Castaldelli-Maia JM, Gorczynski P, et al. Occurrence of mental health symptoms and disorders in current and former elite athletes: a systematic review and meta-analysis. Br J Sports Med 2019;53:700–6.

[6] Rice SM, Gwyther K, Santesteban-Echarri O, et al. Determinants of anxiety in elite athletes: a systematic review and meta-analysis. Br J Sports Med 2019;53:722–30.

[7] American Psychiatric Association. Diagnostic and statistical manual of mental disorders. 5th edition. Arlington (VA): American Psychiatric Publishing; 2013.

[8] Mountjoy M, Brackenridge C, Arrington M, et al. International Olympic Committee consensus statement: harassment and abuse (non- accidental violence) in sport. Br J Sports Med 2016;50:1019–29.

[9] Vella S, Sutcliffe J, Swann C, et al. A systematic review and meta-synthesis of mental health position statements in sport: scope, quality and future directions. Psychol Sport Exerc 2021;55:101946.

[10] Gorczynski P, Fasoli F. LGBTQ+ focused mental health research strategy in response to COVID19. Lancet Psychiatry 2020;7:E56.

[11] US Institute of Medicine. The health of lesbian, gay, bisexual, and transgender people: building a foundation for better understanding. Washington, DC: The National Academies Press; 2011.

[12] Moagi MM, van Der Wath AE, Jiyane PM, et al. Mental health challenges of lesbian, gay, bisexual and transgender people: an integrated literature review. Health SA 2021;26:1487.

[13] Wilson C, Cariola LA. LGBTQI+ youth and mental health: a systematic review of qualitative research. Adolesc Res Rev 2020;5:187–211.

[14] McDonald K. Social support and mental health in LGBTQ adolescents: a review of the literature. Issues Ment Health Nurs 2018;39:16–29.

[15] Bender AK, Lauritsen JL. Violent Victimization among Lesbian, Gay, and Bisexual populations in the United States: findings from the National Crime Victimization Survey, 2017-2018. Am J Public Health 2021;111: 318–26 [published correction appears in Am J Public Health. 2021 Jul;111:e5].

[16] National Sexual Violence Resource Center. Sexual violence & transgender/non-binary communities. Available at: https://www.nsvrc.org/sites/default/files/publications/2019-02/Transgender_infographic_508_0.pdf. Accessed December 23, 2021.

[17] Gruberg S, Mahowald L, Halpin J. The state of the LGBTQ community in 2020. Center for American Progress; 2020. Available at: https://www.americanprogress.org/article/state-lgbtq-community-2020/. Accessed December 23, 2021.

[18] Government Equalities Office. National LGBT survey: research report. July, 2018. Available at: https://assets.publishing.service.gov.uk/government/uploads/system/uploads/attachment_data/file/721704/LGBT-survey-research-report.pdf. Accessed December 23, 2021.

[19] Ojanen TT, Ratanashevorn R, Boonkerd S. Gaps in responses to LGBT issues in Thailand: mental health research, services, and policies. Psychol Sex Rev 2016;7:41–59.

[20] Rutherford K, McIntyre J, Daley A, et al. Development of expertise in mental health service provision for lesbian, gay, bisexual and transgender communities. Med Educ 2012;46:903–13.

[21] McCann E, Sharek D. Challenges to and opportunities for improving mental health services for lesbian, gay, bisexual, and transgender people in Ireland: a narrative account. Int J Ment Health Nurs 2014;23:525–33.

[22] Steele LS, Daley A, Curling D, et al. LGBT identity, untreated depression, and unmet need for mental health services by sexual minority women and trans-identified people. J Womens Health 2017;26:116–27.

[23] Currie A, Blauwet C, Bindra A, et al. Athlete mental health: future directions. Br J Sports Med 2021;55: 1243–4.

[24] Kroshus E, Davoren AK. Mental health and substance use of sexual minority college athletes. J Am Coll Health 2016;64:371–9.

[25] Veliz P, Epstein-Ngo Q, Zdroik, et al. Substance use among sexual minority collegiate athletes: a national study. Subst Use Misuse 2016;51:517–32 [published correction appears in Subst Use Misuse 2016;51: 1074-5].

[26] Oftadeh-Moghadam S, Gorczynski P. Mental health literacy, help-seeking, and mental health outcomes in women rugby players. Women Sport Phys Act J 2021. https://doi.org/10.1123/wspaj.2020-0066.

[27] Kamis D, Glick ID. Improving competition and mental health for transgender athletes. Phys Sportsmed 2021. https://doi.org/10.1080/00913847.2021.1949250.

[28] Jones BA, Arcelus J, Bouman WP, et al. Sport and transgender people: a systematic review of the literature relating to sport participation and competitive sport policies. Sports Med 2017;47:701–16.

[29] Bronfenbrenner U. Toward an experimental ecology of human development. Am Psychol 1977;32:513–31.

[30] McLeroy KR, Bibeau D, Steckler A, et al. An ecological perspective on health promotion programs. Health Educ Q 1988;15:351–77.

[31] Purcell R, Gwyther K, Rice SM. Mental health in elite athletes: increased awareness requires an early intervention framework to respond to athlete needs. Sports Med Open 2019;5:46.
[32] Stambulova N, Wylleman P. Athletes' career development and transitions. In: Papaioannou AG, Hackfort D, editors. Routledge companion to sport and exercise psychology: global perspectives and fundamental concepts. London (UK): Routledge/Taylor & Francis Group; 2014. p. 605–20.
[33] Wylleman P, Reints A, De Knop P. A developmental and holistic perspective on athletic career development. In: Sotiaradou P, Bosscher VD, editors. Managing high performance sport (Foundations of sport Management). London (UK): Routledge; 2013. p. 159–82.
[34] Kuettel A, Larsen CH. Risk and protective factors for mental health in elite athletes: a scoping review. Int Rev Sport Exerc Psychol 2020;13:231–65.
[35] Lee S-M, Lombera JM, Larsen LK. Helping athletes cope with minority stress in sport. J Sport Psychol Action 2019;10:174–90.
[36] Meyer IH. Prejudice, social stress, and mental health in lesbian, gay, and bisexual populations: conceptual issues and research evidence. Psychol Bull 2003;129: 674–97.
[37] Menzel T, Braumüller B, Hartmann-Tews I. The relevance of sexual orientation and gender identity in sport in Europe. Findings from the Outsport survey. Cologne (Germany): German Sport University Cologne, Institute of Sociology and Gender Studies; 2019. Available at: https://leapsports.org/files/1402-Outsport%20Main%20Report.pdf. Accessed December 23, 2021.
[38] Walker NA, Melton EN. The tipping point: the intersection of race, gender, and sexual orientation in intercollegiate sports. J Appl Sport Manag 2015;29:257–71.
[39] Modrakovic D, Way N, Forssell S, et al. Moderating effects of minority stress on the association between adherence to norms of masculinity and psychological well-being in a diverse sample of gay male emerging adults. Psychol Men Masc 2021;22:412–21.
[40] Russell ST, Fish JN. Mental health in lesbian, gay, bisexual, and transgender (LGBT) youth. Annu Rev Clin Psychol 2016;12:465–87.
[41] Cunningham GB. Understanding the experiences of LGBT athletes in sport: a multilevel model. In: Anshel MH, Petrie TA, Steinfeldt JA, editors. APA handbook of sport and exercise psychology, Vol. 1. Sport psychology. Washington, DC: APA Books; 2019. p. 367–83.
[42] Cunningham GB. Diversity and inclusivity in sport organizations: a multilevel perspective. London (UK): Routledge; 2019.
[43] DeFoor MT, Stepleman LM, Mann PC. Improving wellness for LGB collegiate student-athletes through sports medicine: a narrative review. Sports Med Open 2018; 4:48.
[44] Reynolds A, Hamidian Jahromi A. Transgender athletes in sports competitions: how policy measures can be more inclusive and fairer to all. Front Sports Act Living 2021;3:704178.
[45] Lesbian Gay. Bisexual, and Transgender Resource Center. General definitions. Available at: https://lgbt.ucsf.edu/glossary-terms. Accessed December 23, 2021.
[46] Denison E, Kitchen A. Out on the fields: the first international study on homophobia in sport. 2015. Available at: https://outonthefields.com/wp-content/uploads/2020/11/Out-on-the-Fields-Final-Report-1.pdf. Accessed December 23, 2021.
[47] Toomey RB, McGeorge CR, Carlson TS. A mixed-methods pilot study of student athlete engagement in LGBTQ ally actions. JIS 2016;9:247–67.
[48] Cunningham GB. LGBT inclusive athletic departments as agents of social change. JIS 2015;8:43–56.
[49] Maurer-Starks SS, Clemons HL, Whalen SL. Managing heteronormativity and homonegativity in athletic training: in and beyond the classroom. J Athlet Train 2008;43:326–36.
[50] Radio Free Europe/Radio Liberty. Some Olympic athletes just say no – to protests. 2014. Available at: https://www.rferl.org/a/olympics-athletes-protest-homosexual-russia-sochi/25256287.html. Accessed December 23, 2021.
[51] Fredriksen-Goldsen KI, Simoni JM, Kim H-J, et al. The health equity promotion model: reconceptualization of lesbian, gay, bisexual, and transgender (LGBT) health disparities. Am J Orthopsychiatry 2014;84:653–63.
[52] Gorczynski P, Webb T. Developing a mental health research agenda for football referees. Soccer Soc 2021; 22:655–62.
[53] Gorczynski PF, Brittain DR. Call to action: the need for an LGBT-focused physical activity research strategy. Am J Prev Med 2016;51:527–30.
[54] Gouttebarge V, Bindra A, Blauwet C, et al. International Olympic Committee (IOC) Sport Mental Health Assessment Tool 1 (SMHAT- 1) and Sport Mental Health Recognition Tool 1 (SMHRT-1): towards better support of athletes' mental health. Br J Sports Med 2021;55: 30–7.
[55] Castaldelli-Maia JM, Gallinaro JGDME, Falcão RS, et al. Mental health symptoms and disorders in elite athletes: a systematic review on cultural influencers and barriers to athletes seeking treatment. Br J Sports Med 2019;53: 707–21.
[56] Cashmore E, Cleland J. Glasswing butterflies: gay professional football players and their culture. J Sport Soc Issues 2011;35:420–36.
[57] Gorczynski P, Currie A, Gibson K, et al. Developing mental health literacy and cultural competence in elite sport. J Appl Sport Psychol 2021;33:387–401.
[58] Gorczynski P, Gibson K, Thelwell R, et al. The BASES expert statement on mental health literacy in elite sport. Sport Exerc Scientist 2019;59:6–7.
[59] NCAA. Five ways to have an LGBTQ-inclusive athletics department. Available at: https://www.ncaa.org/about/resources/inclusion/five-ways-have-lgbtq-inclusive-athletics-department. Accessed Decembe 23, 2021.

[60] Griffin P, Taylor H. Champions of respect: inclusion of LGBTQ student-athletes and staff in NCAA Programs. NCAA. Available at: https://www.ncaapublications.com/productdownloads/CRLGBTQ.pdf. Accessed December 23, 2021.

[61] Rankin S, Weber G. Mind, body and sport: harassment and discrimination – LGBTQ student athletes. Available at: https://www.ncaa.org/health-and-safety/sport-science-institute/mind-body-and-sport-harassment-and-discrimination-lgbtq-student-athletes. Accessed December 23, 2021.

[62] Chang C, Putukian M, Aerni G, et al. Mental health issues and psychological factors in athletes: detection, management, effect on performance and prevention: American Medical Society for Sports Medicine Position Statement-Executive Summary. Br J Sports Med 2020; 54:216–20.

[63] Knutson D, Koch JM, Goldbach C. Recommended terminology, pronouns, and documentation for work with transgender and non-binary populations. Pract Innov 2019;4:214–24.

[64] Marra J, Law MY, Conlon E. Clinical considerations in caring for transgender athletes. Am Fam Physican 2021; 103:518–20.

[65] McDuff DR, Garvin M. Working with sports organizations and teams. Int Rev Psychiatry 2016;28:95–605.

[66] Baier AL, Kline AC, Feeny NC. Therapeutic alliance as a mediator of change: a systematic review and evaluation of research. Clin Psychol Rev 2020;82:101921.

Advances in Psychiatry and Behavioral Health 2 (2022) 17–28

ADVANCES IN PSYCHIATRY AND BEHAVIORAL HEALTH

Psychiatric Treatment Preferences for the Management of Postconcussion Symptoms

A Survey and Brief Literature Review

Aaron Slone Jeckell, MD[a,b,*], Lydia J. Mckeithan, MD[a,c,1], Aaron M. Yengo-Kahn, MD[a,d], Katherine A. Gifford, PsyD[a,e]

[a]Vanderbilt Sports Concussion Center, Nashville, TN, USA; [b]Department of Psychiatry and Behavioral Health, Vanderbilt University School of Medicine, Nashville, TN, USA; [c]Vanderbilt University School of Medicine, Nashville, TN, USA; [d]Department of Neurological Surgery, Vanderbilt University Medical Center, 1161 21st Avenue South, Medical Center North, Suite T4224, Nashville, TN 37232, USA; [e]Department of Neurology, Vanderbilt University Medical Center, 1207 17th Avenue South, Suite 204, Nashville, TN 37212, USA

KEYWORDS

• Concussion • Mental health • Surveys and questionnaires • Sport concussion • Concussion treatment • Literature review

KEY POINTS

- A small percentage of athletes who experience sport-related concussion (SRC) will go on to develop new or worsened neuropsychiatric symptoms.
- Various interventions including pharmacotherapy can be helpful in managing symptoms that do not resolve within an expected period of time.
- Psychiatrists are uniquely qualified to manage these symptoms which can include cognitive impairment, emotional disturbance, headache/somatic symptoms, and sleep impairment.
- There are no FDA-approved treatments for the management of SRC-related symptoms, but many medications are used off-label.
- Psychiatrists demonstrate a range of confidence in managing these symptoms as well as preferences for various interventions, underscoring the need for future robust studies and evidence-based treatment guidelines.

INTRODUCTION

Concussion is a prevalent form of mild traumatic brain injury (mTBI) affecting millions of individuals every year, with a large proportion of those being youths and/or athletes [1–3]. An estimated 1.6 to 3.8 million sport-related concussions (SRCs) take place every year [2], and as many as 30% of individuals may experience some form of TBI by the age of 25 [4]. These injuries are often accompanied by neuropsychiatric symptoms such as depression, anxiety, sleep disruption, cognitive disturbance, and somatic complaints [5,6]. Furthermore, preinjury psychiatric history has been shown to be associated with prolonged recovery times [7] and an increased risk of developing postconcussion

[1] Present address: 3000 Vanderbilt Place Apartment 411, Nashville, TN 37212.

*Corresponding author. 4599 Northwest 25th Way, Boca Raton, FL 33434. *E-mail address:* aaron.jeckell.md@gmail.com

https://doi.org/10.1016/j.ypsc.2022.03.003
2667-3827/22/

syndrome (PCS) [8], defined as somatic, cognitive, behavioral, and/or emotional symptoms that persist beyond 3 months following mTBI.

It is unclear how a concussion can precipitate a range of neuropsychiatric symptoms, and the pathophysiology is likely different than in those experiencing similar psychiatric symptoms that are not related to concussion [9–13]. While the treatment of affective disorders, sleep issues, and cognitive disorders may be commonplace for a psychiatrist, they often have less exposure to concussion-related pathology. This is notable, as postconcussion-related symptoms typically resolve within a month [11,14], whereas nonconcussion psychopathology can last significantly longer and may be recurrent [15]. This distinction presents a challenge for determining which medications and other treatments are reasonable and for how long patients should be treated [16]. Sports psychiatrists, and particularly those with training in child/adolescent psychiatry, may receive a disproportionate number of these referrals due to the prevalence of SRC among young athletes [1,2,17–20].

Several studies have demonstrated the effectiveness of various medications in managing concussion-related symptoms, such as a retrospective analysis supporting amitriptyline for treating posttraumatic headache [21]. Another nonrandomized, single-blind, placebo run-in study found sertraline to be beneficial when treating depression and cognitive impairment following concussion [22,23]. However, the literature available is inconsistent and not without limitations, ultimately leading to a lack of US Food and Drug Administration (FDA)-approved treatments for concussion-related neuropsychiatric symptoms. Thus, all medications are used "off-label" and under the guidance of limited literature or empirical trials and are frequently driven by anecdotal or extrapolated findings [24]. Although previous surveys have demonstrated that providers agree on the effectiveness of psychological treatment of PCS [25], no consensus exists regarding the usefulness of specific pharmacologic or other interventions for neuropsychiatric symptoms.

The purpose of this study was to understand (i) the comfort level of those identifying as sports psychiatrists in treating concussion-related neuropsychiatric symptoms, (ii) the management preferences for pharmacologic or other interventions to target different subsets of concussion-related neuropsychiatric symptoms, and (iii) whether patient volume is associated with pharmacologic treatment preferences. We hypothesized that comfort level and management preferences would vary based on the psychiatrists' clinical volume of patients with postconcussion symptoms.

METHODS

This survey-based, cross-sectional study assessed (i) provider characteristics (gender, credentials, years in practice, and subspecialty), (ii) experience treating concussion-related symptoms (number of patients treated in the past year and patient demographics), (iii) confidence in managing concussion-related symptoms (100-point scale with 100 representing extremely confident), (iv) pharmacologic treatment preferences for postconcussion-related symptom subsets (including cognitive deficits, fatigue symptoms, sleep issues, headaches, and mood symptoms), (v) typical duration of pharmacotherapy, and (vi) referrals to other specialties. We choose response options based on a review of literature pertaining to the pharmacologic treatment of TBI-related neuropsychiatric symptoms [11,16,26,27]. Respondents had opportunities to provide free text responses indicating other medications or nonpharmacological interventions that they preferred in each scenario. The full survey is available in Supplemental Material.

The survey was sent via email to the listserv of all 87 active members of the International Society for Sports Psychiatry (ISSP) and promoted at an ISSP webinar held on April 25th, 2020. All information included in survey responses was stored anonymously in a secure password-protected database.

Categorial variables are presented as group proportions and counts. Continuous variables demonstrated skew distributions by the inspection of QQ plots and are presented as medians with interquartile ranges (IQR) using Tukey's Hinges. Responses were stratified based on the number of patients (ie, patient volume) treated for postconcussion symptoms in the past year. High and low volume was defined by the median number treated (median = 10), with providers who treated 10 or more patients for concussion symptoms in the past year as *high volume (HV)*, and those who treated less than 10 as *low volume (LV)*. Analysis of categorical variables was performed using Pearson Chi-squared or Fisher exact tests as appropriate based on expected cell counts. Continuous variables were compared across groups using Mann–Whitney U-test. Spearman's rank correlation coefficient (r_s) was calculated to evaluate associations between years in practice, provider confidence level, and number of patients treated for concussion symptoms in the past year. No data were missing, and none were imputed. Statistical significance was set a priori at $P<.05$ without correction for multiple comparisons given the exploratory nature of the study. Statistical analysis was performed using Statistical Package for the Social Sciences (SPSS) version 27 (IBM, Armonk, NY, USA). This study was approved by the Vanderbilt University International Review Board (IRB#: 200274).

RESULTS

Demographics and Experience

A total of 30 individuals (24 male, 80%) completed the survey, 27 of whom were M.D. or equivalent (1 MBChB), and 3 who were D.O. Median years in practice was 11.5 years, with one respondent still in residency. Areas of subspecialization varied, with General Psychiatry (63.3%), Child and Adolescent Psychiatry (CAP) (26.7%), and other (non-NBME accredited) areas of specialization (23.3%) as the 3 most common fields. Adult nonathlete (56.7%), adult professional athlete (50%), and high school athlete (46.7%) were the demographics commonly treated. On average, respondents had treated a median of 10 patients for concussion in the past year. Of all respondents, the median level of confidence caring for concussion-related pathology was 75 and ranged from 10 to 100. Information on respondent training and demographics can be found in Table 1.

When stratified by level of experience, HV providers cared for a median of 10 patients for concussion in the past year, whereas LV providers cared for 3 ($P = .011$), with 3 LV providers having seen none. There was no significant difference in years of practice or confidence between HV and LV providers. However, patient volume was significantly correlated with confidence level among providers ($r_s = 0.38$, $P = .038$). There was no significant correlation between confidence and years in practice ($r_s = 0.17$, $P = .39$) or between years in practice and patient volume ($r_s = 0.00$, $P = 1.00$). HV providers most frequently treated adult patients, with adult nonathlete (78.9% vs 18.2%, $P = .002$) as the most common subgroup (treated for all mental health conditions, not just concussion). This is visualized in Fig. 1.

Treatment Preferences

Across all respondents, there was a preference for stimulant medications (43.3%) for the management of cognitive dysfunction. Some expressed a preference for the use of nonpharmacological intervention (30%), memantine (6.7%), hyperbaric oxygen (3.3%), light therapy (3.3%), and bupropion (3.3%). While there were limited statistical differences between treatment preferences of HV and LV providers, some notable discrepancies are suggested, with *P* values significant in some but not all findings. HV providers more frequently prescribed stimulants (52.6%) relative to LV providers (27.3%, $P = .260$), and LV providers were more likely to rely on other/nonpharmacological treatments (72.7%) than HV providers (21.1%, $P = .009$). For daytime fatigue, respondents indicated preferences for stimulants (30%), selective serotonin reuptake inhibitors (SSRIs) (30%), modafinil (23.3%), and other/nonpharmacological intervention (16.7%). For daytime fatigue, HV providers were more likely to prescribe stimulants (42.1% vs 9.1%, $P = .100$), while LV providers most frequently prescribed SSRIs (45.5% vs 21.05%, $P = .225$). Other treatments for daytime fatigue included the use of nonpharmacological interventions (26.7%, with examples provided by respondents including exercise or psychotherapy), and non-SSRIs such as modafinil (10%) or bupropion (3.3%). Insomnia was managed predominantly with melatonin (40%), followed by trazodone (33.3%), with HV providers more frequently using melatonin (52.6% vs 18.2%, $P = .121$). Respondents frequently prescribed nonsteroidal anti-inflammatory drugs (NSAIDs) (30%) for headache, and many indicated a preference for referring to Neurology. The management of emotional symptoms with SSRIs (n = 24) was preferred by most of both LV and HV respondents (80%). Full treatment preferences are presented in Table 2.

Multiple respondents identified a preference for lifestyle modification and other nonpharmacological interventions as first line for the management of concussion-related neuropsychiatric symptoms. Several indicated efforts to avoid the use of medications if possible. Many comments addressed the need for a multimodal and collaborative treatment plan involving other fields. Physical Therapy (70%) and Neurology (70%) were the most common services to which patients were referred.

Treatment Duration

The duration of treatment ranged across time frames with 3 to 6 months (30%) and 6 to 12 months (40%) being the most common ranges. HV providers were more likely to treat in the 3 to 6 and 6 to 12-month ranges relative to LV providers who were most likely to provide treatment in the 6 to 12-month range ($P = .225$). Two individuals did not identify a particular time frame, noting that this was quite variable based on the patient and other factors.

TABLE 1
Respondent demographics

	Experience groups		*P* value[a]	Overall
	Low volume (n = 11)	**High volume (n = 19)**		**n = 30**
Demographics				
Gender (male)	91 (10)	74 (14)	.372	80 (24)
Years in Practice (median [IQR])	12 [5.5,15.5]	11 [4,22.5]	1.000	11.5 [4,20]
Number of Patients in the last year (median [IQR])	3 [1,5]	10 [10,20]	.011[b]	10 [5, 15]
Confidence (median [IQR])	75 [50,77.5]	80 [70,85]	.142	75 [66, 85]
Degree				
MD or Equivalent	100 (11)	84.2 (16)	.279	90 (27)
DO	0 (0)	15.8 (3)	.279	10 (3)
Subspecialty	Low Volume (n = 11)	High Volume (n = 19)		
Addiction	36.4 (4)	10.5 (2)	.126	20 (6)
Brain Injury Medicine	9.1 (1)	0 (0)	.367	3.3 (1)
Child and Adolescent	18.2 (2)	31.6 (6)	.672	26.7 (8)
Consultation-Liaison	9.1 (1)	10.5 (2)	1.000	10 (3)
Forensic Psychiatry	18.2 (2)	5.3 (1)	.537	10 (3)
Geriatric Psychiatry	0 (0)	5.3 (1)	1.000	3.3 (1)
Sleep Medicine	0 (0)	10.5 (2)	.520	6.7 (2)
General Psychiatry	72.7 (8)	57.9 (11)	.466	63.3 (19)
Other	36.4 (4)	15.8 (3)	.372	23.3 (7)
Type of Patients	Low Volume (n = 11)	High Volume (n = 19)		
Adult Professional	36.4 (4)	57.9 (11)	.256	50 (15)
Adult Recreation	27.3 (3)	47.4 (9)	.279	40 (12)
NCAA	18.2 (2)	47.4 (9)	.140	36.7 (11)
Collegiate Recreational	9.1 (1)	36.8 (7)	.199	26.7 (8)
Adult Nonathlete	18.2 (2)	78.9 (15)	.002	56.7 (17)
High School Athlete	45.5 (5)	47.4 (9)	1.000	46.7 (14)
Adolescent Nonathlete	18.2 (2)	36.8 (7)	.419	30 (9)
Middle School Athlete	9.1 (1)	36.8 (7)	.199	26.7 (8)
Youth Athlete	18.2 (2)	26.3 (5)	1.000	23.3 (7)
Youth Nonathlete	0 (0)	21.1 (4)	.268	13.3 (4)
None	27.3 (3)	0 (0)	.041	10 (3)

[a] Chi-squared or Fisher exact test based on expected cell counts.
[b] Mann–Whitney U-test.

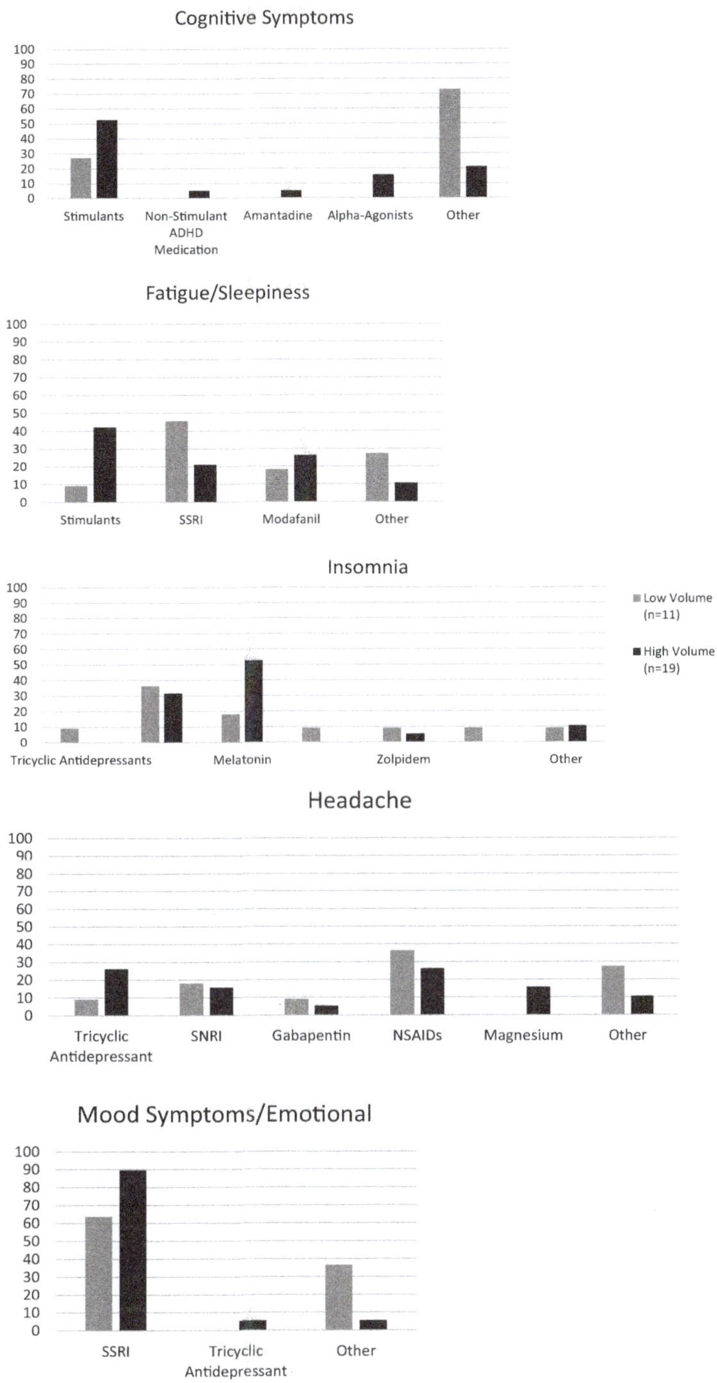

FIG. 1 Treatment preference for symptom clusters by experience (percentage of respondents).

TABLE 2
Treatment preference by experience

	Experience Groups		*P* value[a,b]	Overall
	Low Volume (n = 11)	**High Volume (n = 19)**		
Cognitive Symptoms				
Stimulants	27.3 (3)	52.6 (10)	0.260	43.3 (13)
Nonstimulant ADHD Medication	0 (0)	5.3 (1)	1	3.3 (1)
Amantadine	0 (0)	5.3 (1)	1	3.3 (1)
Alpha-Agonists	0 (0)	15.8 (3)	0.279	10 (3)
Other	72.7 (8)	21.1 (4)	0.009	40 (12)
Fatigue, Sleepiness				
Stimulants	9.1 (1)	42.1 (8)	0.100	30 (9)
SSRI	45.5 (5)	21.1 (4)	0.225	30 (9)
Modafanil	18.2 (2)	26.3 (5)	1	23.3 (7)
Other	27.3 (3)	10.5 (2)	0.327	16.7 (5)
Insomnia				
Tricyclic Antidepressants	9.1 (1)	0 (0)	0.367	3.3 (1)
Trazadone	36.4 (4)	31.6 (6)	1	33.3 (10)
Melatonin	18.2 (2)	52.6 (10)	0.121	40 (12)
Magnesium	9.1 (1)	0 (0)	0.367	3.3 (1)
Zolpidem	9.1 (1)	5.3 (1)	1	6.7 (2)
Benzodiazepine	9.1 (1)	0 (0)	0.367	3.3 (1)
Other	9.1 (1)	10.5 (2)	1	10 (3)
Headache				
Tricyclic Antidepressant	9.1 (1)	26.3 (5)	0.372	20 (6)
SNRI	18.2 (2)	15.8 (3)	1	16.7 (5)
Gabapentin	9.1 (1)	5.3 (1)	1	6.7 (2)
NSAIDs	36.4 (4)	26.3 (5)	0.687	30 (9)
Magnesium	0 (0)	15.8 (3)	0.279	10 (3)
Other	27.3 (3)	10.5 (2)	0.327	16.7 (5)
Emotional (depression/anxiety)				
SSRI	63.6 (7)	89.5 (17)	0.156	80 (24)
Tricyclic Antidepressant	0 (0)	5.3 (1)	1	3.3 (1)
Other	36.4 (4)	5.3 (1)	0.047	16.7 (5)
Treatment Duration				
1–3 mo	18.2 (2)	10.5 (2)	0.611	13.3 (4)
3–6 mo	9.1 (1)	42.1 (8)	0.100	30 (9)
6–12 mo	45.5 (5)	36.8 (7)	0.712	40 (12)

(*continued on next page*)

TABLE 2
(continued)

	Experience Groups		*P* value[a,b]	Overall
	Low Volume (n = 11)	High Volume (n = 19)		
>12 mo	9.1 (1)	10.5 (2)	1	10 (3)
Other	18.2 (2)	0 (0)	0.126	6.7 (2)
Referrals				
Physical Therapy	54.5 (6)	78.9 (15)	0.225	70 (21)
Occupational Therapy	36 (4)	57.9 (11)	0.45	50 (15)
Neurology	71.7 (8)	68.4 (13)	1	70 (21)
Ophthalmology	18.2 (2)	36.8 (7)	0.419	30 (9)
Other	18.2 (2)	36.8 (7)	0.419	30 (9)

[a] Chi-squared or Fisher exact test based on expected cell counts.
[b] Mann–Whitney U-test. For referrals, common "others" were psychology or neuropsychology (5), vestibular or visual rehabilitation (3), [t]referent group is high volume.

DISCUSSION

This study aimed to identify psychiatrist treatment preferences for the management of postconcussive neuropsychiatric symptoms. The ISSP was identified as an ideal target organization, as psychiatrists who specialize in the treatment of the athletic community are assumed to be more likely to be exposed to individuals who have experienced concussion [1,2,19,20]. Our data were stratified by those in the top 50% for patient volume (HV) versus those in the lower 50%. Overall, our findings do not indicate a clear consensus across sports psychiatrists regarding treatment preferences for the management of postconcussive symptoms, even when stratified by provider level of experience. There were, however, several notable differences and similarities in treatment preferences between groups worth identifying.

Treatment Preferences by Patient Volume and Subspecialty

With respect to postconcussive cognitive symptoms, HV providers frequently prescribed stimulant medication for the management of concussion-related cognitive dysfunction. This has some support in the medical literature, and the use of stimulants in TBI has been studied in both human and animal models [28–33]. Nearly half of HV respondents favored stimulants for cognitive deficits and symptoms such as fatigue and sleepiness. As 75% of CAPs included in this survey were in the HV groups, it is possible that these preferences reflect that CAP providers have more comfort with the use of stimulant medications, as childhood attention-deficit/hyperactivity disorder (ADHD) is very frequently treated with this category of medication [34]. Similarly, HV providers may gain more exposure to the use of stimulants for the management of cognitive deficits, and in turn may be more likely to feel comfortable prescribing them to future patients, though we did not specifically assess for this in the survey. Importantly, athletes at elite levels of competition (generally collegiate and above) typically require specific documentation and/or approval to take stimulant medications, which are otherwise often prohibited. Thus, it could also be that it is simply logistically easier to prescribe stimulants for athletes at lower levels of competition (such as child athletes as typically seen by CAP providers).

A somewhat different pattern emerged for sleep-related problems. HV frequently preferred melatonin (52%) for sleep-related issues. A recent study addressed this treatment strategy [35]. Barlow and colleagues found that children who received melatonin following a concussion demonstrated similar persistent postconcussive symptoms as measured on the postconcussion symptom inventory (PCSI), as well as similar cognitive and sleep outcomes, compared with the placebo group. Conversely, the authors reported improvement in externalizing problems such as hyperactivity and aggression with melatonin use. As noted by the authors, the study was underpowered (n = 99, mean age 13.8 years;

SD = 2.6 years, 58% female), and the primary outcome was a change in responses on the PCSI, whereas most providers prescribe it specifically for sleep-related disturbance. Other studies support the use of melatonin in concussion, with studies identifying improvements in subjective sleep quality [36] and potential neuroprotective properties [37,38]. Ultimately, while additional data supporting the use of melatonin in concussion are mixed, melatonin remains a relatively safe and affordable intervention favored by many providers [39].

Providers espoused a more consistent preference for SSRIs to manage postconcussive emotional disturbance, regardless of patient volume. The use of SSRIs in patients who have experienced various forms of traumatic brain injury has been well studied [16,22,23,40]. One consideration when selecting an SSRI is that symptoms related to concussion are typically self-limiting, with the majority resolving within approximately 1 month [11]. SSRIs are known to take anywhere from 2 weeks to 3 months to reach efficacy [41–43]. This temporal overlap makes determining whether symptom resolution is due to pharmacologic intervention or the expected natural course of recovery difficult. However, it is also known that a baseline history of depression and/or family history of depression are risk factors for the development of emotional disturbance after concussion [11,44–46]. It may be the case that a provider finds themselves managing depression after a concussion that otherwise may not have met clinical attention [47–50]. In those situations, the use of SSRIs would be supported [51].

One notable outlier is that the 3 respondents with the most years in practice (average 40 years, confidence level 74.67, patients per year 11.33) all identified preferences for nonpharmacological interventions as much as possible. This may be attributed to the treatment philosophy of using low doses and making changes slowly in young patients and those with recent cerebral injury [16], though it is unclear why this was pronounced in this particular demographic of respondents. Another factor may be that these psychiatrists were trained during a time when psychotherapy was a common aspect of psychiatric practice, whereas psychiatrists being trained now may receive more of an emphasis on pharmacology.

THE NEED FOR CONSENSUS GUIDELINES

Patient volume was only mildly correlated with confidence, whereby greater volume was associated with greater confidence in managing concussion-related symptoms, and a substantial range (10–100) of confidence was reported. While it might be expected that HV providers would feel more confident with the management of concussion, the lack of empirical evidence for treatments remains a serious obstacle. As those with more experience may have seen more treatment failures as well as successes, these providers may rate their confidence lower despite more experience, leading to a weaker than expected degree of correlation. Those with more experience and exposure to mTBI are likely to be more aware of how difficult it can be to manage this condition, whereas an LV provider may be unaware of the challenge and endorse a higher level of confidence, a phenomenon studied by Kruger and Dunning [52]. There may also be a distinction between "comfort" and "confidence" in that while a provider may feel suited to provide care for an individual experiencing postconcussion psychopathology, it may be difficult to feel confident about a treatment plan that is lacking in empirical evidence.

While the treatment of the management of affective disorders, sleep issues, headache, and cognitive dysfunction is always tailored to an individual, there are evidence-based guidelines to guide the management of these conditions in nonconcussed adult and youth patient. For instance, data support the use of SSRIs for 9 to 12 months after achieving depressive symptom remission in adults [53]. However, in nonconcussion depression, one of the primary assumed mechanisms is the "chemical imbalance" in depression hypothesis [54]. What remains to be determined is how closely postconcussive depression mirrors this on a cellular and neurochemical level. Very likely, SRC-related mood disorder is due to a combination of bio-psycho-social changes (including subsequent lifestyle changes, alterations in neuroendocrine changes associated with physical activity, feelings of physical vulnerability, and anxiety relating to uncertain prognosis after a concussion) that may differ from those experienced in nonconcussion depression [9,10,55]. In cases of SRC, particularly at the elite level, psychological (sense of self, identity as an athlete, responsibility to teammates/family, and so forth) and social (isolation during recovery, feedback from teammates/media, and so forth) factors have the potential to be considerable and can impact mood significantly [10,56–60].

Recommendations made by Meehan regarding the initiation of pharmacotherapy after SRC include:

1. The athlete's symptoms have exceeded a typical recovery for SRC.
2. The symptoms are negatively affecting the patient's life to such a degree that the possible benefit of treatment outweighs the potential risks of the medication being considered.

3. The clinician caring for the athlete is knowledgeable and experienced in the general assessment and management of SRC or concussive brain injury in general [16].

Psychopharmacological medications for concussion-related symptoms typically should be deferred until nonpharmacological interventions have proven inadequate [16]. Once a medication is initiated, careful consideration regarding potential side effects and the importance of titration must be given. High rates of exercise may impact the metabolism of various medications, something that should be considered with athletes [61–64], though evidence is not robust in this population. Treatments that increase confusion or cause sedation, fatigue, or drowsiness should be avoided as they may make recovery monitoring difficult [16,27]. Consideration should also be given to the possibility of psychopharmacological medications having an impact on cognitive testing [65].

As mentioned, there are no FDA-approved treatments for the management of symptoms related to concussion [16,26]. There is a lack of detail regarding when to initiate treatment, which treatments have the most evidence, and how long interventions should be maintained. As such, providers are currently largely reliant on indirect and anecdotal evidence and personal experience for the development of treatment plans for concussion. This is likely the main cause of disparity in responses to this survey. Ultimately, our findings strongly reinforce the need for prospective studies to provide evidence-based treatment models. Additionally, in the interim, convening expert consensus panels to provide recommendations would be appropriate.

Limitations to this study include a small sample (n = 30) of providers who self-identify as sports psychiatrists. These individuals may have an interest in concussion but are not necessarily experts in the diagnosis or management of concussion. These findings may be markedly different with a larger sample or with a sample of non-sports psychiatrists who are less likely to manage concussion-related pathology. The decision to stratify respondents as "high volume" based on having treated 10 or more patients for concussion in the past year was based on the median patient volume of our sample. However, having seen 10 patients in the past year for the management of a condition is typically insufficient to confer expertise. The data gathered here highlight purely provider opinion at one point in time and are not intended to be used for the development or guidance of treatment. Rather, this study highlights the need for further study in the field of postconcussion symptoms, particularly in identifying empirically based treatments and pharmacotherapeutic interventions. Our study identifies provider preferences for the management of some neuropsychiatric symptoms but does not identify triggers for the initiation of or indicate treatment duration for any specific intervention. The survey developed was focused on the identification of psychopharmacological preferences for the management of mTBI, as this is a major deficit in the current medical and research literature. While providers were able to write in a preference for nonpharmacological interventions, we did not specifically identify whether providers were more likely to select pharmacologic interventions rather than nonmedication-based approaches.

SUMMARY

Sports psychiatrists have a wide range of confidence in concussion management, and treatment preferences for the management of concussion-related symptoms were not associated with experience level. This may be a result of limited empirical evidence or FDA-approved treatments for neuropsychiatric symptoms following concussion. While it appears small subsets of "high volume" providers agree on some treatments, these are likely based on prescribing models for other conditions or anecdotal evidence. These findings reinforce the need for more robust studies to direct evidence-based pharmacologic and nonpharmacological management with formal guidelines in the future.

CLINICS CARE POINTS

- Management of SRC symptoms should be conducted on a case-by-case basis and symptom-specific basis.
- Pharmacotherapeutic interventions should be considered only after recovery has lapsed beyond a typical or age-appropriate recovery period.
- Medications should be used with caution with careful consideration that treatments do not interfere with the assessment of recovery or neuropsychiatric testing.

DISCLOSURE

The authors have nothing to disclose.

SUPPLEMENTARY DATA

Supplementary data related to this article can be found online at c

REFERENCES

[1] Corrigan JD, Selassie AW, Orman JA. The epidemiology of traumatic brain injury. J Head Trauma Rehabil 2010; 25(2):72–80.

[2] Langlois JA, Rutland-Brown W, Wald MM. The epidemiology and impact of traumatic brain injury: a brief overview. J Head Trauma Rehabil 2006; 21(5):375–8.

[3] McKeithan L, Hibshman N, Yengo-Kahn A, et al. Sport-Related Concussion: Evaluation, Treatment, and Future Directions. Med Sci 2019;7(3):44.

[4] McKinlay A, Grace RC, Horwood LJ, et al. Prevalence of traumatic brain injury among children, adolescents and young adults: prospective evidence from a birth cohort. Brain Inj 2008;22(2):175–81.

[5] McAllister TW, Arciniegas D. Evaluation and treatment of postconcussive symptoms. NeuroRehabilitation 2002; 17(4):265–83.

[6] Busch CR, Alpern HP. Depression after mild traumatic brain injury: a review of current research. Neuropsychol Rev 1998;8(2):95–108.

[7] Guerriero RM, Giza CC, Rotenberg A. Glutamate and GABA imbalance following traumatic brain injury. Curr Neurol Neurosci Rep 2015;15(5):27.

[8] Morgan CD, Zuckerman SL, Lee YM, et al. Predictors of postconcussion syndrome after sports-related concussion in young athletes: a matched case-control study. J Neurosurg Pediatr 2015;15(6):589–98.

[9] Mainwaring L, Bisschop S, Green R, et al. Emotional Reaction of Varsity Athletes to Sport-Related Concussion. J Sport Exerc Psychol 2004;26:119–35.

[10] Mainwaring LM, Hutchison M, Bisschop SM, et al. Emotional response to sport concussion compared to ACL injury. Brain Inj 2010;24(4):589–97.

[11] McCrory P, Meeuwisse W, Dvorak J, et al. Consensus statement on concussion in sport-the 5th international conference on concussion in sport held in Berlin, October 2016. Br J Sports Med 2017;51(11):838–47.

[12] McCrea M, Guskiewicz K, Randolph C, et al. Incidence, clinical course, and predictors of prolonged recovery time following sport-related concussion in high school and college athletes. J Int Neuropsychol Soc 2013; 19(1):22–33.

[13] Ruff RM, Camenzuli L, Mueller J. Miserable minority: Emotional risk factors that influence the outcome of a mild traumatic brain injury. Brain Inj 1996;10(8): 551–65.

[14] Ellis MJ, Ritchie LJ, Koltek M, et al. Psychiatric outcomes after pediatric sports-related concussion. J Neurosurg Pediatr 2015;16(6):709–18.

[15] American Psychiatric Association. Diagnostic and statistical manual of mental disorders : DSM-5. 5th edition. Washington, DC: American Psychiatric Association; 2013.

[16] Meehan WP 3rd. Medical therapies for concussion. Clin Sports Med 2011;30(1):115–24, ix.

[17] Sarmiento K, Thomas KE, Daugherty J, et al. Emergency Department Visits for Sports- and Recreation-Related Traumatic Brain Injuries Among Children - United States, 2010-2016. MMWR Morb Mortal Wkly Rep 2019; 68(10):237–42.

[18] Kerr ZY, Chandran A, Nedimyer AK, et al. Concussion Incidence and Trends in 20 High School Sports. Pediatrics 2019;144(5):e20192180.

[19] Daneshvar DH, Nowinski CJ, McKee AC, et al. The epidemiology of sport-related concussion. Clin Sports Med 2011;30(1):1–17, vii.

[20] Gessel LM, Fields SK, Collins CL, et al. Concussions among united states high school and collegiate athletes. J Athl Train 2007;42(4):495–503.

[21] Tyler GS, McNeely HE, Dick ML. Treatment of post-traumatic headache with amitriptyline. Headache 1980; 20(4):213–6.

[22] Fann JR, Uomoto JM, Katon WJ. Sertraline in the treatment of major depression following mild traumatic brain injury. J Neuropsychiatry Clin Neurosci 2000; 12(2):226–32.

[23] Fann JR, Uomoto JM, Katon WJ. Cognitive improvement with treatment of depression following mild traumatic brain injury. Psychosomatics 2001;42(1):48–54.

[24] Silver JM, McAllister TW, Arciniegas DB. Depression and cognitive complaints following mild traumatic brain injury. Am J Psychiatry 2009;166(6):653–61.

[25] Mittenberg W, Burton DB. A survey of treatments for post-concussion syndrome. Brain Inj 1994;8(5):429–37.

[26] Jeckell AS, Solomon G. Pharmacological Interventions in Sport-Related Concussion. Pract Pain Management 2017; 17(10).

[27] Reddy CC, Collins MW, Gioia GA. Adolescent sports concussion. Phys Med Rehabil Clin N Am 2008;19(2): 247–69, viii.

[28] Chew E, Zafonte RD. Pharmacological management of neurobehavioral disorders following traumatic brain injury–a state-of-the-art review. J Rehabil Res Dev 2009; 46(6):851–79.

[29] Kline AE, Yan HQ, Bao J, et al. Chronic methylphenidate treatment enhances water maze performance following traumatic brain injury in rats. Neurosci Lett 2000; 280(3):163–6.

[30] Plenger PM, Dixon CE, Castillo RM, et al. Subacute methylphenidate treatment for moderate to moderately severe traumatic brain injury: a preliminary double-blind placebo-controlled study. Arch Phys Med Rehabil 1996; 77(6):536–40.

[31] Tramontana MG, Cowan RL, Zald D, et al. Traumatic brain injury-related attention deficits: treatment outcomes with lisdexamfetamine dimesylate (Vyvanse). Brain Inj 2014;28(11):1461–72.

[32] Whyte J, Hart T, Schuster K, et al. Effects of methylphenidate on attentional function after traumatic brain injury. A randomized, placebo-controlled trial. Am J Phys Med Rehabil 1997;76(6):440–50.

[33] Williams SE, Ris MD, Ayyangar R, et al. Recovery in pediatric brain injury: is psychostimulant medication beneficial? J Head Trauma Rehabil 1998;13(3):73–81.
[34] Sharma A, Couture J. A review of the pathophysiology, etiology, and treatment of attention-deficit hyperactivity disorder (ADHD). The Ann Pharmacother 2014;48(2): 209–25.
[35] Barlow KM, Brooks BL, Esser MJ, et al. Efficacy of Melatonin in Children With Postconcussive Symptoms: A Randomized Clinical Trial. Pediatrics 2020; 145(4).
[36] Grima NA, Rajaratnam SMW, Mansfield D, et al. Efficacy of melatonin for sleep disturbance following traumatic brain injury: a randomised controlled trial. BMC Med 2018;16(1):8.
[37] Maldonado MD, Murillo-Cabezas F, Terron MP, et al. The potential of melatonin in reducing morbidity-mortality after craniocerebral trauma. J Pineal Res 2007; 42(1):1–11.
[38] Samantaray S, Das A, Thakore NP, et al. Therapeutic potential of melatonin in traumatic central nervous system injury. J Pineal Res 2009;47(2):134–42.
[39] Osier N, McGreevy E, Pham L, et al. Melatonin as a Therapy for Traumatic Brain Injury: A Review of Published Evidence. Int J Mol Sci 2018;19(5):1539.
[40] Arciniegas DB, Anderson CA, Topkoff J, et al. Mild traumatic brain injury: a neuropsychiatric approach to diagnosis, evaluation, and treatment. Neuropsychiatr Dis Treat 2005;1(4):311–27.
[41] Trivedi MH, Fava M, Wisniewski SR, et al. Medication augmentation after the failure of SSRIs for depression. N Engl J Med 2006;354(12):1243–52.
[42] Machado-Vieira R, Baumann J, Wheeler-Castillo C, et al. The Timing of Antidepressant Effects: A Comparison of Diverse Pharmacological and Somatic Treatments. Pharmaceuticals (Basel) 2010;3(1):19–41.
[43] Rossi A, Barraco A, Donda P. Fluoxetine: a review on evidence based medicine. Ann Gen Hosp Psychiatry 2004; 3(1):2.
[44] Legarreta AD, Brett BL, Solomon GS, et al. The role of family and personal psychiatric history in postconcussion syndrome following sport-related concussion: a story of compounding risk. J Neurosurg Pediatr 2018; 22(3):238–43.
[45] Solomon G, Kuhn A, Zuckerman S. Depression as a Modifying Factor in Sport-Related Concussion: A Critical Review of the Literature. Phys Sportsmed 2015 Early Online: 1–6.
[46] Yang J, Peek-Asa C, Covassin T, et al. Post-concussion symptoms of depression and anxiety in division I collegiate athletes. Dev Neuropsychol 2015;40(1): 18–23.
[47] Iverson GL, Gardner AJ, Terry DP, et al. Predictors of clinical recovery from concussion: a systematic review. Br J Sports Med 2017;51(12):941–8.
[48] Iverson GL, Silverberg ND, Mannix R, et al. Factors Associated With Concussion-like Symptom Reporting in High School Athletes. JAMA Pediatr 2015;169(12): 1132–40.
[49] Lange RT, Iverson GL, Rose A. Depression Strongly Influences Postconcussion Symptom Reporting Following Mild Traumatic Brain Injury. The J Head Trauma Rehabil 2011;26(2):127–37.
[50] Lovell MR, Collins MW, Iverson GL, et al. Recovery from mild concussion in high school athletes. J Neurosurg 2003;98(2):296–301.
[51] March JS, Silva S, Petrycki S, et al. The Treatment for Adolescents With Depression Study (TADS): long-term effectiveness and safety outcomes. Arch Gen Psychiatry 2007;64(10):1132–43.
[52] Kruger J, Dunning D. Unskilled and unaware of it: how difficulties in recognizing one's own incompetence lead to inflated self-assessments. J Pers Soc Psychol 1999; 77(6):1121–34.
[53] National Collaborating Centre for Mental H. National Institute for Health and Clinical Excellence: Guidance. In: Depression: the treatment and Management of depression in adults (Updated Edition). Leicester (UK): British Psychological Society Copyright The British Psychological Society & The Royal College of Psychiatrists; 2010. p. 2010.
[54] Harmer CJ, Duman RS, Cowen PJ. How do antidepressants work? New perspectives for refining future treatment approaches. Lancet Psychiatry 2017;4(5): 409–18.
[55] Zuckerman SL, Yengo-Kahn AM, Brett BL, et al. Benefits of team sport participation versus concerns of chronic traumatic encephalopathy: prioritizing the health of our youth. Concussion 2020;5(2):CNC75.
[56] Brett B, Mummareddy N, Kuhn A, et al. The Relationship Between Prior Concussions and Depression Is Modified by Somatic Symptomatology in Retired NFL Athletes. The J Neuropsychiatry Clin Neurosciences 2019;31(1): 17–24.
[57] Boone EM, Leadbeater BJ. Game on: Diminishing risks for depressive symptoms in early adolescence through positive involvement in team sports. J Res Adolescence 2006;16(1):79–90.
[58] Gorczynski PF, Coyle M, Gibson K. Depressive symptoms in high-performance athletes and non-athletes: a comparative meta-analysis. Br J Sports Med 2017; 51(18):1348–54.
[59] Nixdorf I, Frank R, Beckmann J. Comparison of Athletes' Proneness to Depressive Symptoms in Individual and Team Sports: Research on Psychological Mediators in Junior Elite Athletes. Front Psychol 2016;7:893.
[60] Oler MJ, Mainous AG 3rd, Martin CA, et al. Depression, suicidal ideation, and substance use among adolescents. Are athletes at less risk? Arch Fam Med 1994; 3(9):781–5.
[61] Dossing M. Effect of acute and chronic exercise on hepatic drug metabolism. Clin Pharmacokinet 1985;10(5): 426–31.

[62] Lenz TL. The effects of high physical activity on pharmacokinetic drug interactions. Expert Opin Drug Metab Toxicol 2011;7(3):257–66.

[63] Peng HT, Cheung B. A review of psychophysiological stressors on pharmacokinetics. J Clin Pharmacol 2011; 51(11):1499–518.

[64] Ylitalo P. Effect of exercise on pharmacokinetics. Ann Med 1991;23(3):289–94.

[65] Yengo-Kahn AM, Solomon G. Are psychotropic medications associated with differences in baseline neurocognitive assessment scores for young athletes? A pilot study. Phys Sportsmed 2015;43(3):227–35.

Neurosciences

Advances in Psychiatry and Behavioral Health 2 (2022) 29–36

ADVANCES IN PSYCHIATRY AND BEHAVIORAL HEALTH

Neuropsychiatric Aspect of Posterior Cortical Atrophy

Chuang-Kuo Wu, MD, PhD

Department of Neurology, Brown University Alpert Medical School, Alzheimer's Disease and Memory Disorders Center, Rhode Island Hospital, 593 Eddy Street, APC-7, Providence, RI 02903, USA

KEYWORDS

• Atrophy • Dementia • Alzheimer • Hallucination • Anxiety • Depression • Lewy-body • Agnosia

KEY POINTS

- The diagnosis of Postoria Cortical Atrophy can be made with careful history-taking and cognitive testing accompanied by brain imaging studies.
- The neuropsychiatric issues of Posterior Cortical Atrophy often are unaddressed. Dementia patients with Posterior Cortical Atrophy often experience anxiety and depression initially.
- Through the progressive course of Posterior Cortical Atrophy, patients will further develop self-neglect/Anton's syndrome.
- In the severe stage of dementia due to Posterior Cortical Atrophy, patients frequently present visual hallucination and delusional behavior.
- It is a crucial step to discuss the cognitive deficits as well as neuropsychiatric symptoms with the care-givers for treatment options.

INTRODUCTION

Posterior cortical atrophy (PCA) is an anatomic terminology for a neurodegenerative disease affecting posterior parts of the brain which are associated with a clinical syndrome of difficulty processing visuospatial and visuoperceptual information. The term was created by D. Frank Benson and his colleagues in 1988 [1]. In the recent decade, extensive research has contributed to the promotion of this diagnostic entity. In 2017, a consensus conference was organized and published the guidelines for the diagnostic classification of PCA to raise the awareness of this particular cognitive disorder syndrome. Among the published studies in the recent 3 decades, there are abundant data on the cognitive aspects of PCA and on underlying neuropathological causes of PCA. On the contrary, only a few reports are discussing the neuropsychiatric aspect of PCA. In fact, clinical observations following patients with PCA confirm they can experience all sorts of neuropsychiatric symptoms, ranging from anxiety, depression, suspiciousness, hallucination to delusion throughout the entire course of their illness. Yet there is no effective treatment.

DIAGNOSIS OF POSTERIOR CORTICAL ATROPHY

In general, most symptoms are associated with visual agnosia and apraxia. In the original article published by Benson, and colleagues,[1] the diagnosis of PCA is based on the cognitive deficits of calculation ability, visuoperceptual and visuospatial functions as well as reading and writing skills. According to the published diagnostic criteria, a clinician can be more confident to diagnose PCA by recognizing particular cognitive symptoms and signs [2], Table 1.

E-mail address: cwu6@lifespan.org

https://doi.org/10.1016/j.ypsc.2022.05.001

2667-3827/22/

ABBREVIATIONS

PCA	posterior cortical atrophy
AD	Alzheimer's disease

The patho-anatomic evidence of this clinical syndrome in neuro-imaging studies (either brain MRI or CT scan) demonstrates the regional cerebral cortical atrophy in the posterior portion of the human brain (primarily indicating association cortices of occipital lobes in connection with posterior portions of parietal and temporal lobes, mainly existing *posterior* to the central sulcus of each hemisphere) (Figs. 1 and 2). Therefore, the descriptive term *"posterior cortical atrophy"* is proposed to be used as a diagnostic entity to explain the clinical syndrome of abnormal visual behaviors linked with the anatomic location of brain regional changes.

Based on cognitive neuroscience research, we now know the higher cortical function of visual cortices is based on the 2 connectivity pathways for the information process flow of visual information: the first is focused on the primary visual cortex transmitting visual information to the posterior parietal cortices to provide the "knowing where" cognitive function; the second is described based on the intense connection between occipital and temporal lobes to contribute to the "knowing what" cognitive function [3]. Furthermore, the laterality dominance of cognitive domains–namely, language and spatial cognition–in fact, dictates the predominant function in the posterior portion of either right hemisphere or left hemisphere. For language, left side represents the dominance of reading and writing ability. For spatial cognition, right side primarily controls the visuospatial orientation. When the degeneration of posterior association cortices of occipital, parietal, and temporal lobes is affecting both hemispheres altogether, the most known manifestation would be Balint syndrome. The triad of Balint's syndrome includes 1 optic apraxia (or sticky fixation of both eyes), 2 oculomotor ataxia (or optic dysmetria), 3 simultanagnosia (visual disorientation, seeing trees but not seeing the forest phenomenon). Knowing these details of neurocognitive function should enhance the clinical instinct of diagnosing PCA [3].

Most of these patients with PCA are younger with the onset before 65 years of age (the mean age of onset: 58.9 years) [4]. In the beginning, PCA is an insidious neurocognitive disorder. With a visual compensation mechanism, patients with PCA might or might not be aware of their visual disturbance–such as difficulty recognizing commonly used objects. If they have not known of visual problem, they often complain that they "forget" the location of objects. Moreover, there is not a simple office test that can help clinicians make the diagnosis of PCA (Figs. 3 and 4); and this is an uncommon neurocognitive disorder. Therefore, it commonly takes on average, more than 3 years for the patients with more prominent visual and behavioral symptoms of PCA to receive the correct diagnosis of PCA from an expert [4].

Among published studies of PCA about higher cortical visual cognitive symptoms, inability to recognize visuospatial relation of objects and their surrounding environment causes the most disturbance in daily living activities. Patients can develop compensatory mechanism to cope with inconvenient situations. As the disorder progresses, patients start to experience failure to recognize objects, do simple arithmetical tasks, dress themselves, and drive. Then they often seek for evaluation by the ophthalmologist. Or they believe they have "memory problem" to perform visually

TABLE 1
Diagnostic Criteria

Diagnostic Criteria (Benson et al [1], 1988; Mendez et al [15], 2002; Tang-Wai et al [9], 2004	
• Insidious onset; slow progression	• Visuospatial disorientation
• Visuoperceptual symptoms and signs without ocular explanation-most salient clinical presentation	• Dressing apraxia • Constructional dyspraxia • Dyslexia • Dysgraphia
• Visual agnosia	• Naming deficit
• Balint's syndrome-complete or partial	• Prosopagnosia • Anosognosia
• Gerstmann's syndrome-complete or partial	• Absence of stroke, tumor, TBI, and parkinsonism

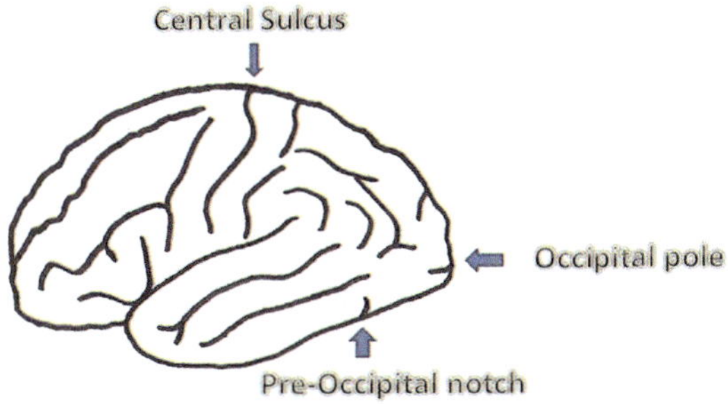

FIG. 1 Drawing of the brain showing the anatomic landmarks for the posterior portion of brain.

guided tasks. At this stage, patients with PCA are nervous as they all have experienced their mistakes in daily chores. Furthermore, as the initial cognitive symptoms cannot be detected by the routine office tests, patients often are told that the findings of their routine examination are within normal limits by primary care physicians and ophthalmologists.

Depression is the most reported psychiatric symptom (more than 50%) [2,5]. The second commonly reported psychiatric symptom is visual hallucination (more than 25%) [6]. In addition, one of the striking features of PCA is the development of unawareness or neglect of the visuoperceptual deficits during the disease course (29% in the initial examination of patients with PCA reported in a clinical data registry) [7].

NEUROPATHOLOGY OF POSTERIOR CORTICAL ATROPHY

To understand the underlying neuropathology of PCA, several studies can be highlighted here for discussion. In 1994, D. Frank Benson et al reported and discussed the neuropathological findings of 2 of the original 5 cases reported in 1988 [5,8]. First case had presented pathologic findings of "progressive subcortical sclerosis," which can be considered as the pathologic findings of reported Pick's disease at that time. The second case exhibited the classic findings of Alzheimer's disease. In addition, they reported a rapidly progressive PCA case with sporadic Creutzfeldt-Jakob disease (CJD); historically, this was called Heidenhain's variant of CJD, the pathologic prion heavily involves occipital lobes and their association cortices in conjunction with parietal lobes. From the viewpoint of behavioral neurology, the authors argued the justification of PCA diagnosis based on the uniform presentation of higher cortical visual cognitive disorder in all 3 cases with different pathologic processes [8].

In the following decade, 2 reports of neuropathology of a larger number of PCA cases based on longitudinal studies reveal that Alzheimer's disease in fact can be demonstrated in two-thirds of patients with PCA [9,10]. The other underlying causes of PCA are corticobasal degeneration (CBD, a tauopathy) and dementia with Lewy bodies (DLB). The UCLA researchers recently report among their collected 65 PCA cases of confirmed neuropathological reports, three quarters of them have Alzheimer's disease and the other have the pathologies of either CBD or DLB [8]. The neuropathological hallmarks of PCA with Alzheimer's exist more in posterior cortical regions and relatively spare the anterior temporal/hippocampal regions. The confirmed PCA cases with CBD show significant motor symptoms. The pathologically DLB in PCA displays visual hallucination more often in addition to motor symptoms (Parkinsonism). As advances in developing the neuro-

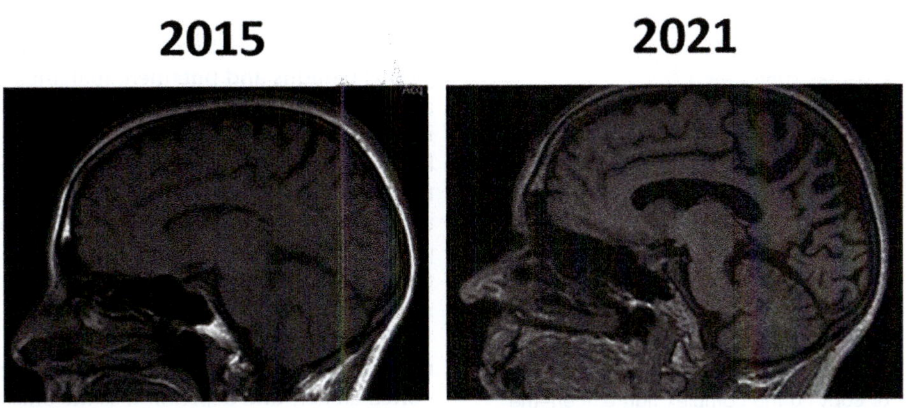

FIG. 2 The evolution of posterior cortical atrophy in the sagittal view of brain MRI, comparing 2015 study with 2021 study.

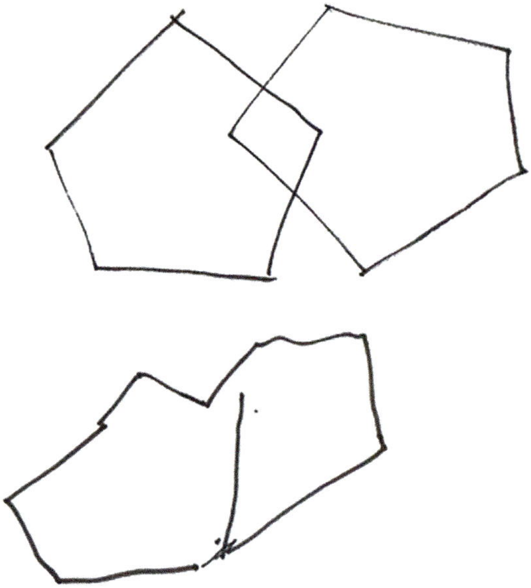

FIG. 3 The test of copying the figures. Upper–normal control; lower–the patient's copying.

imaging biomarkers of Alzheimer's disease (amyloid tracers and tau tracers for brain PET studies), clinicians will be equipped with better diagnostic tools to differentiate the underlying disease pathologies of PCA in the near future [4,11], Figs. 5 and 6.

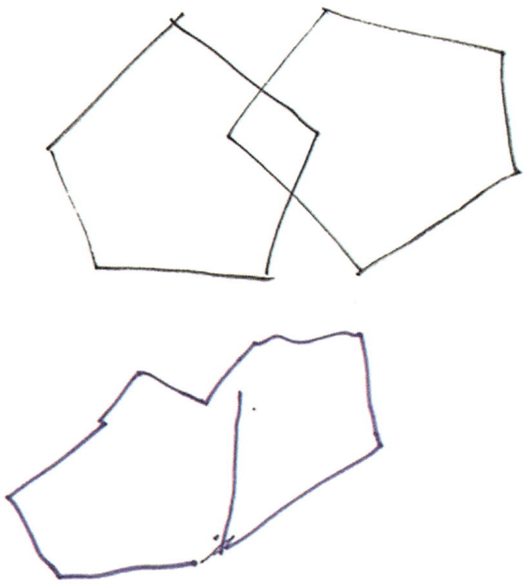

FIG. 4 The test of copying the complex figure. (*Left*–the standard complex figure for copying; *right*–the patient's drawing).

CHALLENGES OF MANAGING POSTERIOR CORTICAL ATROPHY REGARDING ITS NEUROPSYCHIATRIC ISSUES

The value of PCA diagnosis used clinically is to emphasize outstanding and progressive dysfunction in visuospatial and visuoperceptual functions that reflect pathophysiology developing in the posterior cortical regions of the human brain due to various neurodegenerative disorders. By contrast, this diagnostic entity cannot explain the underlying mechanism of neuropsychiatric issues. In providing the care of these patients, caregivers and clinicians in fact note that dealing with different degrees of neuropsychiatric and behavioral issues through the entire course of PCA is more challenging than helping with their cognitive dysfunction.

However, up to date, only a few studies have discussed specific neuropsychiatric symptoms of PCA found in the medical literature after 2004 [2,4,5]. In 2006, Keith A. Josephs,[6] and colleagues of Mayo Clinic reported 13 cases out of total of 59 patients with PCA, who had conducted detailed voxel-based morphometry of MRI study, presented vivid visual hallucination after about 4 years of onset of cognitive symptoms of PCA. All 13 patients were diagnosed with DLB based on the detailed description of their visual hallucinations and neurologic findings of motor symptoms. None of their remaining 46 patients without the presentation of hallucination had fulfilled the diagnosis of DLB, implying that these were all PCA cases of underlying Alzheimer's disease. The volumetric MRI studies showed PCA without hallucination (AD) group found a higher degree of atrophy in temporal and parietal association cortices, posterior cingulate and retro-splenial cortex, and right med-temporal lobe. On the contrary, in PCA with hallucination (DLB) group, more atrophic changes were found in the primary visual cortex, basal forebrain, head of caudate, globus pallidus and putamen, thalamus and hypothalamus, as well as midbrain. These striking differences implied the underlying pathophysiology of visual hallucination in PCA with hallucination could be due to dis-connectivity of primary visual cortex and subcortical structures. As we know, the development of DLB pathology has arisen from the brain stem regions and then progresses into the involvement of subcortical nuclei.

In the following years, comparing PCA cases with typical patients with AD, 2 studies of large group series reported anxiety and depression as the outstanding neuropsychiatric symptoms of PCA. In one study, the authors

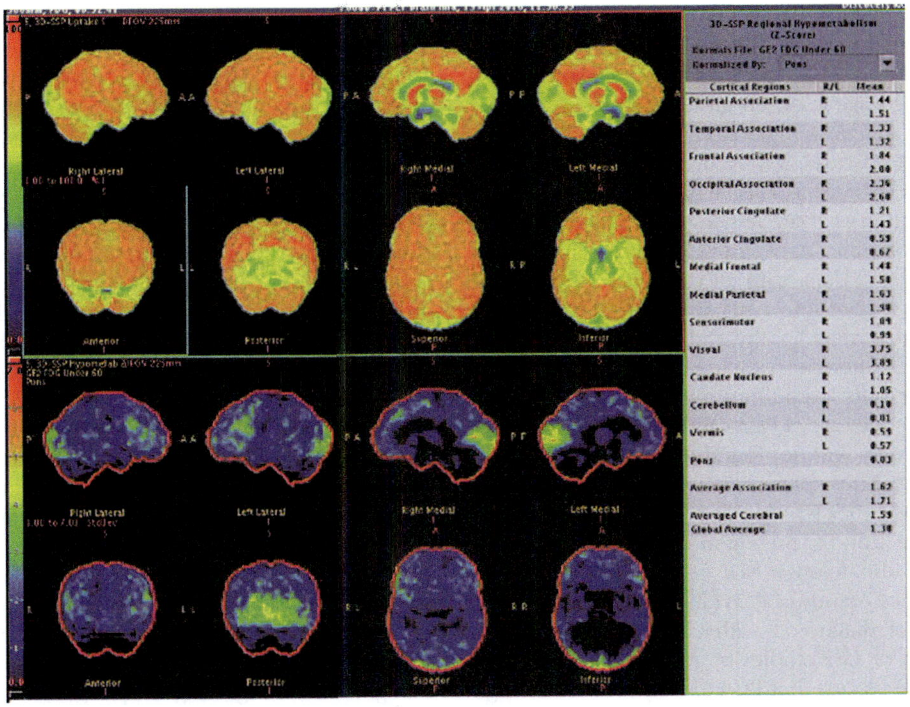

FIG. 5 The pattern of glucose hypometabolism in FDG-PET/CT brain. Upper panel shows decreased metabolism in occipital cortices (in *yellow*); lower panel shows a significant difference in occipital regions compared with normal control data base (in *green*).

excluded patients with PCA with hallucination and compared 20 PCA-AD cases with 20 typical patients with AD by using the neuropsychiatric inventory (NPI) scores of all neuropsychiatric symptoms except hallucination and delusion [12,13]. The onset age of the PCA group was younger than the AD group (mean age: 69.5 vs 75.4). Among 10 items of NPI scores, anxiety was reported most prominent in the PCA-AD group

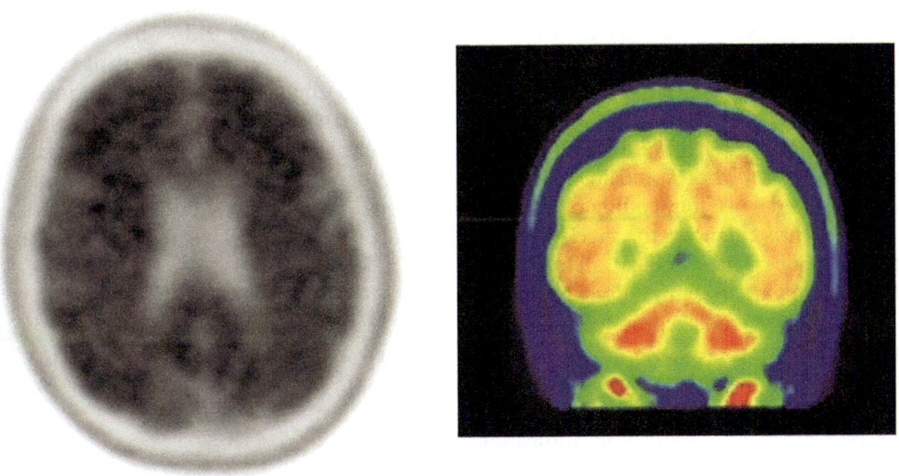

FIG. 6 Positive results of Amyloid tracer–brain PET/CT study (*left* in the original image–a transverse view; *right* in the colored template focused on occipital regions–a coronal view).

(55% in PCA vs 15% in typical AD). Scores of agitation, depression, apathy, and irritability did not show a statistically difference among 2 groups. In the other study, the authors collected age-matched groups of 28 PCA cases and 34 typical AD cases (age onset: 64 vs 66) [14–16]. Among the 28 PCA cases, 3 were already diagnosed with DLB with the presentation of visual hallucination, parkinsonism, fluctuation of awareness, and confirmed positive results of dopamine transporter uptake scan (DAT SPECT). Using NPI data from all cases, the authors reported the most common neuropsychiatric symptoms were depression, anxiety, apathy, and irritability and there was no statistical difference compared the PCA group with the typical AD group. In addition, auditory hallucination was reported in one case of PCA-DLB with visual hallucination. Yet, anxiety was not found to be outstanding in their PCA group. The explanation was that patients with early-onset AD (either typical AD or PCA-AD groups in this study) were found to present more anxiety symptom than patients with late-onset AD.

In a 10-year case study of PCA (2011–2020) with Alzheimer's disease diagnosed with either amyloid-tracer brain PET scan or CSF studies by reviewing the charts, this author here reports that PCA displays the following development of cognitive, behavioral, and psychiatric symptoms in the different stages of the disease course:

Fifteen patients with PCA were collected (8 women; 7 men). The average age of onset was 58. The diagnosis of PCA was made after they had visual/cognitive symptoms ranging from 2 to 4 years of disease onset. All patients with PCA had outstanding cerebral atrophy demonstrated by the brain MRI. In addition, 2 had FDG-PET of brain study, showing severe hypometabolism in the cerebral association cortices of bilateral occipital, parietal, and posterior temporal lobes. Clinically, they all showed characteristics of profound visuoperception/visuospatial dysfunction, including object agnosia, dyslexia, acalculia, and difficulty recognizing the environment. Their cognitive insight was preserved in the early stage. They were afraid of making mistakes on daily routine chores and in their jobs. They were all very frustrated when they could not perform simple routine tasks, such as balancing the checkbook. By the time of diagnosis made by the specialist, all had experienced generalized anxiety mixed with depressive mood and received short-acting benzodiazepine for treatment by their primary care physician.

When PCA progressed, 5 patients presented all cognitive symptoms of Balint's syndrome. Four patients had all cardinal features of Gerstmann's syndrome, indicating more dysfunction of the left hemisphere. The rest of the patients with PCA experienced at least one cognitive symptom of either Balint's syndrome (the most common: failure to track a moving object–optic apraxia) or Gerstmann's syndrome (the most common: acalculia).

In addition, 5 patients with PCA behaved like a blind person and the examination found cortical blindness. Strikingly, they did not think they were blind, even though they were informed that they had severe vision deficit with near blindness. Evidently, they had Anton's syndrome–anosognosia of their profound visual deficit. They also displayed color anomia and/or color blindness. They believed they can "see" the face of their spouses, though they could not describe their hairstyle, characteristics of make-up, and facial expression. To cope with their prosopagnosia, they often used their hands to search for the location of their spouses and paid attention to the source of their voice. For daily living, they believed they can "see" in their houses; yet they were extremely frustrated by the inability to reach wanted objects. By this time, their caregivers reported significant behavioral and psychiatric issues as they all were presenting severe anxiety and paranoia daily. They became very suspicious of family members stealing valuable belongings from them when they could not find them. Moreover, they generated paranoid thoughts–believing things or people threatening them. Afterward, they often became very agitated, presented sundowning syndrome, and at times developed visual illusions and visual hallucinations. For example, one patient mistakenly claimed "seeing water" under the chair and on the living room floor–visual illusion of a new floor carpet; she would scream, hold her cat tightly on the lap and ask for help. Two of these 5 patients with PCA in the severe stage also behaved and presented Capgras delusion (mis-identification delusion syndrome). At the time when they were very agitated, in fact, they not only did not recognize their spouses by looking at face and by hearing voice; but they also believed their spouses in the house were impostors. They were extremely nervous, feeling insecure at home and frantically looking for their spouse.

When following the patients with PCA through stages, these observations suggest that regarding the neuropsychiatric aspect of PCA there are 3 stages:

Mood Symptom Stage

In the early stage, when patients with PCA still have preserved insight and are aware of their visual symptoms, they are anxious about making mistakes and feel depression.

Neglect/Anton's Syndrome Stage

In the moderately progressing stage of worsened visuoperception, patients with PCA lose insight, neglect the profound visual deficit, and visual agnosia. Later on, these patients will likely transition into the next stage and develop thoughts of suspiciousness.

Psychosis Stage

In the behaviorally severe stage, patients with PCA frequently present psychotic behaviors (visual illusions, visual hallucinations, mis-identification delusional syndrome), as their thoughts are occupied by false or distorted images and generate conspiracy theories.

MANAGEMENT

It is disappointing regarding the treatment or therapies of PCA. At the present time, no matter what the underlying pathologies can be, there is NO pharmacologic treatment that can be prescribed for the visuospatial and visuoperceptual dysfunction–the cognitive aspect of PCA. Occupation therapy can be recommended for PCA in the early stage when patients have preserved cognitive insight and can learn strategies to cope with visual cognitive symptoms for daily living. Differentiating the underlying neurodegenerative disorders (AD, DLB, and CBD) is crucial in the treatment of specific cognitive symptoms. For AD, both cholinesterase inhibitors and memantine are indicated for PCA due to AD. However, these medicines often cause more psychiatric and behavioral symptoms, including anxiety, depression, and agitation. Nevertheless, when the amyloid immunotherapy becomes available for the early of AD, the hope is that if diagnosed and treated in the early stage, patients with PCA can avoid the progression of visuospatial/visuoperception dysfunction. Thus, this treatment could potentially prevent the future development of neuropsychiatric symptoms of PCA. For PCA associated with DLB, the dopaminergic drugs might be used to treat outstanding Parkinsonian motor symptoms. However, dopaminergic drugs are known to trigger and worsen visual hallucination. For PCA associated with CBD, an anti-tau therapy to target at abnormal development of tauopathy in the brain at the early stage could be promising so that visual cognitive symptoms would not progress and become detrimental. For unilateral cortical somatosensory loss and limb apraxia of CBD, patients with PCA might benefit from training strategies for daily living activities provided by occupation therapy in the early stage.

Neuropsychiatric symptoms of PCA might be best treated by considering psychopharmacology that targets specific behavioral issues. The effectiveness is often modest and short-lasting. Regarding anxiety and depression, anxiolytics and antidepressants are routinely prescribed to treat patients with PCA in the early stage.

SUMMARY

In sum, the PCA diagnosis is useful clinically to highlight the visuoperception and visuospatial dysfunction of the underlying neurocognitive disorders (AD, DLB, and CBD), which primarily cause the neurodegenerative process of occipital, parietal, and temporal association cortices vividly demonstrated by the neuroimaging studies (head CT scan, brain MRI and PET/CT of brain with FDG tracer). However, the presentation of patients with PCA is not homogeneous. The clinically used cognitive tests are not designed to measure and quantify the visuospatial/visuoperception dysfunction. Unless the clinician pays particular attention to the unique visuospatial/visuoperceptual syndrome, the patients most likely would not receive the correct diagnosis of PCA at the early stage. This is the challenge of diagnosis.

Moreover, after the diagnosis of PCA is made, the major challenge is to manage the behavioral and psychiatric problems of PCA. Only a few clinical research studies recently have described the neuropsychiatric issues of PCA [6,7,12–16]. No study has made recommendations for the management. Through longitudinally observing and managing patients with PCA at the dementia specialty clinic of an academic medical center, this author has observed 3 different stages of developing the neuropsychiatric manifestation throughout the entire disease course. In the end, no matter what the underlying pathologies (AD, CBD, and DLB) are, patients with PCA all experience neuropsychiatric issues. At the present time, we do not have a workable treatment plan. However, awareness of these neuropsychiatric symptoms would provide valuable direction for diagnosis, psychoeducation for the care, and treatment options. In the near future, clinical studies of behavioral intervention and pharmacotherapies should be developed for an effective solution.

CLINICS CARE POINTS

- Posterior Cortical Atrophy is a dementia syndrome that manifests a progressive course of outstanding visuospatial and visuoperception dysfunction.
- Alzheimer's disease is the most common underlying pathology of Posterior Cortical Atrophy. Less often, two other neurodegenerative disorders - dementia with Lewy-bodies and corticobasal degeneration - can also be the cause.

- In addition to cognitive disorder, patients with Posterior Cortical Atrophy have experienced neuropsychiatric symptoms through the course of this dementia syndrome, no matter what kind of underlying pathologies.
- Although there is no cure of Posterior Cortical Atrophy, it is important to recognitive cognitive difficulty and psychiatric symptoms to seek for symptomatic treatments.
- Patients and care-givers can learn from the experienced clinician of the diagnosis of Posterior Cortical Atrophy in order to establish a comprehensive care plan to ensure the safety of daily living and proper intervention of neuropsychiatric issues.

REFERENCES

[1] Benson DF, Davis RJ, Snyder BD. Posterior cortical atrophy. Arch Neurol 1988;45:789–93.

[2] Crutch SJ, Schott JM, Rabinovici GD, et al. Consensus classification of posterior cortical atrophy. Alzheimer's Demen 2017;13(8):870–84.

[3] Ungerleider LG, Mishkin M. Two cortical visual systems. In: Ingle DJ, Mansfield RJW, Goodale MA, editors. The analysis of visual behavior. New York: Academic Press; 1982. p. 549–86.

[4] Schott JM, Crutch SJ. Posterior cortical atrophy. Continuum (Minneap. Minn) 2019;25(1, Dementia):52–75.

[5] Yerstein O, Leia P, Liang L-J, et al. Benson's disease or posterior cortical atrophy, revisited. J Alzheimers Dis 2021;82(2):493–502.

[6] Josephs KA, Whitwell JL, Boeve BF, et al. Visual hallucinations in posterior cortical atrophy. Arch Neurol 2006;63:1427–32.

[7] Olds JJ, Hills WL, Warner J, et al. Posterior cortical atrophy: characteristics from a clinical data registry. Front Neurol 2020;11(June):1–9, Article 358.

[8] Victoroff J, Ross W, Benson DF, et al. Posterior Cortical Atrophy – neuropathologic correlations. Arch Neurol 1994;51:269–74.

[9] Tang-Wai DF, Graff-Radford NR, Boeve BF, et al. Clinical, genetic, and neuropathologic characteristics of posterior cortical atrophy. Neurology 2004;63:1168–74.

[10] Renner JA, Burns JM, Hou CE, et al. Progressive posterior cortical dysfunction: a clinicopathologic series. Neurology 2004;63:1175–80.

[11] Nedelska Z, Josephs KA, Graff-Radford J, et al. 18F-AV-1451 Uptake differs between dementia with Lewy bodies and posterior cortical atrophy. Mov Disord 2019;34(3):344–52.

[12] Isella V, Villa G, Mapelli C, et al. The neuropsychiatric profile of posterior cortical atrophy. J Geriatr Psychiatry Neurol 2015;28(2):136–44.

[13] Everhart DE, Highsmith JM, Davis CE. Posterior cortical atrophy: a case study of Benson's syndrome that initially presented as anxiety disorder. App Neuropsychol Adult 2012;19(3):229–36.

[14] Suarez-Gonzalez A, Crutch SJ, Franco-Macias E, et al. Neuropsychiatric symptoms in posterior cortical atrophy and Alzheimer disease. J Geriatr Psychiatry Neurol 2016; 29(2):65–71.

[15] Mendez MF, Ghajarania M, Perryman KM. Posterior cortical atrophy: Clinical characteristics and differences compared to Alzheimer's disease. Dement Geriatr Cogn Disord 2002;14:33–40.

[16] Wolf R, Schonfeldt-Lecuona C. Depressive symptoms as first manifestation of posterior cortical atrophy. Am J Psych 2006;163(5):939–40.

Advances in Psychiatry and Behavioral Health 2 (2022) 37–46

ADVANCES IN PSYCHIATRY AND BEHAVIORAL HEALTH

Psychedelics for Alzheimer's Disease Palliative Care

Kaitlin R. McManus, BA[a,*], Regan Patrick, PhD[a,b], Meg I. Striepe, PhD[c], Mia J. Drury, BA[a], Rosain Ozonsi, BS[a], Brent P. Forester, MD, MSc[a,b], Marc S. Weinberg, MD, PhD[a,b,d]

[a]McLean Hospital, 115 Mill Street, Belmont, MA 02478, USA; [b]Harvard Medical School, 25 Shattuck Street, Boston, MA 02115, USA; [c]California Institute of Integral Studies, 1453 Mission Street, San Francisco, CA 94103, USA; [d]Massachusetts General Hospital, 55 Fruit Street, Boston, MA 02114, USA

KEYWORDS

• Dementia • Psilocybin • LSD • Ayahuasca • Geriatric • Aging • Quality of life

KEY POINTS

- Psychedelics and psychedelic-assisted psychotherapy may be a consideration across multiple domains relevant to palliative care.
- Alzheimer's disease presents a major challenge and opportunity for incorporating the unmet palliative care needs of patients and their caregivers.
- Developing clinical trials of psychedelics and psychedelic-assisted therapies for palliative care treatment of Alzheimer's disease could foster meaningful benefits for this vulnerable population.

INTRODUCTION

Alzheimer's disease (AD) affects an estimated 6.2 million Americans aged 65 years and older—a number anticipated to double by 2050 [1]. There is no cure for AD, and the clinical promise of the current therapeutic pipeline, at present heavily focused on antiamyloid and anti-tau antibody treatments, remains unclear. In the absence of a cure or effective disease-modifying therapies, palliative approaches are essential and mainstay treatments for improving quality of life in patients and caregivers. Palliative care represents an integral approach to medical practice aiming to alleviate disease-related symptoms and distress. Often initially misconstrued by patient-caregiver dyads as cessation of treatment, palliative care generally gains broad support once its patient-aligned purpose is better understood [2].

Psychedelic-based treatments are a promising but still unexplored approach in palliative medicine. *Psychedelic* means "mind-manifesting," and psychedelic substances include a range of organic and synthetic drugs that have ascribed unusual/transformative psychoactive properties such as changes in sensorium, consciousness state, and interpersonal and intrapersonal connectedness. The classic psychedelics include indoleamines (eg, psilocybin), alkaloids (eg, *N,N*-dimethyltryptamine [DMT], the active constituent of ayahuasca), and ergolines (eg, lysergic acid diethylamide [LSD]), all of which act as agonists at the serotonin $5HT_{2A}$ receptor. Psychedelic-based treatments have appreciated a

*Corresponding author. McLean Hospital, 115 Mill Street, Mailstop 234, Belmont, MA 02478. *E-mail address:* krmcmanus19@gmail.com

https://doi.org/10.1016/j.ypsc.2022.06.001

resurgence of interest in the past decade, with a growing number of high-quality clinical trials marking their collective promise as a paradigm-shifting intervention in psychiatric and palliative care medicine. Of the multiple palliative care domains defined by the National Coalition for Hospice and Palliative Care [3], potential psychedelic-based treatments for patients with AD and their caregivers fall largely under *Psychological and Psychiatric, Social,* and *Spiritual* aspects of care. Herein, the authors review and discuss potential synergies between psychedelic research and these specific palliative care domains in AD, pointing to clinical research evidence largely based on trials of psilocybin, DMT, and LSD.

PSYCHOLOGICAL AND PSYCHIATRIC CARE

Psychiatric Care for Neurobehavioral Symptoms of Alzheimer's Disease

Neurobehavioral symptoms such as apathy, depression, anxiety, agitation, and cognitive-perceptual disturbance (eg, delusions, hallucinations) are highly comorbid along the continuum of AD severity, including the prodromal period [4]. For example, depression and anxiety affect an estimated 40% to 80% of patients, respectively [5,6]. Behavioral symptoms in AD can also exacerbate cognitive deficits, presenting as decline in executive functioning [7], creativity [8], and openness to experiences [9]. These neurobehavioral symptoms confer significant distress and burden on patient-caregiver dyads as well, with caregivers' perceived level of burden and overall quality of life being correlated with symptom severity in patients [10]. Moreover, familial caregivers are rarely adequately trained to manage and cope with chronic agitation and psychosis [11]. Thus, effectively managing neurobehavioral symptoms is a central part of comprehensive AD treatment.

Neurobehavioral symptom management in AD is tailored to the patient and their circumstances and does not solely involve psychotropic medications. Rather, a rounded approach involving treatment of medical conditions and pain, settling into or adjustment of living environment, and treatment of preexisting psychiatric conditions is prioritized. Although there are currently no Food and Drug Administration (FDA)-approved medications for AD neurobehavioral symptoms, geriatric-appropriate doses of common psychotropic medications are routinely prescribed. Drug classes include selective serotonin reuptake inhibitors (SSRIs), atypical antidepressants (eg, trazodone and mirtazapine), nonbenzodiazepine anxiolytics for neurovegetative symptoms and anxiety, and mood stabilizers or atypical antipsychotics for aggressive behaviors. The benefits of such treatments can be clinically meaningful to both patients and caregivers [12]; however, side effects should not be overlooked. These include sedation, increase in risk of falls, and a small but significant increase in risk of strokes and mortality with antipsychotics (leading to clear American Psychiatric Association guidelines [13] and an FDA black box warning).

Psychedelic Effects on Neurobehavioral Symptoms

Many of the recent studies described here were conducted using collectively termed *psychedelic-assisted psychotherapy* (PAP), which emphasizes the drug as a tool to enhance the psychotherapy experience. Some of the earliest and most robust mood-enhancing outcomes have come from psilocybin clinical trials. An early open-label trial of psilocybin-assisted therapy (2 doses 1 week apart) significantly reduced depression scores in a study of treatment-resistant depression (N = 22), with sustained effects for 6 months [14]. Two more recent studies found similarly encouraging outcomes, one of which was a study of intensive psilocybin PAP for major depressive disorder (MDD). Davis and colleagues (2021) enrolled subjects up to age 75 years and observed impressive treatment response and remission for at least 1 month [15]. The other recent study led by Carhart-Harris and colleagues (2021) also found that several outcomes generally favored psilocybin over the SSRI escitalopram in a 6-week trial of 59 adults (up to 80 years old) that used the same therapy setup in both groups, although these differences were not statistically significant [16]. The nuances of these studies are worth further exploration, particularly regarding methods of placebo or comparative drug control and specific PAP protocols.

Several small trials with ayahuasca have shown positive effects of this often-homebrewed N, N-dimethyltryptamine/monoamine oxidase inhibitors (DMT/MAOI) combination treatment of depression and anxiety (the use of an MAOI with DMT prevents peripheral metabolism of the active compound). Two related open-label trials of single-dose ayahuasca on 6 subjects in an inpatient psychiatric unit and 17 nonhospitalized subjects with active MDD saw significant reductions in depression within 1 day and lasting through the 21-day observation period [17,18]. Most recently, a randomized controlled trial of ayahuasca for treatment-resistant depression found a significant difference in response to treatment compared with the placebo group after 1 week [19].

Our understanding of the neural mechanisms of psychedelics and their relationship to neurobehavioral treatment effects remains limited. The indoleamine and ergoline classes of psychedelics confer potent receptor-specific effects in the brain. Although the mechanisms of action of these drugs are unique from traditional psychotropics used in current AD neurobehavioral therapies, there are also important overlapping properties that may provide face validity for their consideration as alternative or supplemental treatments (Box 1). Although a thorough review of the neurobiology of psychedelics is outside the scope of this review, major themes include changes in early sensory gating and processing; decreased activation of subcortical brain regions strongly linked to fear processing, such as the amygdala [20]; induction of plasticity or the measurable restructuring of neuronal communication networks (eg, through synaptogenesis) that underlie learning and memory [21,22]; and complex changes in the awake, resting state activity in the brain (ie, the default mode network [23]).

Psychedelics for Palliation of AD–Related Neurobehavioral Symptoms

One might argue that the promising mood enhancing effects of psychedelics and PAP, as briefly reviewed earlier, provides no stronger a case for application of these novel compounds to AD than toward any affective disorder. In recognition of this fair critique, it is also important to acknowledge the subtle ageism affecting geriatric mental health care, that is, the systemic undertreatment of psychiatric symptoms in older adults; this is true of both community-dwelling and institutionally dwelling individuals [24]. One might therefore flip the question to "why not prioritize this population," given the high prevalence and individual and societal costs of AD-related neuropsychiatric comorbidities.

Still, palliative care of AD-related neurobehavioral symptoms should extend beyond treatment of mood/neurovegetative symptoms. Regarding other neurobehavioral symptoms of AD, there is little recent literature supporting the use of psychedelics for treatment of psychosis; this may be in part due to their prohallucinatory effects, giving rise to their classic label as psychotomimetics. Studies from the 1950s explored the use of LSD in psychotic depression and schizophrenia, with some reports of null effect and others of improved insight and "ventilation of emotion" [25]. An important element of coping with delusional or psychotic symptoms is the degree of insight into the nature of one's thought disorder. Insight scales have been included in several clinical studies investigating the effects of psychedelics on various psychiatric disorders, from depression to addiction [26,27]. Whether the type of insight gained using psychedelic treatment, often described as "emotional breakthroughs" or "peak experiences," is at all related to the clinical insight of patients suffering from primary psychotic disorders [28] is unclear. However, should psychedelic treatments provide an access point for reality testing in delusional or disordered thinking in AD, this may be an avenue to explore for the palliative care of these challenging neurobehavioral features.

Safety of Psychedelics in Individuals with AD

Starting any new pharmacologic intervention in a medically complex and/or frail individual confers several additional challenges, the solutions for which include the well-known mantra "start low, and go slow," as well as thorough safety studies in an appropriately age-matched and comorbid population. In general, the indoleamine and ergoline classes of psychedelics have a relatively mild physiologic safety profile [29]. Risk of dependence or addiction to psilocybin and/or LSD is relatively low [29], as repeated administration builds tolerance, or tachyphylaxis of mental effects, which do not change even with substantial dose increases [30]. Older adults may experience poorer tolerance of the sympathetic changes induced by many psychedelics (eg, short-term tachycardia, hypertension, and hyperthermia). For this reason, use of psychedelics in patients with chronic cardiovascular and neurovascular diseases may be contraindicated. The risk of falls and fractures, already inherent in this population, could also increase with psychedelic treatment, given hyperreflexia, weakness, and possible disorientation. Slower drug metabolism in older individuals may extend the drugs' half-lives, although it is worth noting that there have been no documented human deaths from LSD overdose, and even in extreme overdoses, patients survived without residual consequences [31]. For comparison of safety risk, it is important to point out that electroconvulsive therapy remains the gold-standard treatment of severe depression in the elderly [32], despite many similar risks (eg, sympathetic activation and concerns with use in vascular disease). Safety will continue to be a priority, as psychedelic-based treatments are considered for new patient populations, and less restrictive inclusion criteria may benefit the field. It is encouraging that 2 recent trials of psilocybin [15,16] enrolled patients up to 75 and 80 years old, respectively.

From a mental health risk perspective, the safe and therapeutic setting of drug administration advanced by recent clinical trials promises improved psychiatric

BOX 1
The neurochemistry of Alzheimer's disease neurobehavioral treatments compared with psychedelics

Traditional psychotropics

The monoamine 5-HT, or serotonin, acts on receptors in the brain's limbic system to regulate a wide-range of neurobehavioral functions, from mood and aggression to circadian rhythmicity and appetitive behaviors. Psychotropic compounds, such as selective serotonin reuptake inhibitors (SSRIs) and serotonin-norepinephrine reuptake inhibitors (SNRIs), tricyclic antidepressants, and monoamine oxidase inhibitors, increase synaptic 5-HT levels by blocking reuptake of serotonin into the presynaptic cell. Clinical improvement of mood disorders by SSRIs takes weeks to months of continuous administration to be appreciated, thought to be related to chronically elevated synaptic 5-HT levels leading to decreased postsynaptic serotonin receptors, increases in other neurotransmitters such as norepinephrine, and increased second-messenger activity (eg, cAMP) and target gene expression (eg, brain derived neurotrophic factor—BDNF) [67].

A recent meta-analysis found efficacy of SSRIs in improving a range of neurobehavioral symptoms of dementia (for instance, as seen by improved scores on the multidomain neuropsychiatric inventory), as well as agitation, depression, and perceived care burden [12], noting greater beneficial effects in patients with AD than non-AD dementia. Other serotonin-receptor modulating compounds commonly prescribed for neurobehavioral symptom management in AD include trazodone (5HT2A and 5HT2B receptor antagonist, partial agonist of 5HT1A, along with non-5HT receptor targets), which may improve agitation symptoms [12], buspirone (5HT1A agonist), and mirtazapine (5HT2A and 5HT2C antagonist with non-5HT receptor targets). Commonly prescribed antipsychotics used for neurobehavioral symptoms of AD include quetiapine (5HT1A partial agonist and 5HT2A, -2B, and -2C antagonist among other 5HT and non-5HT receptor targets) and olanzapine (5HT2A inverse agonist among other 5HT and non-5HT receptor targets).

Neurochemical properties of the indolamine and ergoline classes of psychedelics

Indoleamine and ergoline psychedelics have an aromatic indole core akin to serotonin and function as partial agonists to multiple serotonin 5HT receptors. They have particularly high affinity for the 5HT2A receptor, understood as the dominant drug-receptor combination responsible for a multitude of psychedelic-based behavioral and psychological changes in humans [68–70], with lower affinities for other 5HT receptors dependent on the specific compound. Use of the 5HT-2A receptor antagonist ketanserin blocks and reverses all subjective drug effects [68]. Aside from serotonergic activity of these drugs, LSD also targets D1 and D2 dopamine receptors and adrenergic receptors [71], and some of the mood states of euphoria and depersonalization seen with these drug classes may be due to direct or indirect striatal dopamine release [72].

The serotonergic commonalities between SSRI and non-SSRI psychotropics and the indolamine and ergoline psychedelics is cursory and limited by receptor targeting and likely neuroanatomical specificity. Nonetheless, SSRIs and these psychedelics bear common neurobehaviorally supportive downstream pathways. The psychedelic 5HT2A agonism, as continuous use of SSRIs, leads to increased BDNF levels via some of the same transcriptional activation pathways. Psychedelics also increase BDNF levels in the prefrontal cortex. Via interaction with the TrkB receptor, this growth factor can induce changes in neuritogenesis and spinogenesis [73], accounting for BDNF's effects on neuroplasticity—that is, the adaptive changes of neurons thought to underlie many of the beneficial neuropsychiatric effects of SSRIs [74].

well-being as compared with the uncontrolled environment of recreational drug use [33]. A recent meta-analysis of 24 clinical trials of classic psychedelics found no long-term negative psychological effects, although 20.8% of studies did not have available adverse event data [34]. To the AD patient population, psychological risks of psychedelic use are poorly understood. One might imagine, for instance, given the nonlinear trajectory of neurobehavioral and cognitive symptoms in AD, that psychedelic-induced changes in primary sensory processing and association could lead to unpredictable episodes of confusion, disorientation, fear, or aggression, which in turn may not be amenable to therapeutic rationalization depending on disease severity. Another important consideration is the feasibility or value of PAP in this diverse population, wherein depending on degree of cognitive impairment, the patient may or may not be able to fully integrate preparatory or integrative therapy into the psychedelic experience; this may argue for tailored PAP modalities along the continuum of AD staging, such as modifications to PAP that allow for caregiver integration into the process. Should patients be unable to benefit from the preparatory, supportive, and integrative elements, it is possible that the psychological risks of the psychedelic treatment would be different than in a cognitively intact person.

Clarification on PAP-based approaches and thoughtful psychological safety and well-being assessments will be essential in availing this patient population to the potential benefits of psychedelic-based treatments for neurobehavioral symptoms of AD.

SOCIAL CARE

Social Aspects of Care in AD

Cognitive and neurobehavioral symptoms of AD can hinder patients' ability to communicate and interact socially [35], leading to disengagement and isolation. Conversely, decreased social engagement can also increase the risk for developing AD, as individuals with few or no social ties have increased risk of cognitive decline even after adjusting for baseline cognitive status and sociodemographics [36]. Changes in environment, from the common geriatric challenge of diminished social network, to loss of partner, physical relocation, or perhaps disease-specific changes such as institutionalization, all contribute to isolation and loneliness. Caregivers are no more immune to social isolation than patients, particularly if they become more tethered to the ongoing needs of the beneficiary.

Structuring and maintaining social networks emphasizes the development of interpersonal relationships between the patient-caregiver dyad, family, communities, and between the dyad and their medical care team [37]. Many strategies have been used for strengthening social aspects of care. These include physical, art, and music therapy [38], as well as intentional interpersonal communications through one-on-one, group, or family-based practices (eg, reminiscence-based therapy [39]). As with all palliative treatments, strategies should be tailored to the individual. For instance, art therapy can provide a new avenue not only for self-expression but also for communication between patients and peers, caregivers, and family that may circumvent communication deficits inherent with debilitating cognitive function [40]. For individuals at later stages of the disease, more passive forms of social interaction-based therapy, such as collective listening to music, serve not only to reduce neurobehavioral symptoms such as anxiety and depression [41,42] but provide a purposeful passive social opportunity.

Psychedelics and Social Care

Psychedelics and PAP are imbued with potent social connectivity–related properties. Watts and colleagues reported on patients' perceptions of themselves and their relationship to others before and after psilocybin-based PAP [43]. Before treatment, subjects described significant intrapersonal disconnection, using phrases such as feeling "trapped in their minds," and living in a "mental prison," which in turn contributed to profound social detachment, as subjects also reported feeling isolated, having little in common with peers, and sometimes feeling unable to leave their bed. After treatment, however, many responders described a sudden and dramatic reconnection to oneself, with greater openness to new values and perspectives, interest in new activities, and increased desire for connection to others. Several self-report studies of the long-term effects of psychedelics and social interaction have also noted positive effects on social behavior up to and beyond 1 year after initial drug treatment (see [44] for perspective).

Some of the same means for nurturing intrapersonal and interpersonal connectedness in AD have been studied for use alongside of psychedelics. The use of psychedelics recreationally, spiritually, and therapeutically has long been closely linked with the creative arts, including music and visual art, wherein the subjective experience is often dramatically affected and creativity enhanced [45]. Music accompaniment has been written into many clinical psychedelic protocols [46]. Under acute psychedelic influence, sensory processing in the brain is enhanced, whereas sensory association and integrative processing of sensory input is diminished, perhaps allowing for reinterpretation of experience [44].

PAP is an intimate social instrument that provides a safe and therapeutic interaction in the modified setting of psychedelic drug experience. One of the oft-cited goals of PAP is increased connectedness with one's inner sense of self, which nurtures self-compassion and offers an internal locus of healing. PAP involves extensive interpersonal exchange as well, with each step in PAP, from preparation to medication and integration [47], emphasizing a close interpersonal connection between therapist and patient. Preparation, for instance, involves the therapist building a connection with the patient by understanding their life history and intentions for PAP, and integration involves interpretation of the psychedelic experience by patient and therapist, with the intention of enacting long-term change [48]. Thus, connectedness to oneself and to the therapist through the multistep process of PAP offers a direct form of social connectedness.

Psychedelics and Social Care for AD

The bearing of psychedelics on social care in AD blend the vast unmet social needs of this population with the promise of psychedelics for prompting robust changes in desire for connectedness, empathy, creativity, and self-identity. As one example, psychedelic use in the setting of music can lead the individual to connect the song to their own memories [49]. Should similar effects be observed in individuals with AD, in whom autobiographical memory declines along with self-identity, the increased capacity to experience autobiographical scenes while listening to music may offer a novel means of access and reconnection to one's social identity [50].

There are also opportunities to overlay the psychedelic/PAP experience with the existing web of social connectedness programs for AD, including support groups and social recreation programs; this would require significant further development and resources, particularly dependent on the prescribing mechanism. Beyond state and federal restrictions currently in place for most psychedelic compounds, FDA approval is unlikely to mean take-home drugs from the pharmacy, but rather pharmaceutical companies seeking approval for a protocol of drug-assisted therapy—for instance, this may take place on the heels of the successful Phase 3 clinical trial of MDMA for treatment of posttraumatic stress disorder [51,52]. Although such factors apply to the broader scope of purposing psychedelic treatments for AD and other indications, it may have particular significance in the context of social connectedness goals: PAP protocols may require modification to specifically target aspects of social connectedness such as including others outside of the patient-therapist model, such as caregivers and family. Allowing them to interact with the patient while they undergo PAP could help foster connection. Social connection could also be increased by including other patients in group-based treatments, if deemed feasible. Modern group psychedelic-assisted psychotherapy protocols may use group sessions to conserve staff and time resources. These group sessions can resemble formalized group therapy, less formal support groups, or include a group task [53]. In addition, PAP protocols may need to adopt a particular focus, such as the creative arts versus introspective or unstructured therapy.

In prioritizing the needs of patients with AD, the caregiver is commonly overlooked. Caregivers' sense of isolation and loneliness, paired with chronic stress and, for many, grieving, does not meet the diagnostic criteria for a psychiatric disorder *per se,* unless such elements are not managed or alleviated, leading to possible manifestation of a depressive or anxiety disorder. Yet the consideration of including caregivers in PAP sessions or administering PAP to the caregiver themselves is an unexamined territory. One regulatory hurdle is the challenge of prescribing a tightly controlled substance to individuals without diagnostic indication; social isolation and loneliness are not found in the current psychiatric Diagnostic and Statistics Manual (DSM-5). Notwithstanding this and other regulatory challenges, one can envision many meaningful opportunities to use psychedelics to foster greater patient/caretaker self-identity, spurring creativity, fostering empathy, and enhancing the desire for and quality of interpersonal connectedness.

SPIRITUAL, RELIGIOUS, AND EXISTENTIAL ASPECTS OF CARE

Spiritual Care and Well-Being in AD

The degenerative nature of AD can leave affected individuals with a profound sense of existential angst due to the looming and inevitable degradation of cognition and functional independence. These existential concerns can have a devastating effect on emotional and psychological well-being, especially in earlier disease stages when a patient's insight is less likely to be compromised. Therefore, an important facet of AD palliative care across the disease severity spectrum should be aimed at ameliorating the overwhelming and disorienting impact of receiving an Alzheimer's diagnosis. In this vein, spiritual or religious coping may be an effective approach for older adults suffering from progressive or terminal conditions, including dementia [54]; this is relevant in a palliative context, as spiritual coping could help reframe the meaning of such a diagnosis by, for example, shifting one's perspective toward acceptance and reflection and away from perceived loss of control [55]. There are limited empirical data on the use of spiritual care in a palliative context for dementia, and most research examining spirituality as a coping resource for AD is derived from personal anecdotes from patients [54]. However, there is a small body of research suggesting spiritual coping may improve quality of life in patients with AD by facilitating meaning-making and sense of personhood [56]. Effective coping through spirituality may also have indirect palliative benefits through associated stress reduction and improved cognitive function [55]. Thus, using spiritual care to improve the quality of life in this population could be highly effective for those who consider spirituality an important part of their value and belief system.

Psychedelics and Spiritual Care

Psychedelics have often been considered alongside constructs of spirituality due to their historical uses in indigenous spiritual and religious ritual [57]. However, there is also growing contemporary interest in exploring this intersection, given that psychedelic experiences are often described as profoundly moving, transcendent, and transformative. Although such experiences vary depending on the specific compound, situational context, and characteristics of the individual [58,59], they are often associated with an increased sense of well-being [60]; this highlights the potential value of enhancing spiritual care with psychedelics across a range of clinical contexts—an approach sometimes called "psychedelic chaplaincy" when spiritual care providers (eg, priest, rabbi, minister, and so forth) give support or counsel to people preparing for, undergoing, or integrating psychedelic experiences. Moreover, the positive psychotherapeutic outcomes observed across a broad range of PAP studies to date have commonly involved a spiritual dimension. For example, a recent case series examining the use of psilocybin to treat alcohol dependence found that participants reported profound spiritual experiences following treatment, including communion with "a deceased loved one, with a holy figure, and with the Divine" [61]. In addition, a clinical trial on smoking cessation found that psilocybin-facilitated treatment was associated with increased rates of abstinence and that 86% of participants rated their psilocybin sessions as being "among the 5 most spiritually significant experiences" of their lives [62]. In another study of undergraduate students, greater lifetime psychedelic usage was associated with higher levels of spirituality, which in turn predicted better emotional regulation and decreased symptoms of depression, anxiety, and disordered eating [63].

Psychedelics and Spiritual Care for AD

The examples outlined earlier illustrate the promising role for psychedelics in the spiritual care of individuals with AD, particularly those struggling with behavioral and psychological symptoms. Although very little is known about how psychedelics might augment or enhance spiritual care aimed specifically at alleviating existential distress in AD, there is a related literature focused on other terminally ill medical populations (eg, cancer). This research has shown that the spiritual or transcendental effects exerted by psychedelics are often correlated with positive therapeutic outcomes related to existential distress, such as coping with overwhelming changes, death anxiety, and lack of meaning [64]. These psychedelic effects hold significant promise in a palliative context, given the emphasis on existential and spiritual themes [64]. Whether this extends to patients with AD, however, will largely hinge on their level of insight, as the presence of anosognosia—a neurologically mediated impairment in disease self-awareness, and a relatively common feature of AD—would be a clear obstacle in therapeutic efforts aimed at fostering acceptance and reframing the personal and spiritual meaning of an AD diagnosis. That said, other established forms of dementia therapy could be augmented toward similar ends. For example, reminiscence therapy (RT), sometimes referred to as life review therapy, involves and reflection around past activities, events, and life experiences, often with the aid of sensory prompts such as photographs or music recordings from a person's past [65]. A variation of RT known as spiritual reminiscence therapy (SRT) has been developed as an approach to enhancing meaning in life for those with dementia. Some promising recent findings demonstrated that hope, life satisfaction, and spiritual well-being could be significantly improved with a 6-week course of SRT in those with mild *or* moderate dementia [66]. Given the immersive sensory and spiritual/mystical experiences associated with psychedelics, exploring their potential to enhance the therapeutic effects of SRT is an intriguing clinical and research question, especially considering the parallel emphasis on sensory and spiritual elements in SRT.

SUMMARY

As clinical trials of psychedelic-based treatments and PAP expand to new indications over the next several years, their potential value to AD palliative care deserves consideration. Patients suffering from AD can, as other older adults without dementia, suffer from many of the same psychological disorders as younger individuals, although the neurovegetative symptoms may present differently and tend to be overlooked. Some neurobehavioral manifestations of AD (eg, mood-related symptoms) could clearly benefit from psychedelic-based treatment, whereas others (eg, psychotic symptoms and agitation) need further study. The risks of psychedelic use in AD include those generalizable to older adults, as well as the potential depreciation of PAP with worsening cognitive decline and anosognosia in later disease stages. Social connectedness contributes greatly to quality of life, and psychedelic compounds enhance not only self-identity, but empathy, relatedness to others, creativity, and sense of purpose, all of which may benefit patient and caregiver alike. Finally, though AD is not considered an acutely life-threatening illness, the disease course is nevertheless progressive and terminal, thus warranting consideration of the application of psychedelics to AD palliative care, particularly early in disease course, as these compounds have been successful in reducing anxiety, supporting reminiscence, and reducing existential distress in other related populations. Given the recent resurgence in interest in psychedelics for psychiatric disorders and palliative care, we are confident that the continued growth of rigorously designed clinical trials will overcome some of the complex regulatory and practical challenges associated with these promising compounds.

FUNDING

This work was supported by the National Institute of Mental Health (R25 MH094612 to M.S. Weinberg).

CLINICS CARE POINTS

- New palliative care treatments for the evolving neurobehavioral, social, and spiritual needs of persons with Alzheimer's disease and their caregivers are in great necessity.
- A growing number of well-designed clinical trials of psychedelics and psychedelic-assisted therapy for psychiatric illnesses offer encouragement towards extending these compounds' use towards improving the quality of life for persons with Alzheimer's disease.
- Given the vulnerabilities of patients with Alzheimer's disease and related dementias, careful assessment of safety and feasibility of psychedelic compounds in this population will need to be performed. This does not present an insurmountable roadblock, but an opportunity with potentially far-reaching implications.
- For now, addressing some of the great unmet palliative care needs in Alzheimer's disease is a matter of increased screening and clinician and public familiarity with established palliative care strategies, from social and spiritual resources to pharmacological management of neurobehavioral symptoms in patients and caregivers.

DISCLOSURE

R. Patrick receives partial salary support from Biogen, Eisai, NIH/NIA, and Rogers Family Foundation. B.P. Forester receives grant funding from the NIA, Rogers Family Foundation, Spier Family Foundation, Biogen, Eisai, and Lilly and is a consultant for Biogen, Patina Health, and Acadia Pharmaceuticals. M.S. Weinberg receives funding from the NIMH.

REFERENCES

[1] Alzheimer's Association. 2021 Alzheimer's Disease Facts and Figures. Alzheimers Dement 2021;17(3):327–406.

[2] Flieger SP, Chui K, Koch-Weser S. Lack of Awareness and Common Misconceptions About Palliative Care Among Adults: Insights from a National Survey. J Gen Intern Med 2020;35(7):2059–64.

[3] National Consensus Project for Quality Palliative Care. Clinical Practice Guidelines for Quality Palliative Care, 4th edition. Natl Coalit Hosp Palliat Care. 2018. Available at: https://www.nationalcoalitionhpc.org/ncp. Accessed January 9, 2022.

[4] Karttunen K, Karppi P, Hiltunen A, et al. Neuropsychiatric symptoms and Quality of Life in patients with very mild and mild Alzheimer's disease. Int J Geriatr Psychiatry 2011;26(5):473–82.

[5] Steinberg M, Sheppard JM, Tschanz JT, et al. The incidence of mental and behavioral disturbances in dementia: the cache county study. J Neuropsychiatry Clin Neurosci 2003;15(3):340–5.

[6] Kaiser NC, Liang LJ, Melrose RJ, et al. Differences in anxiety among patients with early- versus late-onset Alzheimer's disease. J Neuropsychiatry Clin Neurosci 2014;26(1):73–80.

[7] Baudouin A, Isingrini M, Vanneste S. Executive functioning and processing speed in age-related differences in time estimation: a comparison of young, old, and very old adults. Neuropsychol Dev Cogn B Aging Neuropsychol Cogn 2019;26(2):264–81.

[8] Price KA, Tinker AM. Creativity in later life. Maturitas 2014;78(4):281–6.

[9] Grühn D, Rebucal K, Diehl M, et al. Empathy Across the Adult Lifespan: Longitudinal and Experience-Sampling Findings. Emotion 2008;8(6):753–65.

[10] Mohamed S, Rosenheck R, Lyketsos CG, et al. Caregiver Burden in Alzheimer Disease: Cross-Sectional and Longitudinal Patient Correlates. Am J Geriatr Psychiatry 2010;18(10):917–27.

[11] Chiao CY, Wu HS, Hsiao CY. Caregiver burden for informal caregivers of patients with dementia: A systematic review. Int Nurs Rev 2015;62(3):340–50.

[12] Hsu TW, Stubbs B, Liang CS, et al. Efficacy of serotonergic antidepressant treatment for the neuropsychiatric symptoms and agitation in dementia: A systematic review and meta-analysis. Ageing Res Rev 2021;69:101362.

[13] Reus VI, Fochtmann LJ, Eyler AE, et al. The American Psychiatric Association Practice Guideline on the Use of Antipsychotics to Treat Agitation or Psychosis in Patients With Dementia. Am J Psychiatry 2016;173(5):543–6.

[14] Carhart-Harris RL, Bolstridge M, Rucker J, et al. Psilocybin with psychological support for treatment-resistant depression: an open-label feasibility study. Lancet Psychiatry 2016;3(7):619–27.

[15] Davis AK, Barrett FS, May DG, et al. Effects of Psilocybin-Assisted Therapy on Major Depressive Disorder: A Randomized Clinical Trial. JAMA Psychiatry 2021;78(5):481–9.

[16] Carhart-Harris R, Giribaldi B, Watts R, et al. Trial of Psilocybin versus Escitalopram for Depression. N Engl J Med 2021;384(15):1402–11.

[17] Osório F de L, Sanches RF, Macedo LR, et al. Antidepressant effects of a single dose of ayahuasca in patients with recurrent depression: a preliminary report. Braz J Psychiatry 2015;37(1):13–20.

[18] Sanches RF, de Lima Osório F, Dos Santos RG, et al. Antidepressant Effects of a Single Dose of Ayahuasca in Patients With Recurrent Depression: A SPECT Study. J Clin Psychopharmacol 2016;36(1):77–81.
[19] Palhano-Fontes F, Barreto D, Onias H, et al. Rapid antidepressant effects of the psychedelic ayahuasca in treatment-resistant depression: a randomized placebo-controlled trial. Psychol Med 2019;49(4):655–63.
[20] Barrett FS, Doss MK, Sepeda ND, et al. Emotions and brain function are altered up to one month after a single high dose of psilocybin. Sci Rep 2020;10(1): 2214.
[21] Ly C, Greb AC, Cameron LP, et al. Psychedelics Promote Structural and Functional Neural Plasticity. Cell Rep 2018;23(11):3170–82.
[22] Catlow BJ, Song S, Paredes DA, et al. Effects of psilocybin on hippocampal neurogenesis and extinction of trace fear conditioning. Exp Brain Res 2013;228(4):481–91.
[23] Müller F, Liechti ME, Lang UE, et al. Advances and challenges in neuroimaging studies on the effects of serotonergic hallucinogens: Contributions of the resting brain. Prog Brain Res 2018;242:159–77.
[24] Szczerbińska K, Hirdes JP, Życzkowska J. Good News and Bad News: Depressive Symptoms Decline and Undertreatment Increases With Age in Home Care and Institutional Settings. Am J Geriatr Psychiatry 2012;20(12): 1045–56.
[25] Eisner BG, Cohen S. Psychotherapy with lysergic acid diethylamide. J Nerv Ment Dis 1958;127:528–39.
[26] Carhart-Harris RL, Bolstridge M, Day CMJ, et al. Psilocybin with psychological support for treatment-resistant depression: six-month follow-up. Psychopharmacology (Berl) 2017;235(2):399–408.
[27] Garcia-Romeu A, Davis AK, Erowid F, et al. Cessation and reduction in alcohol consumption and misuse after psychedelic use. J Psychopharmacol Oxf 2019;33(9): 1088–101.
[28] David AS. Insight and psychosis: the next 30 years. Br J Psychiatry 2020;217(3):521–3.
[29] Nichols DE. Psychedelics. Pharmacol Rev 2016;68(2): 264–355.
[30] Vann Jones SA, O'Kelly A. Psychedelics as a Treatment for Alzheimer's Disease Dementia. Front Synaptic Neurosci 2020;12:34.
[31] Passie T, Halpern JH, Stichtenoth DO, et al. The Pharmacology of Lysergic Acid Diethylamide: A Review. CNS Neurosci Ther 2008;14(4):295–314.
[32] Gálvez V, Ho KA, Alonzo A, et al. Neuromodulation Therapies for Geriatric Depression. Curr Psychiatry Rep 2015;17(7):1–15.
[33] Reiff CM, Richman EE, Nemeroff CB, et al. Psychedelics and Psychedelic-Assisted Psychotherapy. Am J Psychiatry 2020;177(5):391–410.
[34] Goldberg SB, Shechet B, Nicholas CR, et al. Post-acute psychological effects of classical serotonergic psychedelics: a systematic review and meta-analysis. Psychol Med 2020;50(16):2655–66.
[35] El Haj M, Jardri R, Larøi F, et al. Hallucinations, loneliness, and social isolation in Alzheimer's disease. Cognit Neuropsychiatry 2016;21(1):1–13.
[36] Bassuk SS, Glass TA, Berkman LF. Social Disengagement and Incident Cognitive Decline in Community-Dwelling Elderly Persons. Ann Intern Med 1999; 131(3):165.
[37] Fazio S, Pace D, Flinner J, et al. The Fundamentals of Person-Centered Care for Individuals With Dementia. Gerontologist 2018;58(suppl_1):S10–9.
[38] Gómez Gallego M, Gómez García J. Music therapy and Alzheimer's disease: Cognitive, psychological, and behavioural effects. Neurol Engl Ed 2017;32(5): 300–8.
[39] Duru Aşiret G, Kapucu S. The Effect of Reminiscence Therapy on Cognition, Depression, and Activities of Daily Living for Patients With Alzheimer Disease. J Geriatr Psychiatry Neurol 2016;29(1):31–7.
[40] Cowl AL, Gaugler JE. Efficacy of Creative Arts Therapy in Treatment of Alzheimer's Disease and Dementia: A Systematic Literature Review. Act Adapt Aging 2014;38(4): 281–330.
[41] Livingston G, Kelly L, Lewis-Holmes E, et al. Non-pharmacological interventions for agitation in dementia: systematic review of randomised controlled trials. Br J Psychiatry 2014;205(6):436–42.
[42] Guétin S, Portet F, Picot MC, et al. Effect of Music Therapy on Anxiety and Depression in Patients with Alzheimer's Type Dementia: Randomised, Controlled Study. Dement Geriatr Cogn Disord 2009;28(1): 36–46.
[43] Watts R, Day C, Krzanowski J, et al. Patients' Accounts of Increased "Connectedness" and "Acceptance" After Psilocybin for Treatment-Resistant Depression. J Humanist Psychol 2017;57(5):520–64.
[44] Vollenweider FX, Preller KH. Psychedelic drugs: neurobiology and potential for treatment of psychiatric disorders. Nat Rev Neurosci 2020;21(11):611–24.
[45] Mason NL, Kuypers KPC, Reckweg JT, et al. Spontaneous and deliberate creative cognition during and after psilocybin exposure. Transl Psychiatry 2021;11(1): 209.
[46] Roseman L, Nutt DJ, Carhart-Harris RL. Quality of Acute Psychedelic Experience Predicts Therapeutic Efficacy of Psilocybin for Treatment-Resistant Depression. Front Pharmacol 2017;8:974.
[47] Nielson EM, Guss J. The influence of therapists' first-hand experience with psychedelics on psychedelic-assisted psychotherapy research and therapist training. J Psychedelic Stud 2018;2(2):64–73.
[48] Grof S, Hofmann A, Weil A. LSD psychotherapy (4th Edition): the healing potential of psychedelic medicine. 4th edition. California: Multidisciplinary Association for Psychedelic Studies; 2008.
[49] Barrett FS, Preller KH, Kaelen M. Psychedelics and music: neuroscience and therapeutic implications. Int Rev Psychiatry Abingdon Engl 2018;30(4):350–62.

[50] Jetten J, Haslam C, Pugliese C, et al. Declining autobiographical memory and the loss of identity: effects on well-being. J Clin Exp Neuropsychol 2010;32(4):408–16.
[51] Mitchell JM, Bogenschutz M, Lilienstein A, et al. MDMA-assisted therapy for severe PTSD: a randomized, double-blind, placebo-controlled phase 3 study. Nat Med 2021; 27(6):1025–33.
[52] Lamkin M. Prescription Psychedelics: The Road from FDA Approval to Clinical Practice. Am J Med 2022; 135(1):15–6.
[53] Trope A, Anderson BT, Hooker AR, et al. Psychedelic-Assisted Group Therapy: A Systematic Review. J Psychoactive Drugs 2019;51(2):174–88.
[54] Beuscher L, Grando VT. Using Spirituality to Cope With Early-Stage Alzheimer's Disease. West J Nurs Res 2009; 31(5):583–98.
[55] Koenig HG. Research on Religion, Spirituality, and Mental Health: A Review. Can J Psychiatry 2009;54(5): 283–91.
[56] Palmer JA, Smith AM, Paasche-Orlow RS, et al. Research Literature on the Intersection of Dementia, Spirituality, and Palliative Care: A Scoping Review. J Pain Symptom Manage 2020;60(1):116–34.
[57] Pedersen W, Copes H, Gashi L. Narratives of the mystical among users of psychedelics. Acta Sociol 2021;64(2): 230–46.
[58] Johnson MW, Hendricks PS, Barrett FS, et al. Classic psychedelics: An integrative review of epidemiology, therapeutics, mystical experience, and brain network function. Pharmacol Ther 2019;197:83–102.
[59] Hartogsohn I. The Meaning-Enhancing Properties of Psychedelics and Their Mediator Role in Psychedelic Therapy, Spirituality, and Creativity. Front Neurosci 2018; 12. Available at: https://www.frontiersin.org/article/10.3389/fnins.2018.00129. Accessed January 18, 2022.
[60] Griffiths RR, Johnson MW, Richards WA, et al. Psilocybin occasioned mystical-type experiences: Immediate and persisting dose-related effects. Psychopharmacology (Berl) 2011;218(4):649–65.
[61] Podrebarac SK, O'Donnell KC, Mennenga SE, et al. Spiritual experiences in psychedelic-assisted psychotherapy: Case reports of communion with the divine, the departed, and saints in research using psilocybin for the treatment of alcohol dependence. Spiritual Clin Pract Wash DC 2021;8(3):177–87.
[62] Johnson MW, Garcia-Romeu A, Griffiths RR. Long-term Follow-up of Psilocybin-facilitated Smoking Cessation. Am J Drug Alcohol Abuse 2017;43(1):55–60.
[63] Lafrance A, Strahan E, Bird BM, et al. Classic Psychedelic Use and Mechanisms of Mental Health: Exploring the Mediating Roles of Spirituality and Emotion Processing on Symptoms of Anxiety, Depressed Mood, and Disordered Eating in a Community Sample. J Humanist Psychol 2021. https://doi.org/10.1177/00221678211048049 00221678211048049.
[64] Schimmel N, Breeksema JJ, Smith-Apeldoorn SY, et al. Psychedelics for the treatment of depression, anxiety, and existential distress in patients with a terminal illness: a systematic review. Psychopharmacology (Berl) 2021. https://doi.org/10.1007/s00213-021-06027-y.
[65] Woods B, Spector A, Jones C, et al. Reminiscence therapy for dementia. Cochrane Database Syst Rev 2005;(2): CD001120.
[66] Wu LF, Koo M. Randomized controlled trial of a six-week spiritual reminiscence intervention on hope, life satisfaction, and spiritual well-being in elderly with mild and moderate dementia. Int J Geriatr Psychiatry 2016;31(2): 120–7.
[67] Martinowich K, Lu B. Interaction between BDNF and Serotonin: Role in Mood Disorders. Neuropsychopharmacology 2008;33(1):73–83.
[68] Preller KH, Herdener M, Pokorny T, et al. The Fabric of Meaning and Subjective Effects in LSD-Induced States Depend on Serotonin 2A Receptor Activation. Curr Biol 2017;27(3):451–7.
[69] Preller KH, Schilbach L, Pokorny T, et al. Role of the 5-HT2A Receptor in Self- and Other-Initiated Social Interaction in Lysergic Acid Diethylamide-Induced States: A Pharmacological fMRI Study. J Neurosci 2018;38(14): 3603–11.
[70] Kraehenmann R, Pokorny D, Aicher H, et al. LSD Increases Primary Process Thinking via Serotonin 2A Receptor Activation. Front Pharmacol 2017;8:814.
[71] Nichols DE. Hallucinogens. Pharmacol Ther 2004; 101(2):131–81.
[72] Ichikawa J, Meltzer HY. The effect of serotonin(1A) receptor agonism on antipsychotic drug-induced dopamine release in rat striatum and nucleus accumbens. Brain Res 2000;858(2):252–63.
[73] Cohen-Cory S, Kidane AH, Shirkey NJ, et al. Brain-derived neurotrophic factor and the development of structural neuronal connectivity. Dev Neurobiol 2010; 70(5):271–88.
[74] Björkholm C, Monteggia LM. BDNF - a key transducer of antidepressant effects. Neuropharmacology 2016;102: 72–9.

Advances in Psychiatry and Behavioral Health 2 (2022) 47–55

ADVANCES IN PSYCHIATRY AND BEHAVIORAL HEALTH

The Therapeutic Potential of Restoring Gamma Oscillations in Alzheimer's Disease

Arianna Ferretti, BS[a], Kassidy Rogers-Healion, BS[b], Aryandokht Fotros, MD, MSc[c,*]

[a]Department of Neuroscience, Brown University, The Alzheimer's Disease and Memory Disorders Center at Rhode Island Hospital, APC Building Room 716, 110 Lockwood Street, Providence, RI 02903, USA; [b]Department of Biology, Tufts University, The Klaus Miczek Lab at the Tufts Graduate School of Biomedical Sciences, 530 Boston Avenue, Medford, MA 02155 USA; [c]Department of Psychiatry and Human Behavior, Brown University, 593 Eddy Street, Potter Building 2, Providence, RI 02903, USA

KEYWORDS

• Gamma oscillations • Alzheimer's disease • Entrainment • Sensory stimulation • EEG • Neurodegeneration • Asynchrony • Amyloid-beta oligomers

KEY POINTS

- Alzheimer's disease (AD) and other neuropsychiatric disorders have disruptions in levels of brain rhythms found on an electroencephalogram (EEG).
- Decreased gamma oscillations in AD suggest decreased connectivity between cortical regions and neuronal circuits due to amyloid-beta-related dysfunction of inhibitory interneurons.
- Optogenetic and sensory stimulation of neurons at gamma frequencies in AD mouse models has showed decreased amyloid-beta aggregation and improved cognitive function.
- Trials of gamma sensory stimulation in humans are limited but have shown decreased atrophy and reduced inflammation overtime in participants with AD. More trials are needed to strengthen these outcomes.

INTRODUCTION

Alzheimer's disease (AD) is a complex neurodegenerative disorder with numerous possible etiologies that have yet to be clearly elucidated. While AD does not have an effective medication to slow disease progression at this time, it remains the most common form of dementia and affects approximately 33 million people in the world [1]. The "amyloid hypothesis" theory of neurodegeneration in AD postulates that increased the formation of amyloid plaques in the brain is the primary cause of increased dementia severity. Based on this hypothesis, aggregation of amyloid-beta protein within and around the hippocampus is believed to cause memory loss associated with neuronal loss and decreased synaptic transmission. AD can affect all domains of cognitive function, including attention, executive function, social cognition, and language. While amyloid-beta pathology is a key diagnostic feature of AD, how and why the protein aggregates are ongoing questions [1].

Identification of a modifiable precipitator for AD has long been of interest to researchers and scientists. Late-onset AD cases represent around 95% of AD, are less likely to be hereditary, and are more likely to have a

*Corresponding author, *E-mail address:* Fotros@brown.edu

https://doi.org/10.1016/j.ypsc.2022.05.002

random cause involving nonfamilial risk factors. Although there have been several possible risk loci identified for late-onset AD, how they influence the development of progressive neurodegeneration is unclear. Early-onset AD is often hereditary and has been linked to mutations in the amyloid precursor protein (APP), presenilin 1, and presenilin 2 genes, all of which play a role in the formation of the amyloid-beta protein [2]. Early-onset cases seem to have a genetic abnormality that directly impacts amyloid production. Meanwhile, late-onset cases may require a "trigger" or certain biological conditions such as inflammation, which start the process of amyloid plaque buildup and neuronal death.

Current treatments for AD are minimally effective and are not disease modifying. Aducanumab was provisionally approved in 2021 as the first disease-modifying treatment of AD. Aducanumab targets the accumulation of amyloid-beta protein, but not other facets of this complex disease. It is still uncertain whether this drug can reduce amyloid-beta plaques, and whether this is sufficient to halt cognitive decline [3]. We are learning that AD might need a multi-targeted treatment, and due to recent advances in AD research, future treatment options for patients with this prognosis are expanding. Clinical trials for AD have focused on tau and amyloid proteins, with uncertainty about the cause of the protein dysfunction. Regardless of what precipitates AD, recent evidence shows that cognitive disruptions go hand-in-hand with alterations in whole-brain dynamics which we will explore further in this article.

There is an established role for the pattern of neuronal oscillation (brainwaves) and their synchronicity in various brain areas in sensory cognitive processing. These oscillations can be captured as frequency bands including alpha, beta, theta, delta, and gamma frequencies measured on electroencephalogram (EEG). A growing body of literature supports an association between changes in neuronal oscillations and neuropsychiatric diseases [4]. The use of brain frequencies as diagnostic biomarkers and modulation of these waves as a treatment tool has been at the forefront of research for AD in recent years [5].

The decreased frequencies on EEGs of patients with AD could represent dysfunction in neural circuits and reduced connectivity between important cortical regions might explain diminished cognitive function. Dysfunction of networks will deteriorate overtime, and segments of the network become increasingly disconnected. This could explain the progressive nature of the disease. As such, studying the electrical activity throughout the brain as a potential biomarker of AD is vital to understanding the disease.

EEG results are often observed as a power spectral analysis. A power spectral analysis views the EEG output as a combination of waves at characteristically different frequencies. For example, the brain waves are divided into groups with distinct frequency ranges, like high-frequency gamma oscillations (around 30–100 Hz). An EEG with high gamma power contains increased content in the gamma range. Gamma power is among the brainwaves that have proven a distinct association with memory function [6]. Theoretically, if decreased gamma oscillations are directly related to cognitive symptoms, then targeting neural networks to restore this activity could provide clinical benefits. This article will focus on providing a review on decreased synchrony between key brain regions involved in cognition is observed in AD, along with decreased gamma power.

ASYNCHRONY AND NETWORK CONNECTIVITY IN ALZHEIMER'S DISEASE: FINDINGS FROM ELECTROENCEPHALOGRAM HUMAN AND ANIMAL STUDIES

An important feature of brain function is connectivity between neurons. Neurons have intrinsic firing rates, so certain frequencies of spikes are more common during bouts of neuronal activation, depending on the type of neuron. For example, the cortex has 3 classifications of neurons based on their firing patterns: intrinsic bursting, fast spiking, and regular spiking [7]. When large groups of neurons are connected with their intrinsic firing rates synchronization of oscillatory activity can occur, signaling connection within or between brain areas. New evidence shows that asynchronous oscillations between 2 functionally linked brain areas present pathologic phenotypes of neurologic dysfunction. For example, patients with tremor show more desynchronized activity between areas of the brain regulating motion [8].

Synchronization of brain activity is represented by oscillations on an EEG. For decades, it has been shown that patients with dementia have EEG results showing slowed rhythms throughout the whole brain, with overall decreases in alpha and beta oscillations [3]. Additionally, increased cognitive impairment in AD has been correlated with increased reduction of these oscillations in the EEG [9]. Diffuse cortical changes in EEG activity recorded in patients with AD are nonspecific to AD and may be present in other neuropsychiatric disorders. Neuroscience research has identified long-range communications in the gamma band range as specifically important in arousal for cognition, particularly attention.

Coherence is a statistical measurement of the relatedness between the amplitude and phase of signals from 2 electrodes placed on one's scalp during an EEG [10]. By simultaneously recording the frequency at 2 electrodes and analyzing their synchrony, it is possible to obtain a measure of coherence between the 2 areas [11]. EEG results from coherence analysis studies looking at the connectivity between electrodes and their interdependencies have found decreased mutual information between distant electrodes in groups of patients with AD compared with control groups. The decreased coherence between electrodes reported in these studies suggests that communication between cortical regions is impaired in AD. [12]. Another study investigating EEG coherence in individuals with mild cognitive impairment (MCI) found decreased alpha-band coherence between electrodes across the temporo-parietal regions. Coherence between long-distance cortical regions was also shown to be more affected in AD than shorter distance recordings, which may be due to AD pathology affecting long axon fibers or the long-range neurons the most. This study shows that connections between cortical areas might be altered early on in AD pathology and that EEG may be a useful noninvasive detection tool to be used in the clinical setting [13].

Experiments using visual stimuli to evoke gamma frequencies show significantly diminished gamma rhythms in individuals with AD compared with controls, suggesting decreased cortical connectivity in AD. Visual stimuli using Cartesian gratings are shown to elicit gamma oscillations in the visual cortex, with an age-dependent decline of power in healthy individuals. Murty and colleagues, 2021, were able to show that stimulus-induced gamma rhythms are also diminished in participants with MCI and AD compared with healthy individuals of the same age and gender. They compared the results of visual flickering with gamma and steady-state visually evoked potentials (SSVEP) in 12 participants with MCI and 5 participants with AD. Both the MCI and AD groups showed no significant difference in static grating SSVEP compared with controls. However, MCI and AD groups showed markedly reduced gamma power in the visual cortex in response to Cartesian grating stimuli. The difference in stimulus-induced gamma power for both MCI and AD groups is significant for the search of reliable and early diagnostic tools for AD. [14].

MECHANISMS OF NETWORK OSCILLATIONS AND ALTERED HIPPOCAMPAL-CORTICAL CONNECTIONS IN ALZHEIMER'S DISEASE

The observations that gamma oscillations are recorded less often in patients with Alzheimer's motivates new research to propose the physiologic mechanism behind the dysregulation of network communications associated with cognitive function. The hippocampus is a key brain region in spatial awareness, arousal, and is whereby neural representations of memories are formed and processed. The cortical dysfunction present in AD may be related to molecular changes and features of signal transmission in hippocampal neurons. The hippocampus is usually the first area affected in people with AD, it is a location of early amyloid-beta aggregation and subsequent neurodegeneration. During disease progression, amyloid-beta oligomers (AβO) proteins can form in the hippocampus and spread throughout the brain. Molecular changes in the hippocampus can even occur before symptoms of AD emerge [15].

The oscillatory activity in subcortical structures, such as the hippocampus, is driven by neurons with intrinsic firing rates. Logically, if the transmission of action potentials between these neurons is altered, so will the phase-locking of spikes in the region. Various intrinsic factors such as the presence of distinct ion channels will contribute to neuronal firing rates. For example, a Ca^{2+}-gated K^+ channel can facilitate rapid Na^+ channel deactivation and a more rapid firing rate. Another aspect of hippocampal neurons that promotes oscillations is the connections between interneurons and pyramidal neurons. Pyramidal neurons in the hippocampus synapse on inhibitory interneurons, which relay the inhibitory GABA neurotransmitter onto other pyramidal neurons in the hippocampus, or other interneurons. There are many types of interneurons in the hippocampus, and throughout the brain that are outside the purview of this review. Due to the intrinsic firing rates of parvalbumin (PV) and somatostatin (SST) expressing interneurons specifically, their respective roles in controlling the theta and gamma oscillations are a focus of related research [16].

Interneurons are essential in forming networks in the brain, by using the activation of one neuron to excite or inhibit the activity of another. PV interneurons in particular may be the drivers of hippocampal gamma oscillations. During persistent firing, the rate is in the gamma range of 30 to 120 Hz and is reduced when voltage-gated Ca^{2+} channels are blocked. PV basket cells in the hippocampus have many postsynaptic connections, onto pyramidal cells, other inhibitory interneurons, and itself [17]. This makes for a complex circuit, whereby it is difficult to pin a sole contributor to hippocampal-cortical network function, when other brain regions are also involved. However, it is important to note the regulatory power these interneurons have in controlling excitation. The focus on PV basket interneurons in promoting synchronous gamma oscillations relates to their structure which facilitates reciprocal linkages between other interneurons and synapses directly onto the soma of excitatory pyramidal neurons. As mentioned previously, PV basket cells have "resonance" for the gamma range. In support of the importance of Ca^{2+} channels for this intrinsic firing rate, AMPAR and NMDAR antagonists eliminate gamma frequency cortical activity, and Ca^{2+} plays an important role in the function of these receptors [16].

To observe the effects of optogenetic stimulation in PV neurons of the hippocampus, one study crossed PV-Cre mice with mice overexpressing APP. These mice showed amyloid deposition in the hippocampus and spatial memory deficits, as well as reduced gamma (30–60 Hz) spectral power. Acute optogenetic stimulation of gamma frequency was effective in controlling hippocampal oscillations and improving the outcomes of memory tasks for an AD mouse model, particularly stimulation during retrieval rather than encoding. This research did not demonstrate whether increased gamma due to optogenetic stimulation was due to artificial or natural oscillations [18].

Alterations to an interneuron's intrinsic firing rate due to disruptions in synaptic connection or insults to the integrity of the neuron may underlie the aberrant hippocampal and cortical oscillations. Mouse models of AD highlight the detrimental effects of AD pathology on these types of neurons. A 2020 study stimulated these interneurons in the hippocampus in a mouse model of AD, to observe the degree that PV and SST interneurons in the hippocampus contribute to the decreased oscillatory activity. Mice injected with AβO had suppressed gamma and theta oscillations; however, optogenetically activating the PV and SST interneurons restored this activity. The activity was recorded with electrodes immunohistochemically confirmed in the CA1 [regions in the hippocampal circuit are numbered CA1-4]. The results also showed increased GABA release from the SST and PV interneurons onto pyramidal neurons in AβO injected mice compared with controls which would suggest a neurochemical mechanism of AβO-related dysfunction [19]. Fig. 1 shows a simplified diagram of amyloid-beta plaques and their potential to disrupt synapses.

The PV and SST inhibitory interneurons in the hippocampus are a salient example of how interneurons contribute to cortical oscillations. In the mouse hippocampus *ex vivo*, an optogenetic approach was used to alter the activity of both PV and SST interneurons. Electrophysiological recordings from the CA3 excitatory pyramidal neurons showed that the disruption of interneuron firing resulted in decreased slow gamma recorded [20]. A specific voltage-gated Na^{+} channel is expressed by the gene Nav1.1 in PV and SST inhibitory interneurons. Hypofunction of Nav1.1 is associated with network dysrhythmias in AD and multiple neuropsychiatric disorders. This effect might be correlated with Nav1.1's role in modulating gamma oscillatory activity. Using this hypothesis, Martinez-Losa and colleagues overexpressed Nav1.1 in a mouse model of AD. Their findings show improved gamma oscillations and improved cognitive functions in human amyloid precursor protein (hAPP)-transgenic mice [21]. There are other interneurons in the hippocampus in addition to SST and PV, including cholecystokinin (CCK) and neuropeptide Y (NPY) expressing interneurons. If circuits with SST and PV are damaged beyond functioning, gamma stimulation may not be an effective treatment of the later stages of AD. The treatment may only have a therapeutic effect if the disease has progressed enough to impede PV and SST inhibition. Further research into hippocampal circuits and AD is required to find the sweet spot for a gamma-stimulating treatment.

NETWORK ABNORMALITIES IN NEUROPSYCHIATRIC DISORDERS

Understanding the network abnormalities of the brain is an important step to understanding and treatment of all neuropsychiatric disorders including dementia. To date, these network abnormalities have been studied in a variety of neuropsychiatric disorders including depression, schizophrenia, autism, and dementia [22].

Several studies have investigated gamma oscillation characteristics in mood disorders and their relation to treatment response. A 2007 study showed that subjects with depression had significantly decreased coherence (a measure of synchronization between brain areas) as well as increased gamma power during baseline and stress conditions. The authors suggest that excess activity on an EEG could be a signal of increased cholinergic activation, which is linked to stress. A possible confounding variable for this study is that subjects with depression were taken off of psychoactive substances

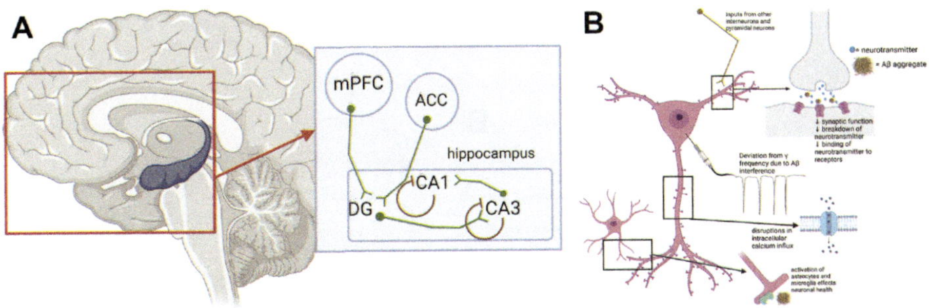

FIG. 1 (**A**) ACC, anterior cingulate cortex; DG, dentate gyrus; mPFC, medial prefrontal cortex. CA1, CA2 = Regions in the hippocampal circuit. Inhibitory interneurons are marked red in the figure. mPFC and ACC are meant to represent inputs to the hippocampus, which begin at the DG. This figure demonstrates the role of interneurons in generating phase-locked electrical activity in the cortex. (**B**) Research has supported that disruptions in APP can affect cortical oscillations. This figure demonstrates how pathologic amyloid-beta plaques could disrupt the circuit. Created with BioRender.

for at least 3 to 5 days, which may have caused some withdrawal effects [23]. Antidepressants alone may impact gamma power. Another article discusses the effects of distinct classes of antidepressants (eg, serotonergic and noradrenergic) on gamma rhythms. Some studies show that antidepressants that increase the levels of serotonin (eg, escitalopram) will decrease gamma power while noradrenergic tricyclics will increase gamma power [24]. Fitzgerald and colleagues suggest that there may be an "optimal," level of gamma that is necessary to allow for healthy brain function, and the possibility for either increased or decreased gamma may explain why some individuals with depression are not responsive to certain antidepressants. The study suggests that gamma oscillations could not only monitor the course of depression but also differentiate between different types of depression [25].

Gamma oscillatory dysfunction is also being studied in schizophrenia. A chronic information processing and integration disorder, schizophrenia is characterized by positive symptoms (presence of new symptoms eg, hallucinations, delusions), negative symptoms (absence or deficit in basic neurosensory features such as anhedonia and avolition), as well as cognitive deficits in working memory and executive functioning. Dysfunction of PV + GABAergic interneurons and NMDA receptors are consistent markers in Schizophrenia [26]. The mechanism of disrupted gamma power may be related to interneuron connections, similar to what is seen in AD. A 2005 study used Dlx5/6 heterozygous mice (Dlx5/6(+/−)) as a model for interneuron dysfunction in schizophrenia. The gene Dlx5/6 regulates GABAergic interneuron development. Cho and colleagues showed that inhibiting interneurons in control mice led to deficits in cognitive flexibility, whereas it was restored to healthy function when mice were stimulated with γ-frequencies of 40 Hz. The improved cognitive flexibility in treated Dlx5/6(+/−) mice was sustained for a month following the treatment [26].

Altered gamma oscillations in schizophrenia could signify decreased synchrony between cortical regions. A 2003 study in humans showed that individuals with predominantly positive symptoms had significantly increased gamma activity while those with predominantly negative symptoms shown decreased gamma activity when compared with controls. In this study, Lee and colleagues further tested these differences by showing that distinct gamma activity was associated with different "symptom dimensions" in participants with schizophrenia. They distinguished 3 dimensions, psychomotor poverty, reality distortion, and disorganization with the respective abnormalities in gamma synchrony: left hemisphere decrease, right hemisphere increase, and diffuse increase [27]. The disconnectivity theory in schizophrenia hypothesizes that cognitive and memory deficits are due to ineffective neuronal communication between brain regions. The implications of gamma activity in neuronal communication suggest that asynchrony of gamma oscillations could be the fundamental neuropathology in schizophrenia [27]. While gamma activity has shown stratification among symptoms, what it illustrates about schizophrenia etiology is still unknown.

POTENTIAL THERAPEUTIC USE OF GAMMA ENTRAINMENT

A potential noninvasive treatment of AD is facilitating cortical gamma oscillations through entrainment. Entrainment in this setting involves synchronizing the

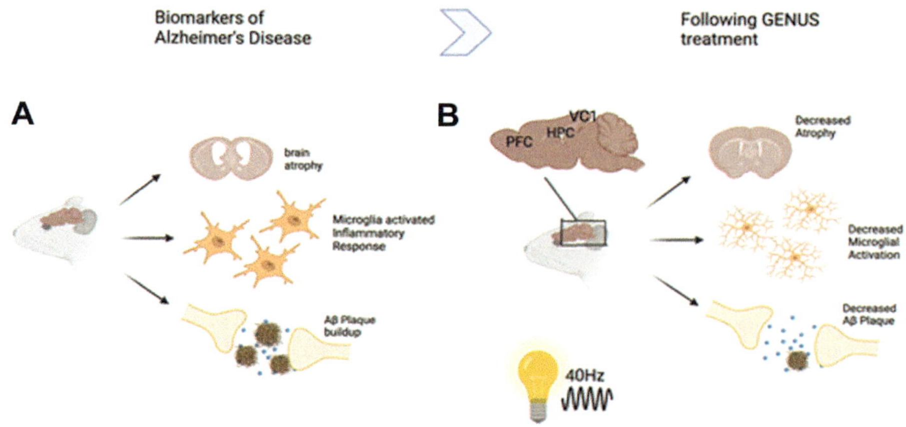

FIG. 2 This figure demonstrates the therapeutic effects of Gamma Entrainment Using Sensory Stimuli (GENUS) on biomarkers of Alzheimer's disease including neuronal atrophy, microglial activated inflammatory response, and amyloid-beta plaque buildup. Images (**A**) and (**B**) show theoretic preliminary and post 40 Hz treatment conditions, respectively. Created with BioRender.

rhythm of brain activity to an exogenous stimulus. Gamma Entrainment Using Sensory Stimulation, or GENUS, has shown promising results in animal models of neuropsychiatric disorders, including AD. The goal of this treatment is to reduce cognitive symptoms and biological markers [28,29]. Several studies in animal models have provided support for this hypothesis. A 2019 study found that entrainment using GENUS on mouse models of neurodegeneration could protect neuronal function as well as cognition [28]. The study used 2 neurodegenerative mouse models of AD, Tau P301S and CK-p25 to look at parameters of neuroprotection after prolonged exposure to GENUS. Tau P301S mimics AD by promoting the formation of tau neurofibrillary tangles in the brain. CK-p25 model causes neurodegeneration by over-expressing p25 (a regulatory subunit of Cyclin-dependent kinase 5 (CdK5)) and overactivation of CdK5. This kinase protein plays an integral role in the regulation of mammalian central nervous system development [30]. Tauopathy and microglial inflammatory response are present in both models, and amyloid buildup is only present in CK-p25. Adaikkan and colleagues found that prolonged exposure to a 40 Hz light flicker during the early ages of P301 and CK-p25 neurodegeneration increased synaptic function and cognitive capabilities while decreasing neuronal loss and microglial activation. Ventricle expansion for GENUS-treated P301S mice was significantly reduced compared with untreated P301S mice. Similarly, CK-p25 showed decreased brain weight while GENUS-treated CK-p25 retained wild-type weight (Fig. 2) [28].

There have only been a few translational studies that sought out to replicate similar results in human participants. In 2021 a clinical study using GENUS for participants with probable AD and mild symptoms, administered high-frequency light and sound for 1-h a day over 4 months. The treatment group showed benefits that included diminished atrophy (characterized by ventricle enlargement) at 3 months compared with baseline [31]. Another 2019 study used healthy volunteers to observe EEG recordings during white light flickers at frequencies of 40, 60, and 80 Hz. The electrical changes were recorded for 30 seconds with the participants' eyes open, staring at the light source. The experiment also tested 60 Hz and 80 Hz light stimulation, and varying degrees of light intensity. Considering promising studies thus far in animal models of AD, this study elected to use healthy subjects, with the goal of fortifying the motif that light stimulation at a specific frequency could drive cortical activation at a synchronous rhythm. The findings could be used in developing a medical device for potential use in AD treatment. They concluded that 40 Hz achieved the most electrodes showing synchronization to light, or entrainment, compared with the 60 Hz and 80 Hz frequencies (at both high and low intensities). Although the highest response at 40 Hz was recorded at occipital electrodes, there was evidence that on average, over half of the electrodes showed a 40 Hz response to the 40 Hz stimuli at the high luminance setting, indicating diffuse entrainment. An important note of the researchers was that each trial was run twice for every participant, and variation between the 2 trials was observed but not statistically analyzed, which would be important to add for future experiments [32].

While these studies show therapeutic uses of gamma entrainment, there is still controversy over whether external stimuli have the power to modulate endogenous gamma oscillations (generated within the brain), and whether gamma oscillations signify increased alertness and cognitive performance as they are believed to. It is possible that using GENUS might coincide with a general increase of EEG signals toward the rhythm of the stimulation and lead to an incorrect assumption that this effect was induced by GENUS. Thus, it is important to identify whether a stimulus-evoked activity, or is showing a response that is separate but coexisting. If the response is the latter, then the GENUS treatment may have an impact on an unintended network or area. Duecker and colleagues conducted an experiment that showed endogenous gamma activity was not entrained by a 40 Hz light flicker. They compared responses to light flicker in the presence and absence of endogenous gamma activity. Endogenous gamma was induced using sinusoidally alternating luminance or "grating," a paradigm that has been shown in several other studies to increase gamma oscillations in the visual cortex. Each person has their own intrinsic frequency in the gamma phase in this cortex, so to optimize the measurement of participants' baseline, their individual "peak" gamma frequency (IGF) was established for comparison. The "grating" stimuli increased IGF activity. If the IGF activity was entrained by the 40 Hz light flicker, then the power of IGF should have decreased when gamma power in response to flicker was produced. When they located the origin of the oscillations, they showed that the gamma response from the "grating" and the gamma response from the "flicker" originated from different locations in the visual cortex. Moreover, the flicker did not entrain the induced gamma activity (the IGF), it induced coexistent gamma activity in another area of the brain. These findings are important for the results of other experiments mentioned in this review and in the future, because they suggest that photic drive alone may not be enough to induce meaningful changes in brain activity. These findings also highlight the importance of measuring entrainment in subjects before starting an experiment, including the estimation of the response's location [33].

While rodents in GENUS experiments don't show sensitivity to variations in light stimulation, the human visual cortex and propagating pathways show more entrainment to light with specific characteristics. There is also evidence that individuals have their own preferred rhythm of resonance that neural networks will be most active at. Lee and Park, and colleagues set out to optimize the light flickering paradigm for human participants by setting up an experiment with white, red, green, and blue light of varying intensities and frequencies ranging from 32 to 50 Hz. They found that oscillations 34 to 38 Hz entrained the most intense gamma oscillations, which spread farther from the visual cortex than other frequencies. Higher luminance and colors with longer wavelengths (red and white) were also found to entrain the strongest oscillations. This study recorded from areas beyond the visual cortex to find that gamma oscillations also increased in these areas due to stimulation, which they described as evidence of entrainment. Lee and Park, and colleagues also note observations from an important connection, that visual and auditory stimuli are likely able to induce entrainment beyond the sensory cortexes. This effect might be associated with modulations to spiking in areas like CA1 of hippocampus, as well as decreased amyloid in the hippocampus [34]. However, evidence supporting this theory has only been found in rodents studies not in human studies [35,36].

A benefit to sensory stimulation as a potential treatment is that the procedure is low risk to participants. In one human study, a combined auditory and visual "flicker" at 40 Hz in patients with MCI due to AD was tolerated in subjects for 8 weeks with 1 hour of stimulation a day. There was 95.5% adherence to the study protocol and low adverse events. Although a short duration, results showed no changes in tau/amyloid ratio and decreased cytokine levels in CSF. After 8 weeks the fMRI showed increased connectivity between the precuneus and posterior cingulate cortex compared with baseline, but no other brain regions. Some limitations of the study include the lack of a control group and limited sample size, as well as the short time period. The treatment group of patients with MCI also does not give insight into the outcome of this treatment in more progressed cases, including feasibility [37].

SUMMARY

If decreased gamma oscillations are directly related to cognitive symptoms, then targeting neural networks to restore this activity could provide benefits. Presently, the effectiveness of AD treatments is measured using biomarkers and assessment of cognitive symptoms. Possible outcomes of a beneficial treatment would be decreased AβO in the brain, which can be studied postmortem or using PET imaging. The marked decrease of gamma power in AD and other dementias offers the possibility of an exciting new parameter for AD diagnosis, progress, and potential treatments. The future of AD treatment calls for a multi-faceted approach. Before the FDA approval of Aducanumab in 2021, there have been no disease-modifying treatments for AD that alter the course of the progressive disease. So far, research coming from the trials of Aducanumab show that this treatment will not be a catch-all for the disease, and additional research must be conducted to find safe and cost-effective treatments that can alleviate symptoms and potentially heal and reverse neuronal damage.

Studies show that the differences between AD EEGs and healthy EEGs may have diagnostic value. However, the length of time needed to capture and interpret an EEG may make this method not particularly useful, especially when other widely used measures such as cognitive scales already exist. However, previous EEG studies were important in emphasizing the potential value from a neuroscience research perspective and a neural dynamics approach to understanding AD. The characteristic differences between AD EEGs and others might serve as a guide to specific network dysfunction in hippocampus and cortical areas and allow more targeted treatment.

So far, amyloid-beta levels have been a key feature of AD pathology, and dementia symptoms are usually linked to decreased connectivity between brain areas. In rodent models, stimulation of the visual and auditory cortex using GENUS, and more specific stimulation of brain areas using optogenetic stimulation at around 40 Hz, has been shown to increase functional connectivity and decrease amyloid-beta protein. While in-depth analyses of gamma entrainment in humans have not yet shown the elimination of amyloid from the brain areas, it demonstrated downregulation of cytokines in the CSF of patients with AD after GENUS intervention, which could suggest a reduction in inflammation [37]. The targeted benefits of optogenetic stimulation in rodent studies could suggest a potential for gamma frequencies with deep brain stimulation in humans.

A limitation of most studies so far includes small sample sizes and the duration of treatment. Additionally, studies that have investigated the optimal stimulation using GENUS such as light intensity and frequency are conducted in healthy participants, and may not be applicable in patients with AD due as their network dynamics might be different. Nevertheless, the application of noninvasive light flicker and its safety features in AD mouse models has been an area of interest to researchers and might provide a guide for similar work in humans [35]. In summary, the reviewed growing body of research in neural dynamics provides strong evidence that gamma oscillations can be considered not only as a diagnostic tool and biomarker of AD but also used for monitoring severity and as the basis of new treatments.

CLINICS CARE POINTS

- Using a light flicker or other sensory stimulation to elicit gamma oscillations is non-invasive and is safe to use as a treatment.
- Initial research findings are promising, but more research needs to be done on the long term effects and efficacy of sensory stimulation in Alzheimer's patients.

DISCLOSURE

The authors report no commercial or financial conflicts of interest. No funding source was used for writing this article.

REFERENCES

[1] Sheppard O, Coleman M. Alzheimer's disease: etiology, neuropathology and pathogenesis. Exon Publications; 2020. p. 1–21.

[2] Sevigny J, Chiao P, Bussière T, et al. The antibody aducanumab reduces Aβ plaques in Alzheimer's disease. Nature 2016;537(7618):50–6.

[3] Liu KY, Howard R. Can we learn lessons from the FDA's approval of aducanumab? Nat Rev Neurol 2021;17(11):715–22.

[4] Başar E. Brain oscillations in neuropsychiatric disease. Dialogues Clin Neurosci 2013;15(3):291.

[5] Zhang H, Geng X, Wang Y, et al. The significance of EEG alpha oscillation spectral power and beta oscillation phase synchronization for diagnosing probable Alzheimer disease. Front Aging Neurosci 2021;13:291.

[6] Jensen O, Kaiser J, Lachaux J-P. Human gamma-frequency oscillations associated with attention and memory. Trends Neurosci 2007;30(7):317–24.

[7] Connors BW, Gutnick MJ. Intrinsic firing patterns of diverse neocortical neurons. Trends Neurosciences 1990;13(3):99–104.

[8] Schnitzler A, Gross J. Normal and pathological oscillatory communication in the brain. Nat Rev Neurosci 2005;6(4):285–96.
[9] Jeong J. EEG dynamics in patients with Alzheimer's disease. Clin Neurophysiol 2004;115(7):1490–505.
[10] Bowyer SM. Coherence a measure of the brain networks: past and present. Neuropsychiatr Electrophysiol 2016; 2(1):1–12.
[11] French CC, Beaumont JG. A critical review of EEG coherence studies of hemisphere function. Int J Psychophysiol 1984;1(3):241–54.
[12] Jeong J, Gore JC, Peterson BS. Mutual information analysis of the EEG in patients with Alzheimer's disease. Clin Neurophysiol 2001;112(5):827–35.
[13] Locatelli T, Cursi M, Liberati D, et al. EEG coherence in Alzheimer's disease. Electroencephalogr Clin Neurophysiol 1998;106(3):229–37.
[14] Murty DV, Manikandan K, Kumar WS, et al. Stimulus-induced gamma rhythms are weaker in human elderly with mild cognitive impairment and alzheimer's disease. Elife 2021;10.
[15] Mufson EJ, Mahady L, Waters D, et al. Hippocampal plasticity during the progression of Alzheimer's disease. Neuroscience 2015;309:51–67.
[16] Cardin JA. Inhibitory interneurons regulate temporal precision and correlations in cortical circuits. Trends Neurosciences 2018;41(10):689–700.
[17] Pelkey KA, Chittajallu R, Craig MT, et al. Hippocampal GABAergic inhibitory interneurons. Physiol Rev 2017; 97(4):1619–747.
[18] Etter G, van der Veldt S, Manseau F, et al. Optogenetic gamma stimulation rescues memory impairments in an Alzheimer's disease mouse model. Nat Commun 2019; 10(1):1–11.
[19] Chung H, Park K, Jang HJ, et al. Dissociation of somatostatin and parvalbumin interneurons circuit dysfunctions underlying hippocampal theta and gamma oscillations impaired by amyloid β oligomers in vivo. Brain Struct Funct 2020;225(3):935–54.
[20] Antonoudiou P, Tan YL, Kontou G, et al. Parvalbumin and somatostatin interneurons contribute to the generation of hippocampal gamma oscillations. J Neurosci 2020;40(40):7668–87.
[21] Martinez-Losa M, Tracy TE, Ma K, et al. Nav1.1-overexpressing interneuron transplants restore brain rhythms and cognition in a mouse model of Alzheimer's disease. Neuron 2018;98(1):75–89. E75.
[22] Yener GG, Başar E. Brain oscillations as biomarkers in neuropsychiatric disorders: following an interactive panel discussion and synopsis. Supplements Clin Neurophysiol 2013;62:343–63.
[23] Strelets V, Garakh ZV, Novototskii-Vlasov VY. Comparative study of the gamma rhythm in normal conditions, during examination stress, and in patients with first depressive episode. Neurosci Behav Physiol 2007;37(4): 387–94.
[24] Papp N, Vas S, Bogáthy E, et al. Acute and chronic escitalopram alter EEG gamma oscillations differently: relevance to therapeutic effects. Eur J Pharm Sci 2018;121: 347–55.
[25] Fitzgerald PJ, Watson BO. Gamma oscillations as a biomarker for major depression: an emerging topic. Translational Psychiatry 2018;8(1):1–7.
[26] Cho KK, Hoch R, Lee AT, et al. Gamma rhythms link prefrontal interneuron dysfunction with cognitive inflexibility in Dlx5/6+/− mice. Neuron 2015;85(6):1332–43.
[27] Lee K-H, Williams L, Haig A, et al. Gamma (40 Hz) phase synchronicity" and symptom dimensions in schizophrenia. Cogn Neuropsychiatry 2003;8(1):57–71.
[28] Adaikkan C, Middleton SJ, Marco A, et al. Gamma entrainment binds higher-order brain regions and offers neuroprotection. Neuron 2019;102(5):929–43. E928.
[29] Iaccarino HF, Singer AC, Martorell AJ, et al. Gamma frequency entrainment attenuates amyloid load and modifies microglia. Nature 2016;540(7632):230–5.
[30] Cruz JC, Tseng H-C, Goldman JA, et al. Aberrant CDK5 activation by P25 triggers pathological events leading to neurodegeneration and neurofibrillary tangles. Neuron 2003;40(3):471–83.
[31] Chan D, Suk H-J, Jackson B, et al. 40hz sensory stimulation induces gamma entrainment and affects brain structure, sleep and cognition in patients with Alzheimer's dementia. medRxiv 2021.
[32] Jones M, McDermott B, Oliveira BL, et al. Gamma band light stimulation in human case studies: Groundwork for potential Alzheimer's disease treatment. J Alzheimer's Dis 2019;70(1):171–85.
[33] Duecker K, Gutteling TP, Herrmann CS, et al. No evidence for entrainment: endogenous gamma oscillations and rhythmic flicker responses coexist in visual cortex. J Neurosci 2021;41(31):6684–98.
[34] Lee K, Park Y, Suh SW, et al. Optimal flickering light stimulation for entraining gamma waves in the human brain. Scientific Rep 2021;11(1):1–10.
[35] Singer AC, Martorell AJ, Douglas JM, et al. Noninvasive 40-Hz light flicker to recruit microglia and reduce amyloid beta load. Nat Protoc 2018;13(8):1850–68.
[36] Martorell AJ, Paulson AL, Suk H-J, et al. Multi-sensory gamma stimulation ameliorates Alzheimer's-associated pathology and improves cognition. Cell 2019;177(2): 256–71. E222.
[37] He Q, Colon-Motas KM, Pybus AF, et al. A feasibility trial of gamma sensory flicker for patients with prodromal Alzheimer's disease. Alzheimer's & Dementia. Translational Res Clin Interventions 2021;7(1):e12178.

Psychotherapeutics

Advances in Psychiatry and Behavioral Health 2 (2022) 57–70

ADVANCES IN PSYCHIATRY AND BEHAVIORAL HEALTH

Advances in Psychotherapy with Internet-Based Cognitive Behavioral Therapy for Anxiety and Obsessive-Compulsive Disorder

Allie N. Townsend, MA[a,b], Alyssa G. Hertz, MS[a,c], Johann M. D'Souza, MA[a,d,e], Andrew D. Wiese, PhD[a,*]

[a]Department of Psychiatry and Behavioral Sciences, Baylor College of Medicine, 1977 Butler Boulevard, Houston, TX 77030, USA; [b]The Chicago School of Professional Psychology, 1015 15th Street NW, Washington, DC 20005 USA; [c]Philadelphia College of Osteopathic Medicine, 4170 City Avenue, Philadelphia, PA 19131 USA; [d]Department of Psychology, University of Houston, 4800 Calhoun Road, Houston, TX 77004 USA; [e]Texas Institute for Measurement, Evaluation, and Statistics, University of Houston, 4800 Calhoun Road, Houston, TX 77004 USA

KEYWORDS

• ICBT • Internet treatment • Cognitive behavioral therapy • Anxiety • OCD

KEY POINTS

- Virtual therapy addresses barriers to treatment access through self-help, videoconferencing, and Internet-based cognitive behavioral therapy modalities.
- ICBT is an efficacious and effective method for delivering treatment across anxiety disorders and obsessive-compulsive disorder. Patient engagement is an important factor impacting response to treatment.
- ICBT treatment modalities incorporate principles of traditional in-person cognitive behavioral therapy; however, they are delivered using different methods including video conferencing, self-help apps, and messaging services between patients and providers.
- ICBT is an effective treatment option and improves access to care, but additional research is needed to better understand and address individual differences that may prevent response to treatment and to improve access to care.

BACKGROUND

Treatment of psychiatric conditions has historically relied on the use of individual in-person treatment [1]. The evolution of modern technology has influenced health care at large by increasing patient access, exchange of information, assessment, and treatment implementation. In recent years, there has been a growing trend to use technology in the provision of mental health treatment to improve access to care [2]. Anxiety and obsessive-compulsive disorders (OCD) are two related but distinct presentations with growing emphasis on incorporating modern technologies. These technology-enhanced treatments share similar principles with traditional in-person treatment.

According to the World Health Organization, approximately 264 million people are affected by anxiety disorders [3], making them the most prevalent domain of psychiatric disorders [4]. Each anxiety disorder exhibits unique characteristics, although a common symptom across all anxiety disorders is persistent and excessive worry or fear disproportionate to real threat [5]. There are several types of anxiety disorders, with

*Corresponding author, *E-mail address:* Andrew.Wiese@bcm.edu

https://doi.org/10.1016/j.ypsc.2022.05.003

2667-3827/22/

social anxiety disorder (SAD) and specific phobia being the most common [4]. SAD is characterized by a marked and enduring fear that persists in social settings where scrutiny and judgment from others is possible [3], whereas specific phobia is characterized by fear of exposure to a specific stimulus, including but not limited to: heights, animals, and needles [6]. Additional anxiety disorders include generalized anxiety disorder (GAD), where individuals exhibit uncontrollable and irrational worry about several events and activities, and panic disorder (PD), which is characterized by a future-oriented concern of unexpected and reoccurring panic attacks [4,7]. In 2013, the diagnostic classification of anxiety disorders experienced several adjustments, resulting in the removal of OCD as an anxiety disorder, and reclassification in its own diagnostic category of obsessive-compulsive spectrum disorders, which also include body-focused repetitive behaviors, such as trichotillomania and excoriation, and hoarding disorder [3]. Although OCD is now considered diagnostically separate from anxiety disorders, they share characteristics, such as excessive and exaggerated anxiety in response to specific stimuli. Because of the diagnostic similarity the treatments are also similar.

OCD is a debilitating psychiatric condition that is characterized by unwanted and distressing thoughts, images, or impulses known as obsessions [8]. Importantly, affected persons recognize obsessions as ego dystonic, or starkly contrary to the individual's values/desires (eg, "I will hit someone with my car"). Obsessions and associated distress are often followed by compulsions, which are repetitive physical or mental rituals that the individual feels compelled to perform to prevent or mitigate distress [8,9]. The cyclical nature of OCD is maintained and/or exacerbated through negative reinforcement given that compulsions temporarily alleviate anxiety and distress [8]. Although compulsions may facilitate immediate relief, this is short-lived because the thoughts are recurrent. The OCD cycle, shown in Fig. 1, is characterized by (1) obsessions, (2) anxiety/distress, (3) compulsive behavior, and (4) temporary relief until the next obsession. OCD is common with a lifetime prevalence of 2% and typically has a chronic illness duration [10].

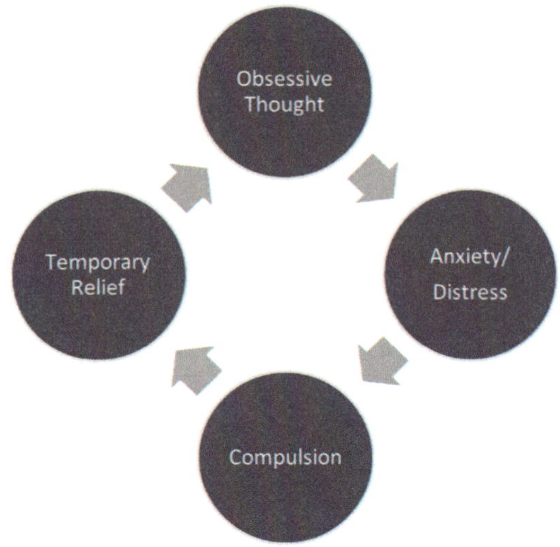

FIG. 1 The OCD cycle.

COGNITIVE BEHAVIORAL THERAPY

Cognitive behavioral therapy (CBT) is the first-line treatment of individuals with anxiety disorders and OCD [11,12]. CBT purports the onset and maintenance of psychopathology is attributed to maladaptive thoughts and behaviors that then have a dysfunctional relationship to emotions [13]. Traditional CBT includes psychoeducation, symptom self-monitoring, hierarchy development, exposure and response prevention (ERP), anxiety management skills, and cognitive restructuring [12]. CBT is administered as a monotherapy or in combination with psychotropic medications, although CBT is as or more effective than medication alone for anxiety and OCD [12,14]. Pharmacologic treatments, such as selective serotonin reuptake inhibitors, are often recommended for moderate to severe pathology and significantly decrease symptoms and improve functioning [12,15].

For anxiety disorders and OCD, CBT attributes pathology to an overestimation of threat followed by avoidance, a cycle that is established and maintained through fear conditioning [11,16,17]. Fear conditioning is an association-based learning in which an individual learns that a neutral stimulus is dangerous based on its association with a negative experience [12]. Consequently, fear conditioning is negatively reinforced through avoidance and/or compulsions, because these behavioral responses provide temporary relief and prohibit new learning from occurring [11,14,18]. For example, if an individual who experienced public embarrassment while giving a speech subsequently avoids any opportunities for speeches in the future, they remove the possible presence of anxiety related to public speaking. Although this effectively prevents anxiety in the short-term, the individual loses the opportunity to experience neutral or positive speaking experiences, and therefore, their fear of public speaking is maintained and oftentimes generalized (talking in a group setting, speaking to individuals of authority). In the context of OCD, if an individual with contamination fears avoids touching doorknobs perceived to be "contaminated," they prevent/minimize the onset of anxiety symptoms, and through continued avoidance, can develop generalized fears of other surfaces resulting in impairments of basic daily functioning.

ERP is a specific cognitive-behavioral intervention and is the gold standard treatment of OCD [12,19]. ERP modifies learned fear associations by intentionally confronting internal and/or external triggers that activate anxiety [18,20]. While confronted with feared stimuli, individuals are encouraged to refrain from performing compulsions and avoidant behaviors [20]. Repeating this process allows the individual to integrate new information that disconfirms pathologic associations, resulting in a reduction of anxiety. Exposure exercises are categorized as in vivo, imaginal, and interoceptive, yet all serve as methods of approaching feared stimuli [18]. In vivo exposures involve in-person, physical confrontation with a feared stimulus (eg, touching a contaminated object), which most directly targets learned fears. When in vivo exposures are difficult to access or unsafe to perform, imaginal exposure is used. Here the individual vividly pictures the feared situation. Although imaginal exposure is used for any fear, it is particularly useful for fears that are difficult to recreate, such as hitting a person with a car, going to hell, or having a terminal diagnosis. Lastly, for individuals who fear the physiologic symptoms of anxiety, interoceptive exposures are used to intentionally induce feared physical sensations, such as elevated heart rate, shortness of breath, sweating, and/or nausea [18]. Exposure to these sensations allows the individual to learn that despite their discomfort, the physiologic symptoms are not dangerous or permanent; this further encourages the individual to engage in previously avoided situations that could bring about physiologic discomfort, such as exercise or driving.

An extensive body of literature provides robust evidence for CBT as an effective and efficacious treatment modality for anxiety disorders [21–23]. Compared with waitlist or other psychotherapies, CBT exhibits superiority in reducing worrying and anxiety, and improved quality of life for persons diagnosed with GAD [24,25]. Moreover, individuals with specific phobia who received CBT, compared with waitlist, placebo, and nonexposure interventions, reported a significant reduction in symptoms [26]. Although findings from these individual studies are encouraging, data from multiple meta-analytic studies provide further support for CBT demonstrating significant symptom reduction and increased quality of life for various anxiety disorders, including GAD, SAD, PD, and specific phobia [17,27,28]. Although there is clear evidence that CBT results in symptom change, there is also evidence demonstrating long-term treatment gains, with evidence for sustained symptoms reduction 1 year out from treatment [21,29]. Taken together, there is extensive literature providing support for CBT as a first-line treatment of anxiety disorders.

CBT with ERP is also a highly effective treatment of OCD [30–32]. Researchers have found that CBT leads to long-term, clinically significant treatment gains, despite symptom presentation, severity, and psychological comorbidities for those with OCD [23,33]. Meta-analytic reviews have demonstrated a 43% reduction on the Yale-Brown Obsessive-Compulsive Scale (Y-BOCS), the gold standard assessment tool for OCD symptom severity, after receiving ERP [34]. In addition to long-term symptom improvement, ERP demonstrates superiority relative to medication alone. Foa and colleagues [35] found participants randomized into ERP only or ERP plus clomipramine had greater symptom reduction relative to clomipramine alone. Additional research has since supported this finding, highlighting the effectiveness of ERP or ERP plus medication over medication alone [36,37]. In sum, research has clearly established ERP as the front-line, efficacious, and enduring treatment of OCD.

INTERNET-BASED TREATMENT

Although the annual cost of medical expenses associated with anxiety disorders in the United States has been estimated at $33 billion, the health care system suffers from reduced access to effective treatment options for anxiety disorders and OCD [38,39]. Despite substantial research support for its effectiveness, CBT is poorly disseminated, underused, and difficult to access for persons affected by these psychiatric conditions [40]. Studies have reported that the average delay between onset of diagnosis and initial treatment contact is 10 years [22]. Furthermore, less than 10% of individuals receive appropriate, evidence-based psychological treatment of the respective conditions for which they meet criteria [40]. Gaining access to CBT, specifically ERP, is attributed to treatment barriers, such as location, cost, time restraints, and stigmatization [22,41]. Limited access to treatment can significantly exacerbate symptoms and contribute to higher dysfunction [42]. Therefore, there has been a demand for and major focus on improving access to appropriate treatment, such as ERP.

Recent decades have seen a steady increase in the use of Internet-based interventions for anxiety disorders and OCD because of greater accessibility, affordability, and portability as compared with in-person treatments [39,43,44]. Internet treatment can vary widely regarding level of therapist involvement and whether or not the treatment is delivered in a synchronous fashion. The Internet-based treatment that is most similar to traditional CBT is real-time, individual interaction with a therapist via videoconferencing to allow for maximal provider support and observation of verbal and nonverbal communication. On the other end of the spectrum, some Internet-based treatments allow patients to work independently through guided treatment modules with limited, or absent, therapist support.

Videoconferencing

Therapy delivered via videoconferencing, commonly termed telehealth, telemental health, and telemedicine, is most similar to traditional therapy given the real-time interactive sessions. Videoconference services address dissemination issues by decreasing travel time, schedule conflicts, and reluctance to meet in person because of stigma. However, there are costs to having sufficient videoconferencing technology for patients and providers alike [45]. Furthermore, required therapist time is not less than traditional therapy, because both modalities require provider and patient to be present and engaged during the therapy visit. Regarding treatment outcomes, videoconferencing has been found to be an efficacious and safe treatment option for a broad range of diagnoses, including anxiety and OCD [46–48]. In sum, videoconferencing has been found to be an appropriate treatment option that addresses some barriers to care. Although it is most similar to in-person individual therapy, therapists should consider for whom this modality is appropriate and which barriers videoconferencing will mitigate relative to in-person services.

Self-help

Self-help interventions are another Internet-based approach that addresses barriers to receiving evidence-based treatment [49,50]. Several controlled clinical trials that compared Internet-based self-help interventions have found moderate to large effect sizes in SAD, PD, posttraumatic stress disorder, and GAD [51]. Similarly, studies have demonstrated large pretreatment to post-treatment effects on OCD compared with treatment as usual or waitlist [52,53]. Self-help is categorized into two groups: unguided or guided [49]. Unguided self-help is characterized as engagement with treatment without clinician support. Guided self-help is defined as participation in treatment that involves some clinician contact, ranging from minimal guidance via email to considerable time reviewing material and proving feedback [49,54,55]. Although both forms of self-help are useful, there is strong empirical support demonstrating the superiority of guided self-help [55,56]. Spek and colleagues [56] postulated that the presence of therapist support is a main factor in distinguishing large from small effect sizes for treatment response.

In 2016, the US Census Bureau reported 76% of individuals owned a smartphone, 77% a computer, and 58% owned a tablet [57]. The ubiquity of personal devices has greatly increased accessibility to self-help treatments including ERP [39,44]. A considerable amount of research has also focused on smartphone apps. One study found 70.6% of people use smartphone apps to self-monitor symptoms [58]. Smartphone apps, particularly those that adapt interventions from evidence-based treatments, were found to be more effective in reducing anxiety symptoms [59,60].

Despite these benefits, there are limitations to technology-based self-help. A primary concern involves lack of regulation, which can lead users to receive inaccurate information about their psychiatric conditions and/or treatment [43,61]. Additionally, many apps do not have the storage capacity to incorporate manualized treatments, such as CBT. Consequently, individuals may only be receiving condensed aspects of treatment [62]. Lastly, research suggests treatment benefits are limited to persons with mild symptomology [63]. This may discourage those with moderate-to-severe symptoms from seeking Internet-based self-help treatment or may result in them receiving an inadequate dose of CBT, further perpetuating their psychopathology. On a higher level, this could be problematic, because it may leave recipients of insufficient CBT interventions questioning the effectiveness of CBT. In sum, it is essential to consider the fit of a respective CBT intervention modality to the specific individual, because misjudgment may have iatrogenic effects.

INTERNET-BASED COGNITIVE BEHAVIORAL THERAPY

Internet-based CBT (ICBT) typically involves a patient following a therapeutic treatment program available on the Internet while receiving therapist support via telephone, email, and/or videoconferencing [52]. ICBT allows for an individualized approach to virtual therapy as patients work with a therapist who gradually introduces therapy materials, self-guided assignments, and provides homework feedback. In this approach, the clinician's support is often provided in an asynchronous fashion. There are multiple benefits to this type of therapy because it can be accessed at any time of day by the patient, can occur regardless of geographic or transportation status, and is less time-demanding on the therapist [64]. The efficacy of ICBT for anxiety disorders and OCD is detailed next.

Internet-based cognitive behavioral therapy for anxiety disorders

Research has generally found ICBT to be an efficacious treatment of adults with anxiety disorders [65].When compared with face-to-face treatment, ICBT for anxiety disorders does not seem to produce significantly different findings at posttreatment or follow-up [65,66]. ICBT has been studied for multiple anxiety disorders including PD, SAD, GAD, and health anxiety.

Trials assessing PD have revealed that ICBT is superior compared with waitlist controls [67–69]. Allen and colleagues [67] evaluated the efficacy of ICBT for PD in primary care settings and found the treatment to be effective, although there were lower completion and adherence rates compared with those found in clinical trial. Low adherence rates were found to be related to the amount of therapist contact, highlighting the importance of practitioner education, presence, and regular communication with patients. Despite the empirical basis for ICBT for PD, one study failed to find support for ICBT treatment of mild panic symptoms [70]. This could potentially indicate limitations in the effectiveness of ICBT for subclinical symptomatology.

Among anxiety disorders, ICBT has some of the strongest empirical support in treating SAD [71,72]. Findings have demonstrated that ICBT can yield significant improvements in social anxiety symptoms and accompanying depressed mood [73–76]. Studies comparing ICBT with traditional group CBT have found similar outcomes at posttreatment and follow-up [77,78]. Direct comparisons of ICBT and traditional CBT for SAD have failed to reveal significant differences in treatment response [78–80]. Despite the large empirical literature, a notable portion of patients do not achieve clinically significant improvement from ICBT for SAD [72].

ICBT for GAD has been shown to be an efficacious treatment option [81–83]. Multiple studies have shown ICBT to be superior to waitlist conditions [81–83]. These findings do not seem specific to young- and middle-aged adults either, with one study finding evidence for symptom reduction in older adults (age 60+) with GAD following a course of ICBT [84].

Health anxiety has additionally been studied for ICBT treatment. Hedman and colleagues [85–87] have repeatedly demonstrated the efficaciousness of ICBT for health anxiety. Their work found ICBT to be superior to control groups, including behavioral stress management, for the treatment of severe health anxiety [86]. Additional research comparing ICBT with an online psychoeducation program found ICBT to be superior in reducing illness anxiety symptoms [88]. Results from a recent study by Axelsson and colleagues [89] revealed that ICBT was noninferior to traditional face-to-face CBT for the treatment of health anxiety within a primary care setting. This finding is particularly relevant, because ICBT may help alleviate barriers to treatment that are present in the context of face-to-face CBT. Overall, ICBT is an appropriate treatment option across anxiety disorders that produces similar outcomes to traditional CBT.

Internet-based cognitive behavioral therapy for obsessive-compulsive disorder

The first randomized-controlled trial assessing ICBT for OCD compared ICBT with online supportive therapy [52]. ICBT consisted of self-help text materials for the main treatment components, which are psychoeducation, cognitive restructuring, ERP, and relapse prevention. Participants completed text-material, worksheets, and self-rating forms that were communicated to therapists via email, with no synchronic interactions. Results revealed a clinically significant decrease in symptom severity for ICBT over the attention control group, as reflected by Y-BOCS [90] scores that were maintained at 4-month follow-up. The authors found that the time commitment of the therapists was 129 minutes per participant, which is roughly a quarter of what is typically involved in traditional CBT treatment of OCD.

Subsequent studies have been conducted to further evaluate ICBT's efficacy in treating OCD compared with other interventions. ICBT has been shown to be superior to waitlist and pharmacologic treatment as usual [91,92]. A study comparing ICBT and progressive relaxation training found that roughly half of the ICBT group achieved symptom improvement and one-third achieved symptom recovery compared with 29% and 11% in the relaxation group, respectively [93]. The relaxation group was offered ICBT after they completed their course of relaxation training, and results from this sample indicated that the combined relaxation/ICBT was no more effective than the ICBT only group.

Additional research has further supported the enduring effects of ICBT for up to 2 years posttreatment [94,95]. Andersson and colleagues [94] tested the impact of booster ICBT sessions on the long-term effects of ICBT for OCD. Participants who completed an initial trial of ICBT for OCD [52] were split to receive a 3-week ICBT booster or no booster as they were followed for enduring effects. Results revealed that both groups had large enduring effects [94]. The ICBT booster group showed initial superiority at the 7-month follow-up; however, these differences disappeared in the 12- and 24-month follow-ups. In sum, ICBT for OCD is efficacious and effective and is a safe treatment option for individuals with limited access to traditional in-person delivery of ERP.

Outcome-associated variables

Although evidence is clear that ICBT is generally effective in treating OCD and anxiety disorders, there are important individual differences that may help explain why some individuals do and do not respond to ICBT treatments. Treatment adherence in ICBT refers to the extent of engagement individuals have with the online content, often defined by the number of modules or lessons completed [96,97]. Association between treatment adherence and outcomes has been inconsistent, with some studies reporting a clear positive association [98,99] and others failing to find a clear association between adherence and outcomes (Table 1) [100,101]. Despite inconsistent and disparate research findings linking adherence and outcome, many individuals do not complete ICBT programs [96,102], indicating a need for further research aimed at increasing adherence to ICBT.

Treatment effectiveness may also depend on such factors as symptom severity and pretreatment beliefs about the effectiveness of ICBT. Higher baseline severity has been associated with greater response to ICBT for OCD [52]. A few studies have revealed that higher perceived credibility of ICBT at pretreatment is associated with faster symptom reduction for GAD and health anxiety [84,86]. However, findings on the association between expectancy beliefs and treatment outcomes have been mixed, possibly because of varied timings of assessment [83,84,86,103].

Although somewhat inconsistent, multiple meta-analyses have revealed that therapist-guided ICBT is superior to self-guided ICBT in regard to treatment adherence, dropout rates, and overall treatment efficacy [56,104]. It is hypothesized that therapist support increases accountability, thus reducing treatment dropout, while facilitating patient learning. Oromendia and colleagues [68] found that scheduled therapist support was associated with greater symptom improvement for ICBT for PD compared with nonscheduled therapist support. The nonscheduled support that depended on patient-demand resulted in lower patient time with therapist. A meta-analysis of virtual CBT for OCD found self-led treatment without therapist involvement to have moderate effect sizes and high levels of outcome variability [105]. When comparing low therapist involvement with absent therapist involvement, superior treatment response has been found in therapist-involved treatment [105].

The therapeutic alliance has been long-established as a critical part of the therapeutic process. In ICBT, the alliance is formed between the therapist and patient; however, the alliance does not seem to be associated with treatment outcomes [106,107]. In fact, a lenient therapist approach to homework completion has been shown to be associated with poorer outcomes in ICBT for GAD [108]. A causal relationship between these two variables should not be inferred given potential impacting variables (ie, patient motivation); however, other therapist variables should be assessed as they relate to ICBT treatment outcomes.

Recent work evaluating the therapeutic alliance in ICBT differentiates the patient's alliance with the therapist from their alliance with the program [109]. This

TABLE 1
Advantages and disadvantages of ICBT for the treatment of anxiety disorders and OCD

Advantages	Disadvantages
Decrease barriers (ie, travel, costs, time off from work)	Poor treatment adherence
Improved access to evidence-based treatments	May be less effective for milder symptoms
Can access treatment throughout the day	Less individualized
Less time demanding on therapist	Lack of trained clinical providers
Superior to waitlist (ie, PD, GAD, health anxiety, OCD)	Negative attitudes toward Internet interventions
Superior to waitlist and pharmacologic treatment (ie, OCD)	

research demonstrated that these separate measures of alliance were associated with different treatment outcomes for patients with PD. Specifically, patient program alliance was associated with symptom change but not adherence or dropout, whereas patient therapist alliance was associated with adherence but not symptom change. Therefore, it is suggested that future research on the working alliance in ICBT recognizes these components as distinct constructs that uniquely impact outcomes.

One clear benefit of ICBT is the reduction in therapist and health care resources required. Andrews and colleagues [79] stated that therapists in face-to-face treatment spend 13 times longer communicating with patients compared with ICBT. Therefore, ICBT reduces health care costs and allows therapists to dedicate more attention to patients with increased severity [110]. Although therapists have positive opinions toward telehealth generally, less is known about their opinions toward ICBT specifically [111,112].

Intensive Internet-based cognitive behavioral therapy

Increasing attention in the literature has been placed on more condensed, accelerated ERP treatment options to facilitate faster symptom improvement, maximize patient motivation and therapeutic momentum, and encourage a timely return to daily activities [113–115]. Time-intensive CBT treatments have been studied for various anxiety disorders, including SAD, PD, and agoraphobia, and OCD [113,114,116,117]. The recent rise in ICBT research has contributed preliminary studies on the feasibility and acceptability of intensive ICBT [115,118].

One study evaluated an intensive treatment of ICBT for 10 participants with PD and agoraphobia [115]. This included six online lessons that were completed over 7 days, accompanied by clinician support via telephone and email. Results yielded reductions in panic, agoraphobic, and impairment symptoms that maintained at 2-month follow-up. Jain and colleagues [118] investigated intensive ICBT for SAD. Comparable with the previous study, 15 participants with SAD completed five online lessons over 7 days, with clinician support available via telephone and email. Significant reductions in social anxiety and functional impairment symptoms were found at posttreatment and 1-month follow-up. These preliminary studies have revealed promising results for the feasibility and acceptability of intensive ICBT for PD and SAD, although continued trials are needed to draw stronger conclusions on the efficacy of intensive ICBT.

Treatment perception

Patient perception of treatment is an important variable that can impact treatment effectiveness. In recent meta-analyses of ICBT, patients report ICBT to be highly acceptable [119,120]. Despite this, not all patients respond to or complete treatment, and some find the process of engaging in self-led treatment to be difficult. To further understand differing patient perspectives and outcomes, some research has qualitatively analyzed patient experiences in ICBT [121–123]. Halmetoja and colleagues [122] examined patient experience 4 years after completing ICBT for SAD. Results indicated that patients who were able to independently engage in the treatment modules and overcome barriers while working through the course of treatment had superior sustainability compared with patients who were more passive in their treatment. A recent study by Pedersen and colleagues [123] highlighted that generalizing the treatment content to real-world applications was difficult for some patients. The telephone check-ins from therapists were perceived by some as too infrequent and broad to be effective. Noncompleters of the ICBT treatment generally emphasized a desire for additional support, including face-to-face support, from therapists on an as-needed basis.

CLINICAL IMPLICATIONS, LIMITATIONS, FUTURE DIRECTIONS

Perhaps the most important clinical implication of ICBT is that it is generally as efficacious as traditional CBT and can greatly increase the availability of services to those in need because it requires less time from providers. One study estimated a full-time psychologist who normally treats 20 to 30 patients a week using traditional CBT could see 80 patients a week using ICBT with no increase in provider time [124]. There are potential limitations to consider, such as reduced quality of care when treating such a notable number of patients per week; however, the concept of increased provider availability remains, nonetheless. Reduced therapist time could also reduce the cost burden on the patient. Furthermore, ICBT is superior to CBT in some ways because ICBT facilitates ongoing data collection of patient safety, progress, and outcomes, which could yield subsequent research benefits [54]. Additionally, the highly structured nature of ICBT makes protocol adherence much more likely than with CBT. However, this rigid structure can also have consequences in that ICBT may not offer the flexibility to adapt to individual patient presentations in the way traditional CBT can. As more advanced techniques, such as machine learning, are incorporated into Internet protocols, ICBT can become increasingly tailored to the individual [125].

Despite the benefits, there are several limitations associated with ICBT. One limitation to ICBT, specifically for interventions requiring videoconferencing of regular patient-provider interaction, is the lack of clinicians who are trained to provide, oversee, or even recommend ICBT. That said, there are promising models for therapist training in ICBT [124,126]. However, the greatest barrier is that many patients will not be interested in receiving services through the Internet versus in person. One study found that among patients interested in behavioral treatment, 91.9% would consider face-to-face treatment, whereas only 48.0% would consider Internet-based treatment [127]. The acceptability of ICBT did not increase with the increase in remote working because of COVID-19 policies [128].

Much research shows the effectiveness of ICBT when it is properly implemented to individuals receptive to the idea of receiving treatment through nontraditional means [129]. Future research should focus on increasing patient acceptability and use of ICBT. Advances in this area thus far have been more difficult than anticipated. One study found that providing an 800-word treatment rationale increased self-reported acceptability of ICBT, that is, a positive attitude toward the intervention [130]. Contrary to expectation, the increase in acceptability was not accompanied by an increase in self-reported willingness to use ICBT or an increase in seeking out ICBT services. Other studies have looked at patient attitude toward computerized therapy, but the implication of these studies may be limited if positive attitudes are not associated with greater use of ICBT [131]. Therefore, future research should focus on increasing participant's use of ICBT and not just enhancing their attitude toward it.

A recent large-scale study focused explicitly on increasing use of, and adherence to, ICBT using a 5-minute multimedia presentation [132]. However, the study found that the presentation did not significantly increase either the use of or adherence to ICBT. The most common reasons for nonadherence cited by participants were lack of time (34%), forgetting to use the program (14.6%), technical issues (12.5%), and difficulty concentrating (10.4%). Additional research has highlighted an association between poor computer literacy and nonadherence including drop-out following Internet-related problems and stress related to the computer format [96]. This could be particularly relevant for populations that are at-risk for poor computer literacy, such as elderly populations, low socioeconomic status, and rural communities with less access. Several of the reasons for nonadherence could be addressed by the personal follow-up associated with traditional CBT. If so, future studies could investigate the effectiveness of combining ICBT with a personal follow-up.

Along the same lines, future research can clarify the impact of lack of human contact as a reason for not using ICBT. Because human contact in therapy is associated with greater motivation, it is thought that participants would be more willing to use therapist-assisted ICBT over self-guided ICBT [133]. However, the results in the research are mixed [131]. If human contact is indeed an important motivation in willingness to use ICBT, therapist time could still be saved with the involvement of ICBT technicians. One study found that assistance by a technician was as effective as assistance from a clinician [134].

Given that the question of how to increase patient engagement in ICBT continues to remain unanswered, a humbler more exploratory approach may be warranted. Perhaps a future study should simply interview patients resistant to ICBT use and ask them what their barriers to use are and how to overcome those barriers. A small study ($n = 24$) took this approach by asking participants how to increase participation in World Wide Web–based mental health services [135]. The participants suggested identifying and addressing individual barriers to engagement. One way of implementing this feedback would be for patients to meet with a therapist or nontherapist collaborator who would listen to and address the individual's barriers to treatment. Once the barriers are resolved, the individual could begin a course of ICBT.

Additional ways to increase use of ICBT are higher monetary incentives and targeting specific demographics that are more willing to express interest, such as those with greater psychopathology [128]. Given the difficulty in accessing evidence-based care in many places, ICBT could be offered for those waiting for traditional CBT and in this way benefit those who are more motivated for treatment. Another approach to increase implementation could be a hybrid model of traditional CBT and ICBT where the ICBT sessions are slowly phased in throughout the course of treatment [136]. In sum, ICBT is an effective treatment, and its biggest challenge is the unwillingness of patients to use it. Future research should understand personal barriers to using ICBT to collaborate with patients to help them overcome their challenges.

SUMMARY

Existing literature makes clear that cognitive-behavioral interventions are first-line and effective treatments for anxiety disorders and OCD [11,12]. With noted examples of barriers limiting patient access to care, and the detrimental impact of leaving psychopathology untreated, it is essential that clinicians and researchers alike examine how technologies can be used to effectively deliver CBT interventions to those in need. With rapid proliferation and technological advances, many providers are now equipped with tools (ie, ICBT) to help those in need. It is clear ICBT can help individuals with anxiety disorders and OCD, and that the treatment is superior to control conditions or no treatment. Limitations to the treatment exist, most notably regarding limited patient acceptance, efficacy for subclinical presentations, training for providers, and a less individualized treatment approach. ICBT is a suitable treatment option that is likely to gain increasing support in years to come, therefore continued research and practice is indicated to address treatment limitations.

CLINICS CARE POINTS

- Advantages of ICBT for the treatment of anxiety disorders and OCD include increased patient access to evidence-based treatment, decreased barriers (ie, travel, costs, time off from work), and decreased time demand for providers.
- Disadvantages of ICBT for the treatment of anxiety disorders and OCD include poor patient attitudes and adherence, limited effectiveness for mild symptomatology, lack of provider training, and a nontailored approach to care.

DISCLOSURE

The authors have no relevant finanical interst or affilications with any commercial intersts related to the subjects discussed in this article. The authors recieved no specific grant or finanical support for this manuscript, authorship, and/or publication of this article.

REFERENCES

[1] Fernandez E, Woldgabreal Y, Day A, et al. Live psychotherapy by video versus in-person: a meta-analysis of efficacy and its relationship to types and targets of treatment. Clin Psychol Psychother 2021. https://doi.org/10.1002/cpp.2594.
[2] Andersson G. Internet-delivered psychological treatments. Annu Rev Clin Psychol 2016;12:157–79.
[3] Garakani A, Murrough JW, Freire RC, et al. Pharmacotherapy of anxiety disorders: current and emerging treatment options. Front Psychiatry 2021;11. https://doi.org/10.3389/fpsyt.2020.595584.
[4] Thibaut F. Anxiety disorders: a review of current literature. Dialogues Clin Neurosci 2017;19:87–8.
[5] American Psychiatric Association. Diagnostic and statistical manual of mental disorders. 5th ed. Washington D.C.; 2013.
[6] Jefferies P, Ungar M. Social anxiety in young people: a prevalence study in seven countries. PLoS One 2020;15:e0239133.
[7] Konnopka A, Konig H. Economic burden of anxiety disorders: a systematic review and meta-analysis. Pharmacoeconomics 2019;38:5–37.
[8] Brauer L, Lewin AB, Storch EA. A review of psychotherapy for obsessive-compulsive disorder. M & B 2011;2:38–44.
[9] Wheaton MG, Chen SR. Homework completion in treating obsessive-compulsive disorder with exposure and ritual prevention: a review of the empirical literature. Cogn Ther Res 2021;45(2):236–49.
[10] Jaisoorya TS, Janardhan Reddy YC, Nair BS, et al. Prevalence and correlates of obsessive-compulsive disorder and subthreshold obsessive-compulsive disorder among college students in Kerala, India. Indian J Psychiatry 2017;59:56–62.
[11] Grebe SC, Bergez KC, Lee EB, et al. Chapter 6: Evidence-based treatment of pediatric obsessive-compulsive and related disorders. In: Steele RG, Roberts MC, editors. Handbook of evidence-based therapies for children and adolescents. 2nd edition. Cham: Springer; 2020. p. 71–84.
[12] McGuire JF, Storch EA. An inhibitory learning approach to cognitive-behavioral therapy for children and adolescents. Cogn Behav Pract 2019;26:214–24.
[13] Hofmann SG, Asnaani A, Vonk IJ, et al. The efficacy of cognitive behavioral therapy: a review of meta-analysis. Cognit Ther Res 2012;36:427–40.
[14] Abramowitz JS, Blakey SM, Reuman L, et al. New directions in the cognitive-behavioral treatment of OCD: theory, research, and practice. Behav Ther 2018;49:311–22.
[15] Simpson HB, Foa EB, Liebowitz MR, et al. Cognitive-behavioral therapy vs risperidone for augmenting serotonin reuptake inhibitors in obsessive-compulsive disorder: a randomized clinical trial. JAMA Psychiatry 2013;70:1190–9.
[16] Beck AT, Haigh EAP. Advances in cognitive theory and therapy: the generic cognitive model. *Annu Rev Clin Psychol* 2014;10:1–24.
[17] Carpenter JK, Andrews LA, Witcraft SM, et al. Cognitive-behavioral therapy for anxiety and related disorders: a

meta-analysis of randomized placebo-controlled trials. Depress Anxiety 2018;35:502–14.
[18] Kaczkurkin AN, Foa EB. Cognitive-behavioral therapy for anxiety disorders: an update on the empirical evidence. Dialogues Clin Neurosci 2015;17:337–46.
[19] Guzick AG, Reid AM, Balkhi AM, et al. That was easy! Expectancy violations during exposure and response prevention for childhood obsessive-compulsive disorder. Behav Modif 2020;44:319–42.
[20] McGuire JF, Lewin AB, Storch EA. Enhancing exposure therapy for anxiety disorders, obsessive-compulsive disorder and post-traumatic stress disorder. Expert Rev Neurother 2014;14:893–910.
[21] DiMauro J, Domingues J, Fernandez G, et al. Long-term effectiveness of CBT for anxiety disorders in an adult outpatient clinic sample: a follow-up study. Behav Res Ther 2013;51:82–6.
[22] Law C, Boisseau CL. Exposure and response prevention in the treatment of obsessive-compulsive disorder: current perspective. Psychol Res Behav Manag 2019;12: 117–1174.
[23] Olatunji BO, Davis ML, Powers MB, et al. Cognitive-behavioral therapy for obsessive-compulsive disorder: a meta-analysis of treatment outcome and moderators. J Psychiatr Res 2013;47:33–41.
[24] Hanrahan F, Field AP, Jones FW, et al. A meta-analysis of cognitive therapy for worry in generalized anxiety disorder. Clin Psychol Rev 2013;33:120–32.
[25] Hirsch CR, Beale S, Grey N, et al. Approaching cognitive behavior therapy for generalized anxiety disorder from a cognitive perspective. Front Psychol 2019;10:1–14.
[26] Roth A, Fonagy P. What works for whom?: a critical review of psychotherapy research. 2nd edition. New York: Guilford Press; 2009.
[27] Cuijpers P, Sijbrandij M, Koole S, et al. Psychological treatment of generalized anxiety disorder: a meta-analysis. Clin Psychol Rev 2014;34:130–40.
[28] Mayo-Wilson E, Dias S, Mavranezouli I, et al. Psychological and pharmacological interventions for social anxiety disorder in adults: a systematic review and network meta-analysis. Lancet Psychiatry 2014;1: 368–76, d.
[29] Watanabe N, Furukawa TA, Chen J, et al. Change in quality of life and their predictors in the long-term follow-up after group cognitive behavioral therapy for social anxiety disorders: a prospective cohort study. BMC Psychiatry 2010;81:1–10.
[30] Janardhan-Reddy YC, Sudhir PM, Manjula M, et al. Clinical practice guidelines for cognitive-behavioral therapies in anxiety disorders and obsessive-compulsive and related disorders. Indian J Psychiatry 2020;62:S230–50.
[31] Reid JE, Laws KR, Drummond L, et al. Cognitive behavioural therapy with exposure and response prevention in the treatment of obsessive-compulsive disorder: a systematic review and meta-analysis of randomised controlled trials. Compr Psychiatry 2021;2:152223.
[32] Skapinakis P, Caldwell DM, Hollingworth W, et al. Pharmacological and psychotherapeutic interventions for management of obsessive-compulsive disorder in adults: a systematic review and network meta-analysis. Lancet Psychiatry 2016;3:730–9.
[33] Rector NA, Richter MA, Katz D, et al. Does the addition of cognitive therapy to exposure and response prevention for obsessive compulsive disorder enhance clinical efficacy? A randomized controlled trial in a community setting. Br J Clin Psychol 2018;58:1–18.
[34] Abramowitz J, Franklin M, Foa E. Empirical status of cognitive-behavioral therapy for obsessive-compulsive disorder: a meta-analytic review. Rom J Cogn Behav Psychotherapies 2002;2(2):89–104.
[35] Foa EB, Liebowitz MR, Kozak MJ, et al. Randomized, placebo-controlled trial of exposure and ritual prevention, clomipramine, and their combination in the treatment of obsessive-compulsive disorder. Am J Psychiatry 2005;162:151–61.
[36] Ferrando C, Selai C. A systematic review and meta-analysis on the effectiveness of exposure and response prevention therapy in the treatment of obsessive-compulsive disorder. J Obsessive-Compulsive Relat Disords 2021;100684. https://doi.org/10.1016/j.jocrd.2021.100684, Published online.
[37] Romanelli RJ, Wu FM, Gamba R, et al. Behavioral therapy and serotonin reuptake inhibitor pharmacotherapy in the treatment of obsessive-compulsive disorder: a systemic review and meta-analysis of head-to-head randomized controlled trials. Depress Anxiety 2014;31(8):641–52.
[38] Shirneshan E, Bailey J, Relyea G, et al. Incremental direct medical expenditures associated with anxiety disorders for the U.S. adult population: evidence from the medical expenditure panel survey. J Anxiety Disord 2013;27(7):720–7.
[39] Van Ameringen M, Turna J, Khalesi Z, et al. There is an app for that! the current state of mobile applications (apps) for DSM-5 obsessive-compulsive disorder, post-traumatic stress disorder, anxiety and mood disorders. Depress Anxiety 2016;34:526–39.
[40] Gunter RW, Whittal ML. Dissemination of cognitive-behavioral treatments for anxiety disorders: overcoming barriers and improving patient access. Clin Psychol Rev 2010;30:194–202.
[41] Mancebo MC, Eisen JL, Sibrava NJ, et al. Patient utilization of cognitive-behavioral therapy for OCD. Behav Ther 2011;42:399–412.
[42] McIngvale E, Bordnick PS, Hart J. A self-help website for obsessive compulsive disorder: who is accessing the website? J Technology Hum Serv 2015;33:191–203.
[43] Donker T, Petrie K, Proudfoot J, et al. Smartphones for smarter delivery of mental health programs: a systematic review. J Med Internet Res 2013;15:e247.
[44] Haug T, Nordgreen T, Öst LG, et al. Self-help treatment of anxiety disorders: a meta-analysis and meta-regression of effects and potential moderators. Clin Psychol Rev 2012;32:425–45.

[45] Matsumoto K, Hamatani S, Makino T, et al. Guided Internet-based cognitive behavioral therapy for Japanese patients with obsessive-compulsive disorder: a protocol of the randomized controlled trial (preprint). JMIR Res Protoc 2020. https://doi.org/10.2196/18216.
[46] Rees CS, Maclaine E. A systematic review of videoconference-delivered psychological treatment for anxiety disorders. Aust Psychol 2015;50(4):259–64.
[47] Storch EA, Caporino NE, Morgan JR, et al. Preliminary investigation of web-camera delivered cognitive-behavioral therapy for youth with obsessive-compulsive disorder. Psychiatry Res 2011;189(3): 407–12.
[48] Tuerk PW, Keller SM, Acierno R. Treatment for anxiety and depression via clinical videoconferencing: evidence base and barriers to expanded access in practice. FOCUS 2018;16(4):363–9.
[49] Mehrotra S, Sudhir P, Rao G, et al. Development and pilot testing of an Internet-based self-help intervention for depression for Indian users. Behav Sci 2018;8:36.
[50] Schroder J, Berger T, Westermann S, et al. Internet interventions for depression: new developments. Dialogues Clin Neurosci 2016;18:203–12.
[51] Berger T, Boettcher J, Caspar F. Internet-based guided self-help for several anxiety disorders: a randomized controlled trial comparing a tailored with a standardized disorder-specific approach. Psychotherapy 2014; 51:207–19.
[52] Andersson E, Enander J, Andrén P, et al. Internet-based cognitive behaviour therapy for obsessive–compulsive disorder: a randomized controlled trial. Psychol Med 2012;42(10):2193–203.
[53] Wootton BM, Titov N, Dear BF, et al. The acceptability of Internet-based treatment and characteristics of an adult sample with obsessive compulsive disorders: an Internet survey. PLoS One 2011;6:E20548.
[54] Andersson G, Titov N. Advantages and limitations of Internet-based interventions for common mental disorders. World Psychiatry 2014;13(1):4–11.
[55] Cuijpers P, Riper H. Internet interventions for depression disorder: an overview. Revista de Psicopatología y Psicología Clínica 2014;19:209–16.
[56] Spek V, Cuijpers P, Nyklicek I, et al. Internet-based cognitive behaviour therapy for symptoms of depression and anxiety: a meta-analysis. Psychol Med 2007; 37(03):319.
[57] Marley J, Farooq S. Mobile telephone apps in mental health practice: uses, opportunities and challenges. BJPsych Bull 2015;39:288–90.
[58] Chan S, Torous J, Hinton L, et al. Towards a framework for evaluating mobile mental health apps. elemed e-Health 2015;21:1038–41.
[59] Firth J, Torous J, Nicholas J, et al. The efficacy of smartphone-based mental health interventions for depressive symptoms: a meta-analysis of randomized controlled trials. World Psychiatry 2017; 16:287–98.
[60] Newman MG, Jacobson NC, Rackoff GN, et al. A randomized controlled trial of a smartphone-based application for the treatment of anxiety. Psychotherapy Res 2021;31:443–54.
[61] Stoyanov SR, Hides L, Kavanagh DJ, et al. Mobile app rating scale: a new tool for assessing the quality of health mobile apps. JMIR mHealth and uHealth 2015;3:e27.
[62] Dagöö J, Asplund RP, Bsenko HA, et al. Cognitive behavior therapy versus interpersonal psychotherapy for social anxiety disorder delivered via smartphone and computer: a randomized controlled trial. J Anxiety Disord 2014;28(4):410–7.
[63] Newman MG, Szkodny LE, Llera SJ, et al. A review of technology-assisted self-help and minimal contact therapies for anxiety and depression: is human contact necessary for therapeutic efficacy? Clin Psychol Rev 2011;31(1):89–103.
[64] Holmes EA, Ghaderi A, Harmer CJ, et al. The Lancet Psychiatry Commission on psychological treatments research in tomorrow's science. Lancet Psychiatry 2018;5(3):237–86.
[65] Olthuis JV, Watt MC, Bailey K, et al. Therapist-supported Internet cognitive behavioural therapy for anxiety disorders in adults. Cochrane Database Syst Rev 2016. https://doi.org/10.1002/14651858.cd011565.pub2.
[66] Carlbring P, Andersson G, Cuijpers P, et al. Internet-based vs. face-to-face cognitive behavior therapy for psychiatric and somatic disorders: an updated systematic review and meta-analysis. Cogn Behav Ther 2018; 47(1):1–18.
[67] Allen AR, Newby JM, Mackenzie A, et al. Internet cognitive–behavioural treatment for panic disorder: randomised controlled trial and evidence of effectiveness in primary care. BJPsych Open 2016;2(2): 154–62.
[68] Oromendia P, Orrego J, Bonillo A, et al. Internet-based self-help treatment for panic disorder: a randomized controlled trial comparing mandatory versus optional complementary psychological support. Cogn Behav Ther 2016;45(4):270–86.
[69] Wims E, Titov N, Andrews G, et al. Clinician-assisted Internet-based treatment is effective for panic: a randomized controlled trial. Aust N Z J Psychiatry 2010; 44(7):599–607.
[70] van Ballegooijen W, Riper H, Klein B, et al. An Internet-based guided self-help intervention for panic symptoms: randomized controlled trial. J Med Internet Res 2013;15(7):e154.
[71] Boettcher J, Carlbring P, Renneberg B, et al. Internet-based interventions for social anxiety disorder: an overview. Verhaltenstherapie 2013;23(3):160–8.
[72] Chen H, Rodriguez MA, Qian M, et al. Predictors of treatment outcomes and adherence in Internet-based cognitive behavioral therapy for social anxiety in China. Behav Cogn Psychother 2020;1–13.

[73] Berger T, Hohl E, Caspar F. Internet-based treatment for social phobia: a randomized controlled trial. J Clin Psychol 2009;65(10):1021–35.
[74] Furmark T, Carlbring P, Hedman E, et al. Guided and unguided self-help for social anxiety disorder: randomised controlled trial. Br J Psychiatry 2009;195(5): 440–7.
[75] Tillfors M, Carlbring P, Furmark T, et al. Treating university students with social phobia and public speaking fears: Internet delivered self-help with or without live group exposure sessions. Depress Anxiety 2008;25(8):708–17.
[76] Titov N, Andrews G, Schwencke G, et al. Shyness 1: Distance treatment of social phobia over the Internet. Aust N Z J Psychiatry 2008;42(7):585–94.
[77] Andersson G, Carlbring P, Holmström A, et al. Internet-based self-help with therapist feedback and in vivo group exposure for social phobia: a randomized controlled trial. J Consult Clin Psychol 2006;74(4): 677–86.
[78] Hedman E, Andersson G, Ljótsson B, et al. Internet-based cognitive behavior therapy vs. cognitive behavioral group therapy for social anxiety disorder: a randomized controlled non-inferiority trial. In: García AV, editor. PLoS One6. 2011. 2011. p. e18001.
[79] Andrews G, Davies M, Titov N. Effectiveness randomized controlled trial of face to face versus Internet cognitive behaviour therapy for social phobia. Aust N Z J Psychiatry 2011;45(4):337–40.
[80] Botella C, Gallego MJ, Garcia-Palacios A, et al. An Internet-based self-help treatment for fear of public speaking: a controlled trial. Cyberpsychol Behav Soc Netw 2010;13(4):407–21.
[81] Paxling B, Almlöv J, Dahlin M, et al. Guided Internet-delivered cognitive behavior therapy for generalized anxiety disorder: a randomized controlled trial. Cogn Behav Ther 2011;40(3):159–73.
[82] Robinson E, Titov N, Andrews G, et al. Internet treatment for generalized anxiety disorder: a randomized controlled trial comparing clinician vs. technician assistance. García AV. PLoS One 2010;5(6):e10942.
[83] Titov N, Andrews G, Robinson E, et al. Clinician-assisted Internet-based treatment is effective for generalized anxiety disorder: randomized controlled trial. Aust N Z J Psychiatry 2009;43(10):905–12.
[84] Jones SL, Hadjistavropoulos HD, Soucy JN. A randomized controlled trial of guided Internet-delivered cognitive behaviour therapy for older adults with generalized anxiety. J Anxiety Disord 2016;37:1–9.
[85] Hedman E, Andersson G, Andersson E, et al. Internet-based cognitive–behavioural therapy for severe health anxiety: randomised controlled trial. Br J Psychiatry 2011;198(3):230–6.
[86] Hedman E, Axelsson E, Görling A, et al. Internet-delivered exposure-based cognitive–behavioural therapy and behavioural stress management for severe health anxiety: randomised controlled trial. Br J Psychiatry 2014; 205(4):307–14.
[87] Hedman E, Axelsson E, Andersson E, et al. Exposure-based cognitive–behavioural therapy via the Internet and as bibliotherapy for somatic symptom disorder and illness anxiety disorder: randomised controlled trial. Br J Psychiatry 2016;209(5):407–13.
[88] Newby JM, Smith J, Uppal S, et al. Internet-based cognitive behavioral therapy versus psychoeducation control for illness anxiety disorder and somatic symptom disorder: a randomized controlled trial. J Consult Clin Psychol 2017;86(1):89–98.
[89] Axelsson E, Andersson E, Ljótsson B, et al. Effect of Internet vs face-to-face cognitive behavior therapy for health anxiety. JAMA Psychiatry 2020;13. https://doi.org/10.1001/jamapsychiatry.2020.0940:Published online May.
[90] Goodman WK, Price LH, Rasmussen SA, et al. The Yale-Brown Obsessive Compulsive Scale. I. Development, use, and reliability. Arch Gen Psychiatry 1989;46(11):1006–11.
[91] Wootton BM, Dear BF, Johnston L, et al. Remote treatment of obsessive-compulsive disorder: a randomized controlled trial. J Obsessive-Compulsive Relat Disord 2013;2(4):375–84.
[92] Mahoney AEJ, Mackenzie A, Williams AD, et al. Internet cognitive behavioural treatment for obsessive compulsive disorder: a randomised controlled trial. Behav Res Ther 2014;63:99–106.
[93] Kyrios M, Ahern C, Fassnacht DB, et al. Therapist-assisted Internet-based cognitive behavioral therapy versus progressive relaxation in obsessive-compulsive disorder: randomized controlled trial. J Med Internet Res 2018;20(8):e242.
[94] Andersson E, Steneby S, Karlsson K, et al. Long-term efficacy of Internet-based cognitive behavior therapy for obsessive–compulsive disorder with or without booster: a randomized controlled trial. Psychol Med 2014;44(13):2877–87.
[95] Wootton BM, Dear BF, Johnston L, et al. Self-guided Internet-delivered cognitive behavior therapy (iCBT) for obsessive–compulsive disorder: 12 month follow-up. Internet Interventions 2015;2(3):243–7.
[96] Beatty L, Binnion C. A systematic review of predictors of, and reasons for, adherence to online psychological interventions. Int J Behav Med 2016;23(6):776–94.
[97] Christensen H, Griffiths KM, Farrer L. Adherence in Internet interventions for anxiety and depression. J Med Internet Res 2009;11(2):e13.
[98] El Alaoui S, Hedman E, Kaldo V, et al. Effectiveness of Internet-based cognitive–behavior therapy for social anxiety disorder in clinical psychiatry. J Consult Clin Psychol 2015;83(5):902–14.
[99] Hilvert-Bruce Z, Rossouw PJ, Wong N, et al. Adherence as a determinant of effectiveness of Internet cognitive behavioural therapy for anxiety and depressive disorders. Behav Res Ther 2012;50(7–8):463–8.
[100] Nordgreen T, Havik OE, Öst LG, et al. Outcome predictors in guided and unguided self-help for social anxiety disorder. Behav Res Ther 2012;50(1):13–21.

[101] Schulz A, Stolz T, Vincent A, et al. A sorrow shared is a sorrow halved? A three-arm randomized controlled trial comparing Internet-based clinician-guided individual versus group treatment for social anxiety disorder. Behav Res Ther 2016;84:14–26.
[102] Farrer LM, Griffiths KM, Christensen H, et al. Predictors of adherence and outcome in Internet-based cognitive behavior therapy delivered in a telephone counseling setting. Cogn Ther Res 2014;38(3):358–67.
[103] Hedman E, Andersson E, Ljótsson B, et al. Clinical and genetic outcome determinants of Internet- and group-based cognitive behavior therapy for social anxiety disorder. Acta Psychiatrica Scand 2012;126(2):126–36.
[104] Baumeister H, Reichler L, Munzinger M, et al. The impact of guidance on Internet-based mental health interventions: a systematic review. Internet Interventions 2014;1(4):205–15.
[105] Wootton BM. Remote cognitive–behavior therapy for obsessive–compulsive symptoms: a meta-analysis. Clin Psychol Rev 2016;43:103–13.
[106] Becker E, Amdersson G. Internet-and computer-based treatmetn of generalized anxiety disroder (GAD). In: Gerlach A, Gloster A, editors. Generalized Anxiety Disorder & Worrying. Hoboken NJ: Wiley-Blackwell; 2020. p. 319–34.
[107] Sucala M, Schnur JB, Constantino MJ, et al. The therapeutic relationship in e-therapy for mental health: a systematic review. J Med Internet Res 2012;14(4):e110.
[108] Paxling B, Lundgren S, Norman A, et al. Therapist behaviours in Internet-delivered cognitive behaviour therapy: analyses of e-mail correspondence in the treatment of generalized anxiety disorder. Behav Cogn Psychother 2013;41(3):280–9.
[109] Zalaznik D, Strauss AY, Halaj A, et al. Patient alliance with the program predicts treatment outcomes whereas alliance with the therapist predicts adherence in Internet-based therapy for panic disorder. Psychotherapy Res 2021;31(8):1022–35.
[110] Mewton L, Smith J, Rossouw P, et al. Current perspectives on Internet delivered cognitive behavioral therapy for adults with anxiety and related disorders. Psychol Res Behav Manag 2014;37. https://doi.org/10.2147/prbm.s40879:Published online January.
[111] Békés V, Aafjes-van Doorn K. Psychotherapists' attitudes toward online therapy during the COVID-19 pandemic. J Psychotherapy Integration 2020;30(2):238–47.
[112] Shklarski L, Abrams A, Bakst E. Navigating changes in the physical and psychological spaces of psychotherapists during Covid-19: when home becomes the office. Pract Innov 2021;6(1):55–60.
[113] Jonsson H, Kristensen M, Arendt M. Intensive cognitive behavioural therapy for obsessive-compulsive disorder: a systematic review and meta-analysis. J Obsessive-Compulsive Relat Disord 2015;6:83–96.
[114] Knuts IJ, Esquivel G, Overbeek T, et al. Intensive behavioral therapy for agoraphobia. J Affect Disord 2015;174:19–22.
[115] Stech EP, Grierson AB, Chen AZ, et al. Intensive one-week Internet-delivered cognitive behavioral therapy for panic disorder and agoraphobia: a pilot study. Internet Interventions 2020;20:100315.
[116] Oldfield VB, Salkovskis PM, Taylor T. Time-intensive cognitive behaviour therapy for obsessive-compulsive disorder: a case series and matched comparison group. Br J Clin Psychol 2011;50(1):7–18.
[117] Wootton BM, MacGregor A. Accelerated outpatient individual cognitive-behaviour therapy for panic disorder: a case study. Clin Psychol 2016;22(1):92–8.
[118] Jain N, Stech E, Grierson AB, et al. A pilot study of intensive 7-day Internet-based cognitive behavioral therapy for social anxiety disorder. J Anxiety Disord 2021;84:102473.
[119] Andrews G, Basu A, Cuijpers P, et al. Computer therapy for the anxiety and depression disorders is effective, acceptable and practical health care: an updated meta-analysis. J Anxiety Disord 2018;55:70–8.
[120] Etzelmueller A, Vis C, Karyotaki E, et al. Effects of Internet-based cognitive behavioral therapy in routine care for adults in treatment for depression and anxiety: systematic review and meta-analysis. J Med Internet Res 2020;22(8):e18100.
[121] Advocat J, Lindsay J. Internet-based trials and the creation of health consumers. Soc Sci Med 2010;70(3):485–92.
[122] Halmetoja CO, Malmquist A, Carlbring P, et al. Experiences of Internet-delivered cognitive behavior therapy for social anxiety disorder four years later: a qualitative study. Internet Interventions 2014;1(3):158–63.
[123] Pedersen MK, Mohammadi R, Mathiasen K, et al. Internet-based cognitive behavioral therapy for anxiety in an outpatient specialized care setting: a qualitative study of the patients' experience of the therapy. Scand J Psychol 2020;61(6):846–54.
[124] Hedman E, Ljótsson B, Rück C, et al. Effectiveness of Internet-based cognitive behaviour therapy for panic disorder in routine psychiatric care. Acta Psychiatrica Scand 2013;128(6):457–67.
[125] Lenhard F, Sauer S, Andersson E, et al. Prediction of outcome in Internet-delivered cognitive behaviour therapy for paediatric obsessive-compulsive disorder: a machine learning approach. Int J Methods Psychiatr Res 2018;27(1):e1576.
[126] Hadjistavropoulos HD, Thompson MJ, Klein B, et al. Dissemination of therapist-assisted Internet cognitive behaviour therapy: development and open pilot study of a workshop. Cogn Behav Ther 2012;41(3):230–40.
[127] Mohr DC, Siddique J, Ho J, et al. Interest in behavioral and psychological treatments delivered face-to-face, by telephone, and by Internet. Ann Behav Med 2010;40(1):89–98.
[128] Molloy A, Anderson PL. Increasing acceptability and outcome expectancy for Internet-based cognitive behavioral therapy during the COVID-19 pandemic. Telemed e-Health 2021;7.

[129] Andersson G, Titov N, Dear BF, et al. Internet-delivered psychological treatments: from innovation to implementation. World Psychiatry 2019;18(1):20–8.

[130] Molloy A, Ellis DM, Su L, et al. Improving acceptability and uptake behavior for Internet-based cognitive-behavioral therapy. Front digital Health 2021;3.

[131] Knechtel LM, Erickson CA. Who's logging on? Differing attitudes about online therapy. J Technology Hum Serv 2020;39(1):24–42.

[132] Batterham PJ, Calear AL, Sunderland M, et al. A brief intervention to increase uptake and adherence of an Internet-based program for depression and anxiety (enhancing engagement with psychosocial interventions): randomized controlled trial. J Med Internet Res 2021;23(7):e23029.

[133] Titov N, Andrews G, Davies M, et al. Internet treatment for depression: a randomized controlled trial comparing clinician vs. technician assistance. PLoS One 2010;5(6):e10939.

[134] Johansson R, Andersson G. Internet-based psychological treatments for depression. Expert Rev neurotherapeutics 2012;12(7):861–70.

[135] Gulliver A, Calear AL, Sunderland M, et al. Consumer-guided development of an engagement-facilitation intervention for increasing uptake and adherence for self-guided web-based mental health programs: focus groups and online evaluation survey. JMIR formative Res 2020;4(10):e22528.

[136] Topooco N, Riper H, Araya R, et al. Attitudes towards digital treatment for depression: a European stakeholder survey. Internet interventions 2017;8:1–9.

Advances in Psychiatry and Behavioral Health 2 (2022) 71–78

ADVANCES IN PSYCHIATRY AND BEHAVIORAL HEALTH

Advances in Psychotherapy for Older Adults Using Video-to-Home Treatment

Jennifer Freytag, PhD[a,b,*], Hilary N. Touchett, PhD, RN[a,b], Jennifer L. Bryan, PhD[a,b,e], Jan A. Lindsay, PhD[a,b,c], Christine E. Gould, PhD[d,e]

[a]Houston VA HSR&D Center for Innovations in Quality, Effectiveness and Safety, Michael E. DeBakey VA Medical Center, (MEDVAMC 152), 2002 Holcombe Boulevard, Houston, TX 77030, USA; [b]VA South Central Mental Illness Research, Education and Clinical Center, 2200 Fort Roots Drive, Bldg. 58, North Little Rock, AR 72114, USA; [c]Menninger Department of Psychiatry and Behavioral Sciences, Baylor College of Medicine, Lee and Joe Jamail Specialty Care Center, 1977 Butler Boulevard, Houston, TX 77030, USA; [d]Geriatric Research Education and Clinical Center (GRECC), Veterans Affairs Palo Alto Health Care System, 3801 Miranda Avenue, Palo Alto, CA 94304-1207, USA; [e]Department of Psychiatry & Behavioral Sciences, Stanford University School of Medicine, 291 Campus Drive, Li Ka Shing Building, Stanford, CA 94305-5101, USA

KEYWORDS

• Telemedicine • Geriatrics • Telemental health • Video-to-home

KEY POINTS

- Video-to-home (VTH) is an effective means of providing telemental health to older adults.
- Older adults are willing to use telemedicine for mental health and in some cases prefer it.
- Barriers to using VTH with older adults include technology acceptance, access, and physical and cognitive limitations.
- Providers have used new and innovative methods to address barriers.

INTRODUCTION/BACKGROUND

Video-to-home (VTH) telemedicine allows providers to conduct synchronous clinical encounters over secure video connections (eg, VA Video Connect, thera-LINK, doxy.me). VTH for mental health care has grown rapidly over the past decade due in part to advances in telehealth platforms and digital infrastructure, as well as the availability of smartphones [1,2]. However, access to VTH is inconsistent geographically (rural and frontier communities), demographically (age, race, education), and institutionally (under-resourced health care systems) [3]. The rush to convert face-to-face to remote clinical encounters during the COVID-19 pandemic has only heightened disparities in VTH use [4]. Older adults have become a population of particular concern—not only do they risk serious complications of the virus if they are exposed during face-to-face clinical care; but they are also less likely to use telemedicine for remote health care [5].

There is an urgent need to address the wide range of barriers that prevent older adults from using VTH, from age-related physical and cognitive decline to attitudes toward technology. Telehealth provides opportunities to improve care; VTH has improved access to providers, such as specialists, and helped patients obtain timelier diagnoses [6]. It can also cut drive time and provide access for patients who live at a distance from facilities, have physical barriers to attending visits, or behavioral

*Corresponding author. (MEDVAMC 152), 2002 Holcombe Boulevard, Houston, TX 77030. *E-mail address:* Jennifer.freytag@va.gov

https://doi.org/10.1016/j.ypsc.2022.03.004
2667-3827/22/ Published by Elsevier Inc.

issues that make in-person care difficult [7]. Incorporating VTH into routine care is important to providing high-quality health care for older adults, who make up the largest group of health care consumers in the United States. Because of shifts in demographics, the population of older adults grows considerably each year. More than 54 million people over 65 live in the United States; within the next 2 decades, the number of older adults is expected to double [8].

Although the barriers to older adults' use of VTH pose a challenge to health care systems, the landscape of current research is filled with innovative ways to address barriers and, importantly, is beginning to address negative stereotypes about older adults' ability to use VTH technology. In this article, we will discuss some barriers to using VTH with older adults and approaches to addressing those barriers. See Table 1 for a summary of barriers and strategies to address them.

VIDEO-TO-HOME AS A TREATMENT MODALITY FOR OLDER ADULTS

Although face-to-face visits are most common, a growing body of evidence shows that VTH is as effective as face-to-face for treating a variety of conditions in adults of all ages (Box 1) [9–12]. For example, noninferiority studies comparing VTH to in-person clinic visits for posttraumatic stress disorder in Veterans have shown that VTH can successfully function as a substitute for face-to-face care [9,13–16]. When compared with telephone visits, VTH has been shown to be more successful, with positive outcomes in treating conditions such as depression [17] and smoking cessation [18]. VTH is also a feasible treatment of obsessive-compulsive disorder [19], panic disorder [20], social anxiety disorder [21,22], and smoking cessation [18]. Reduced lengths of hospitalization, better medication adherence, symptom reduction, lower attrition, and more effective therapy have also been reported [23,24]. Additionally, when used as a treatment modality, VTH has had positive effects on symptoms [25,26].

Until recently, comparatively less research has focused on the effectiveness of VTH for treating older adults. Among the 3 modalities for clinic visits, face-to-face, telephone, and video conferencing, VTH requires skills that are still novel for some older adults, such as checking Internet connections and troubleshooting audio and video issues. Thus, older patients tend to prefer in-person interactions, which are most familiar [27]. Throughout the pandemic, more older adults received telephone visits than VTH [28]. Because of the ubiquity of telephones and comfort with that technology, much of the telemedicine research involving older adults has focused on telephone-based interventions, many with positive outcomes [29]. However, VTH has been shown to be as effective as telephone interventions in screening for and treating depression in older adults [17,30]. Additionally, when used as a treatment modality, VTH has positively affected the quality of life; social isolation; and symptoms of anxiety, social isolation, and depression [25,26].

Both older patients and providers have generally responded positively to VTH. Older adults are receptive to receiving both medical and psychiatric services via VTH [31,32]. Older adults have positive attitudes toward technology's benefits that are consistent across age groups, and older adults have reported high levels of satisfaction with participating in telemedicine visits [6,31,33]. Provider attitudes toward providing telemental health treatment of older adults are positive or neutral on the whole [34,35]. Providers believe that improved access to care, flexibility, cost-saving, and efficiency enabled by VTH are particularly valuable [36].

DISCUSSION

Addressing Barriers to Widespread Use of Video-to-Home

Acceptance of video-to-home

The successful adoption of VTH relies on the willingness of patients and providers to use it. Many older adults experience anxiety when using new technologies and feel less comfort, self-efficacy, and control when using communication technology specifically [33,37]. However, when new technology is introduced in a way that connects it to familiar experiences, it is more likely to be accepted by older adults [2,38]. The senior technology acceptance model (STAM) is the most widely used framework for understanding older adults' willingness to use new technologies. It includes factors that influence the adoption of new technologies such as VTH and takes into account social-cognitive variables (self-efficacy and computer anxiety), as well as attitudes (perceived usefulness and perceived ease of use), and usage behavior [39]. Additionally, the model captures characteristics unique to older adults, including age-related health conditions, self-reported health conditions, functional abilities, cognitive abilities, attitude toward aging, and life satisfaction [40].

Applications of the STAM model have found that different variables account for older adults' acceptance of technology. Many have found that acceptance of technologies such as telemedicine is explained best by

TABLE 1
Strategies for addressing barriers to VTH use with older adults

Barrier	Strategies
Acceptance of VTH	Provide effective training to both patients and providers • Emphasize *usefulness* and *ease of use* when introducing VTH. • Highlight *benefits* of using VTH regularly. • Teach troubleshooting and emphasize the *usefulness* of learning those strategies for general use of technology. • Train providers in documentation and reimbursement.
Physical and cognitive limitations	Educate patients and providers on a variety of adaptive strategies • Keep up to date on innovations in adaptive equipment. • Adopt adaptive equipment tailored to patient. • Focus on VTH repetition and practice. • Use simple analogies and metaphors. • Provide paper copies of instructions.
Access	Understand factors affecting equitable access • Assess availability of broadband, Internet, and equipment. • Understand that attitudes toward VTH are influenced by experience with technology. • Understand and address cultural barriers to using VTH • Adapt VTH programs for varying levels of health literacy.
Establishing rapport	Use rapport-building strategies during VTH visits • Encourage more patient participation in VTH visits. • Slow speech during visits to help with understanding. • Train providers in interpersonal communication strategies using VTH. • Practice technical troubleshooting strategies in advance.
Privacy	Train providers in methods of maintaining privacy during VTH • Provide training on issues such as HIPAA compliance, maintaining a secure virtual environment, and dealing with multiple participants during VTH visits.
Safety	Train providers in possible safety issues during VTH visits • Create a safety plan for medical emergencies. • Provide training in identifying abuse and neglect using VTH. • Practice methods of separating multiple participants during VTH visits for private interviews.
Reimbursement	Be aware of documentation and reimbursement • Document VTH visits in compliance with reimbursement rules. • Advocate for reimbursement parity for VTH visits.

specific attitudes (perceived usefulness and perceived ease of use) [41–43]. Others have found stronger relationships between social-cognitive variables and acceptance [44]: older adults may not accept communication technologies such as VTH that they do not perceive to be useful or have clear benefits [45–47]. This same concept applies to technical help—if the assistance provided (eg, possible troubleshooting methods) does not appear useful, older adults are less likely to accept it [48,49]. Studies have shown that repeated behavior, or habit, fits into the STAM model, and emphasize that acceptance and adoption are also driven by repeated use, which explains why acceptance typically changes once an individual uses a communication technology multiple times [50,51].

It is also important to consider the role of providers in VTH acceptance; provider resistance to using technology not only affects the use of VTH but also can influence the perceptions of patients [52]. Providers in some instances have been more deterred by technical

BOX 1
Video-to-home as a treatment modality

Key Points

- Has been shown more successful than telephone for treatment.
- Feasible for screening for and treating a range of conditions.
- Outcomes include
  - Reduced hospitalization
  - Better medication adherence
  - Symptom reduction
  - Lower attrition
  - Positive change in the quality of life
  - Reduced social isolation

difficulties than patients, and patients are more satisfied with VTH, despite these difficulties [52,53]. Similar to older adults, provider acceptance of telemedicine is highly dependent on usefulness and ease of use. One difference for physicians is the effect of self-efficacy on the use of telemedicine—providers who were not able to successfully use telemedicine tended to be resistant to using it. The study suggests that training and education are essential to provider adoption of these technologies [52]. Finally, the ability to easily document visits inpatient records and receive reimbursement positively influences acceptance and adoption.

Physical and cognitive limitations

Telemedicine visits can be challenging for older adults because of age-related physical conditions, such as hearing impairment and vision loss, as well as progressive cognitive decline [53–55]. These challenges are complicated by a patient's psychological and behavioral issues, including the severity of symptoms, diagnosis, and lack social skills [56]. Physical conditions that can create challenges to the use of VTH include hearing impairment [5], visual impairment [49], touch sensitivity [57,58], and neurologic symptoms, such as tremors [58]. Adaptive equipment and techniques can assist with many of these challenges [59]. When the immediate challenges to the use of VTH platforms can be overcome, for patients with physical impairments that require transportation assistance, VTH can save time, energy, and money because patients can avoid commuting to facilities [60].

Older adults also face cognitive decline, which also impacts their ability to use VTH for psychotherapy. The limitations caused by cognitive decline affect patients' ability to participate in telemental health through VTH [61]. For example, older adults are less able to learn new information (eg, instructions for using VTH), retain information (eg, to repeat the same kind of troubleshooting in VTH), and pay attention (eg, watching a video on features of VTH) [26,62]. Research suggests several methods for addressing these challenges, many of which include repetition and practice [50,51]. Others include drawing on semantic memory, where many of the earliest memories are stored, by making analogies and using metaphor (eg, explaining the way talking through VTH is similar to a phone conversation) and providing paper copies of simple written instructions [63]. VTH programs can and should be tailored to levels and types of cognitive decline, including advanced dementia [64]. VTH has been used successfully to treat patients with dementia and their caregivers. VTH delivery of psychosocial and cognitive behavioral therapy (including problem-solving training), has shown improvement in caregiver outcomes [65]. For example, caregivers benefitted from group therapy, with a decrease in anxiety and depression [66].

Access

Discussion of equitable access to telemedicine for older adults underscores the heterogeneity of the group. While there are characteristics common to older adults, research involving equitable access to VTH must also take into account the intersection of social characteristics and abilities [67]. For example, older adults from racial or ethnic minority backgrounds or Medicaid beneficiaries were less likely to use VTH [68]. Inequitable access to telemedicine is often associated with the *digital divide,* a term that describes the division between those who are able to access technology and those who are not, based on characteristics such as socioeconomic status, age, and race [69]. The digital divide refers to several factors that inhibit the use of telehealth. First is a lack of the equipment and Internet connectivity to participate in VTH, which affects many older adults [70]. More than 25% of Medicare beneficiaries did not have Internet access at home. People with low socioeconomic status, those 85 years or older, and those in communities of color were also less likely to have digital access [28].

The digital divide also refers to the skills, interests, and emotional and psychological conditions associated with an inability to access technology [71]. The digital divide affects older adults in unique ways; for example, although older adults recognize the power of communication technologies to help ameliorate social isolation, the inability to successfully use this technology makes them feel more isolated [72]. Their attitudes toward technology such as VTH are also colored by their lack of experience with technology, cultural barriers, and lack of health literacy [72]. These complex issues must be addressed for VTH to be successfully implemented.

Using VTH with older adults in rural areas underscores the complexities of the digital divide. Rural-dwelling adults have less access to broadband and less willingness to participate in VTH than their nonrural counterparts [73]. This population tends to be in poorer health, more socially isolated, and more affected by unmet mental health needs [74]. Moreover, there is a shortage of mental health professionals in these areas [6]. Successful efforts to implement VTH in these areas must not only address the lack of digital infrastructure in these communities but also the attitudes, cultural beliefs, and literacy of rural older adults. If these barriers can be surmounted, patients who use VTH have access to a range of mental health services that may be unavailable in their own community [73,75].

Establishing patient–provider rapport

Patients and providers have expressed concern about establishing therapeutic relationships through VTH. Although they find telehealth effective, both providers and patients perceive face-to-face interactions more positively [74]. In most patient–provider relationships, the provider is the dominant communicator, and that dominance makes the therapeutic relationship asymmetric, with the provider having more control in the relationship. In an analysis of psychotherapy sessions, one study found that some asymmetries in online relationships involved characteristics unique to VTH, including interruptions caused by technology failures, and privacy [76,77]. Other factors that influence relationship building during all therapeutic modalities include cultivating mutual trust [78], equitable participation in the visit [79], communication skills [80], and interpersonal competence [81]. Undoubtedly, developing therapeutic relationships can be challenging for both older adults and providers during VTH visits. Recent work has shown that providers have developed a rapport with older adults during VTH using adaptive strategies, such as slowing their speech and communicating with patience during technical difficulties [35]. Additionally, rapport can be developed as both providers and older adults become more comfortable with telemental health [82].

Privacy, ethics, and policy

Privacy concerns often affect older adults' willingness to use VTH. Older adults who are less familiar with technologies such as VTH can have concerns about the privacy of psychotherapy visits. A lack of trust in communication technology can fuel older adults' resistance to using telemedicine platforms [2,65]. Older adults from under-resourced populations tend to have less trust in privacy when using communication technologies; however, trust tends to improve with greater use [23]. Mental health providers also face privacy concerns that involve both HIPAA compliance and patient privacy. Providers can be trained in methods to address privacy concerns specific to VTH.

A related concern is a patient safety during a remote visit. Because providers are unable to physically assist a patient if, for example, the patient has a medical emergency during a visit, a safety plan specifies a procedure for whom to contact and what to document [83]. Additionally, a safety plan should specify procedures for patients who contact their provider while in distress. Providers must also have training in identifying potential safety issues, such as signs of self-harm, as well abuse, and neglect by conducting virtual physical examinations and speaking separately with patients and caregivers.

Finally, concern for the growth of VTH visits for older adults hinges on Medicare reimbursement [6]. Reimbursement schemes that promote the use of telehealth generally help break down barriers to use, such as rurality and lack of infrastructure [3]. Before the pandemic, low reimbursement rates limited the use of telemedicine [84]. Although reimbursement for VTH has become common during the pandemic, issues persist in systematizing coding, billing, and clinic workflows. As support for VTH grows, continued parity in VTH reimbursement rates and clearer guidance on reporting will help ensure its use.

SUMMARY

Mental health providers have played an important role in the adoption of VTH since the beginning of the pandemic; providers have been early adopters of telemedicine and videoconferencing in particular [85]. Two studies note that mental health and psychiatry departments in large medical centers were among the first to shift completely to telehealth once the pandemic began [85,86]. Research into psychotherapeutic VTH must continue to discover ways to reach more patients, implement novel uses of VTH, and improve the quality of remote mental health care.

CLINICS CARE POINTS

- Clinicians should consider video-to-home a viable format for mental health treatment.
- Clinicians must consider factors that influence patients' use of video-to-home telehealth.
- Successful clinical use of video-to-home telehealth requires attention to boundaries to use.

DISCLOSURE

This work is supported by a grant from the VA Office of Rural Health, Veterans Rural Health Resource Center-Salt Lake City and partly the result of the use of facilities and resources of the Houston VA HSR&D Center for Innovations in Quality, Effectiveness and Safety (CIN13-413) and the VA South Central Mental Illness Research, Education and Clinical Center, which played no role in the design and conduct of the work; in the collection, analysis and interpretation of the data; and in the preparation, editing or censuring of the manuscript. The opinions expressed are those of the authors and do not necessarily reflect those of the Department of Veterans Affairs, the US government, or Baylor College of Medicine.

REFERENCES

[1] Weil AR. Telehealth. Health Aff (Millwood) 2018; 37(12):1915.

[2] Jimison H, Gorman P, Woods S, et al. Barriers and drivers of health information technology use for the elderly, chronically ill, and underserved. Evid Rep Technol Assess (Full Rep 2008;175:1–1422.

[3] Lin CC, Dievler A, Robbins C, et al. Telehealth In health centers: Key adoption factors, barriers, and opportunities. Health Aff (Millwood) 2018;37(12):1967–74.

[4] Wosik J, Fudim M, Cameron B, et al. Telehealth transformation: COVID-19 and the rise of virtual care. J Am Med Inform Assoc 2020;27(6):957–62.

[5] van den Berg N, Schumann M, Kraft K, et al. Telemedicine and telecare for older patients–A systematic review. Maturitas 2012;73(2):94–114.

[6] Lum HD, Nearing K, Pimentel CB, et al. Anywhere to anywhere: Use of telehealth to increase health care access for older, rural veterans. Public Policy Aging Rep 2020; 30(1):12–8.

[7] Kruse C, Fohn J, Wilson N, et al. Utilization barriers and medical outcomes commensurate with the use of telehealth among older adults: Systematic review. JMIR Med Inform 2020;8(8):e20359.

[8] World Health Organization. *10 Facts on Ageing and the Life Course.* 2017. Available from URL: www.who.int/features/factfiles/ageing/ageing_facts/en Retrieved 2022.

[9] Knowlton CN, Nelson KG. PTSD telehealth treatments for veterans: Comparing outcomes from in-person, clinic-to-clinic, and home-based telehealth therapies. J Rural Ment Health 2021;45(4):243–55. https://doi.org/10.1037/rmh0000190.

[10] Hersh WR, Helfand M, Wallace J, et al. Clinical outcomes resulting from telemedicine interventions: A systematic review. BMC Med Inform Decis Mak 2001;1:5.

[11] Ekeland AG, Bowes A, Flottorp S. Effectiveness of telemedicine: A systematic review of reviews. Int J Med Inform 2010;79(11):736–71.

[12] Fletcher TL, Hogan JB, Keegan F, et al. Recent advances in delivering mental health treatment via video to home. Curr Psychiatry Rep 2018;20(8):1–9.

[13] Acierno R, Gros DF, Ruggiero KJ, et al. Behavioral activation and therapeutic exposure for posttraumatic stress disorder: A noninferiority trial of treatment delivered in person versus home-based telehealth. Depress Anxiety 2016;33(5):415–23.

[14] Morland LA, Mackintosh MA, Glassman LH, et al. Home-based delivery of variable length prolonged exposure therapy: A comparison of clinical efficacy between service modalities. Depress Anxiety 2020;37(4):346–55.

[15] Egede LE, Acierno R, Knapp RG, et al. Psychotherapy for depression in older veterans via telemedicine: A randomised, open-label, non-inferiority trial. Lancet Psychiatry 2015;2(8):693–701.

[16] Morland LA, Mackintosh MA, Rosen CS, et al. Telemedicine versus in-person delivery of cognitive processing therapy for women with posttraumatic stress disorder: A randomized noninferiority trial. Depress Anxiety 2015;32(11):811–20.

[17] Choi NG, Marti CN, Wilson NL, et al. Effect of Telehealth Treatment by Lay Counselors vs by Clinicians on Depressive Symptoms Among Older Adults Who Are Homebound: A randomized clinical trial. JAMA Netw Open 2020;3(8):e2015648.

[18] Kim SS, Darwish S, Lee SA, et al. A randomized controlled pilot trial of a smoking cessation intervention for US women living with HIV: Telephone-based video call vs voice call. Int J Womens Health 2018;10:545–55.

[19] Goetter EM, Herbert JD, Forman EM, et al. An open trial of videoconference-mediated exposure and ritual prevention for obsessive-compulsive disorder. J Anxiety Disord 2014;28(5):460–2.

[20] Bouchard S, Paquin B, Payeur R, et al. Delivering cognitive-behavior therapy for panic disorder with agoraphobia in videoconference. Telemed J E Health 2004;10(1):13–25.

[21] Nauphal M, Swetlitz C, Smith L, et al. A preliminary examination of the acceptability, feasibility, and effectiveness of a telehealth cognitive-behavioral therapy group for social anxiety disorder. Cogn Behav Pract 2021; 28(4):730–42.

[22] Yuen EK, Herbert JD, Forman EM, et al. Acceptance based behavior therapy for social anxiety disorder through videoconferencing. J Anxiety Disord 2013; 27(4):389–97.

[23] Adams SM, Rice MJ, Jones SL, et al. Telemental health: Standards, reimbursement, and interstate practice. J Am Psychiatr Nurses Assoc 2018;24(4):295–305.
[24] Simon GE, Ludman EJ, Tutty S, et al. Telephone psychotherapy and telephone care management for primary care patients starting antidepressant treatment: A randomized controlled trial. JAMA 2004;292(8):935–42.
[25] Hirani SP, Beynon M, Cartwright M, et al. The effect of telecare on the quality of life and psychological well-being of elderly recipients of social care over a 12-month period: The Whole Systems Demonstrator cluster randomised trial. Age Ageing 2014;43(3):334–41.
[26] Merchant RA, Liu SG, Lim JY, et al. Factors associated with social isolation in community-dwelling older adults: A cross-sectional study. Qual Life Res 2020; 29(9):2375–81.
[27] Bujnowska-Fedak MM, Mastalerz-Migas A. Usage of medical internet and e-health services by the elderly, . Environment Exposure to Pollutants843. New York: Springer; 2014. p. 75–80.
[28] Roberts ET, Mehrotra A. Assessment of disparities in digital access among Medicare beneficiaries and implications for telemedicine. JAMA Intern Med 2020;180(10): 1386–9.
[29] Bashshur RL, Shannon GW, Bashshur N, et al. The empirical evidence for telemedicine interventions in mental disorders. Telemed J E Health 2016;22(2):87–113.
[30] Şahin E, Yavuz Veizi BG, Naharci MI. Telemedicine interventions for older adults: A systematic review. J Telemed Telecare 2021 1357633X211058340.
[31] Grubaugh AL, Cain GD, Elhai JD, et al. Attitudes toward medical and mental health care delivered via telehealth applications among rural and urban primary care patients. J Nerv Ment Dis 2008;196(2):166–70.
[32] Hantke N, Lajoy M, Gould CE, et al. Patient satisfaction with geriatric psychiatry services via video teleconference. Am J Geriatr Psychiatry 2020;28(4):491–4.
[33] Czaja SJ, Sharit J. Age differences in attitudes toward computers. J Gerontol B Psychol Sci Soc Sci 1998; 53B(5):P329–40.
[34] Hoffmann M, Wensing M, Peters-Klimm F, et al. Perspectives of psychotherapists and psychiatrists on mental health care integration within primary care via video consultations: Qualitative preimplementation study. J Med Internet Res 2020;22(6):e17569.
[35] Goldberg EM, Jiménez FN, Chen K, et al. Telehealth was beneficial during COVID-19 for older Americans: A qualitative study with physicians. J Am Geriatr Soc 2021; 69(11):3034–43.
[36] Connolly SL, Miller CJ, Lindsay JA, et al. A systematic review of providers' attitudes toward telemental health via videoconferencing. Clin Psychol (New York) 2020;27(2): e12311.
[37] Mitzner TL, Savla J, Boot WR, et al. Technology adoption by older adults: findings from the PRISM trial. Gerontologist 2019;59(1):34–44.
[38] Mahmood A, Yamamoto T, Lee M, et al. Perceptions and use of gerotechnology: Implications for aging in place. J Hous Elder 2008;22(1–2):104–26.
[39] Chen K, Chan AH. Gerontechnology acceptance by elderly Hong Kong Chinese: A senior technology acceptance model (STAM). Ergonomics 2014;57(5):635–52.
[40] Chen K, Lou VWQ. Measuring senior technology acceptance: Development of a brief, 14-Item scale. Innov Aging 2020;4(3). https://doi.org/10.1093/geroni/igaa016.
[41] Hauk N, Hüffmeier J, Krumm S. Ready to be a silver surfer? A meta-analysis on the relationship between chronological age and technology acceptance. Comput Hum Behav 2018;84:304–19.
[42] De Veer AJ, Peeters JM, Brabers AE, et al. Determinants of the intention to use e-Health by community dwelling older people. BMC Health Serv Res 2015;15(1):1–9.
[43] Wang L, Rau P-LP, Salvendy G. Older adults' acceptance of information technology. Educ Gerontol 2011;37(12): 1081–99.
[44] Niehaves B, Plattfaut R. Internet adoption by the elderly: Employing IS technology acceptance theories for understanding the age-related digital divide. Eur J Inf Syst 2014;23(6):708–26.
[45] Lorenzen-Huber L, Boutain M, Camp LJ, et al. Privacy, technology, and aging: A proposed framework. Ageing Int 2011;36(2):232–52.
[46] Czaja S, Beach S, Charness N, et al. Older adults and the adoption of healthcare technology: Opportunities and challenges. Tech Active Aging 2013;27–46.
[47] Peek ST, Wouters EJ, Van Hoof J, et al. Factors influencing acceptance of technology for aging in place: A systematic review. Int J Med Inform 2014;83(4):235–48.
[48] Thielke S, Harniss M, Thompson H, et al. Maslow's hierarchy of human needs and the adoption of health-related technologies for older adults. Ageing Int 2012;37(4): 470–88.
[49] Fisk AD, Czaja SJ, Rogers WA, et al. Designing for older adults: principles and creative human factors approaches. Florida: CRC press; 2019.
[50] Kadylak T, Cotten SR. United States older adults' willingness to use emerging technologies. Inf Commun Soc 2020;23(5):736–50.
[51] Berkowsky RW, Rikard R, Cotten SR. Signing off: Predicting discontinued ICT usage among older adults in assisted and independent living. In Zhou J, Salvendy G, editors. Human Aspects of IT for the Aged Population. Design for Everyday Life. ITAP 2015. Lecture Notes in Computer Science, vol. 9194. Springer, Cham (Switzerland). https://doi.org/10.1007/978-3-319-20913-5_36.
[52] Rho MJ, Choi Iy, Lee J. Predictive factors of telemedicine service acceptance and behavioral intention of physicians. Int J Med Inform 2014;83(8):559–71.
[53] Stronge AJ, Rogers WA, Fisk AD. Human factors considerations in implementing telemedicine systems to accommodate older adults. J Telemed Telecare 2007; 13(1):1–3.

[54] Heart T, Kalderon E. Older adults: Are they ready to adopt health-related ICT? Int J Med Inform 2013; 82(11):e209–31.

[55] Freese J, Rivas S, Hargittai E. Cognitive ability and Internet use among older adults. Poetics 2006;34(4–5):236–49.

[56] Sugarman DE, Horvitz LE, Greenfield SF, et al. Clinicians' perceptions of rapid scale-up of telehealth services in outpatient mental health treatment. Telemed J E Health 2021;27(12):1399–408.

[57] Armbrüster C, Sutter C, Ziefle M. Notebook input devices put to the age test: The usability of trackpoint and touchpad for middle-aged adults. Ergonomics 2007;50(3): 426–45.

[58] Cheong Y, Shehab RL, Ling C. Effects of age and psychomotor ability on kinematics of mouse-mediated aiming movement. Ergonomics 2013;56(6):1006–20.

[59] Stowers J, Verduzco-Gutierrez M. Parking meters to touch screens: The unforeseen barriers that expansion of telemedicine presents to the disability community. Am J Phys Med Rehabil 2021;100(11):1105–8.

[60] Bashshur RL, Shannon GW, Krupinski EA, et al. National telemedicine initiatives: essential to healthcare reform. Telemed J E Health 2009;15(6):600–10.

[61] Gentry MT, Lapid MI, Rummans TA. Geriatric telepsychiatry: Systematic review and policy considerations. Am J Geriatr Psychiatry 2019;27(2):109–27.

[62] Lesch H, Burcher K, Wharton T, et al. Barriers to healthcare services and supports for signing deaf older adults. Rehabil Psychol 2019;64(2):237.

[63] Mayhorn CB, Stronge AJ, McLaughlin AC, et al. Older adults, computer training, and the systems approach: A formula for success. Educ Gerontol 2004;30(3):185–203.

[64] Harris MT, Rogers WA. Developing a healthcare technology acceptance model (H-TAM) for older adults with yhypertension. Aging Soc 2021;1–21. https://doi.org/10.1017/S0144686X21001069.

[65] Chi N-C, Demiris G. A systematic review of telehealth tools and interventions to support family caregivers. J Telemed Telecare 2015;21(1):37–44.

[66] Austrom MG, Geros KN, Hemmerlein K, et al. Use of a multiparty web based videoconference support group for family caregivers: Innovative practice. Dementia 2015;14(5):682–90.

[67] Johnson D, Clarkson J, Huppert F. Capability measurement for inclusive design. J Eng Des 2010;21(2–3): 275–88.

[68] Schifeling CH, Shanbhag P, Johnson A, et al. Disparities in video and telephone visits among older adults during the COVID-19 pandemic: Cross-sectional analysis. JMIR Aging 2020;3(2):e23176.

[69] van Dijk J, Hacker K. The digital divide as a complex and dynamic phenomenon. Inf Soc 2003;19(4):315–26.

[70] DiMaggio P, Hargittai E, Celeste C, et al. Digital inequality: From unequal access to differentiated use. Social Inequality 2004;355–400.

[71] Francis J, Ball C, Kadylak T, et al. Aging in the digital age: Conceptualizing technology adoption and digital inequalities. Aging and Digital Technology. Singapore: Springer; 2019. p. 35–49.

[72] Ball C, Francis J, Huang K-T, et al. The physical–digital divide: Exploring the social gap between digital natives and physical natives. J Appl Gerontol 2019;38(8):1167–84.

[73] Bujnowska-Fedak M, Grata-Borkowska U. Use of telemedicine-based care for the aging and elderly: Promises and pitfalls. Smart Homecare Technol Telehealth 2015. https://doi.org/10.2147/shtt.S59498.

[74] Williams IC, Mattos MK. We're Still Here: Addressing the Diverse Healthcare Needs of Older Adults in Rural Areas. Pub Policy & Aging 2021;31(4):126–8. https://doi.org/10.1093/ppar/prab017.

[75] Richardson LD, Norris M. Access to health and health care: How race and ethnicity matter. Mt Sinai J Med 2010;77(2):166–77.

[76] Armas A, Meyer SB, Corbett KK, et al. Face-to-face communication between patients and family physicians in Canada: A scoping review. Patient Educ Couns 2018; 101(5):789–803.

[77] Cipolletta S, Frassoni E, Faccio E. Construing a therapeutic relationship online: An analysis of videoconference sessions. Clin Psychol 2018;22(2):220–9.

[78] Cook KS, Kramer RM, Thom DH, et al. Trust and distrust in patient-physician relationships: perceived determinants of high-and low-trust relationships in managed-care settings, . *Trust and distrust in organizations: Dilemmas and approaches*. New York: Russell Sage Foundation; 2004. p. 65–98.

[79] Roter D. The enduring and evolving nature of the patient–physician relationship. Patient Educ Couns 2000;39(1):5–15.

[80] DiMatteo MR. A social-psychological analysis of physician-patient rapport: toward a science of the art of medicine. J Social Issues 1979;35(1):12–33.

[81] Duffy FD, Gordon GH, Whelan G, et al. Assessing competence in communication and interpersonal skills: The Kalamazoo II report. Acad Med 2004;79(6):495–507.

[82] Brooks E, Turvey C, Augusterfer EF. Provider barriers to telemental health: obstacles overcome, obstacles remaining. Telemed J E Health 2013;19(6):433–7.

[83] Luxton DD, Sirotin AP, Mishkind MC. Safety of telemental healthcare delivered to clinically unsupervised settings: A systematic review. Telemed e-Health 2010; 16(6):705–11.

[84] Devore PA, Paulich MJ, Talkington SG, et al. The slow pace of interactive video telemedicine adoption: the perspective of telemedicine program administrators on physician participation. Telemed e-Health 2007;13(6).

[85] Rosen CS, Morland LA, Glassman LH, et al. Virtual mental health care in the Veterans Health Administration's immediate response to coronavirus disease-19. Am Psychol 2021;76(1):26.

[86] Understanding Telemedicine's "New Normal": Variations in Telemedicine Use by Specialty Line and Patient Demographics. Telemed e-Health 2022. https://doi.org/10.1089/tmj.2021.0041.

Advances in Psychiatry and Behavioral Health 2 (2022) 79–93

ADVANCES IN PSYCHIATRY AND BEHAVIORAL HEALTH

Recent Advances in Psychotherapy with Virtual Reality

Closing the Research-to-Practice Gap

Joey Ka-Yee Essoe, PhD[a,*], Ainsley K. Patrick, BS[a], Katlyn Reynolds, BS[a,b], Abigael Schmidt, BS[a,c], Kesley A. Ramsey, PhD[a], Joseph F. McGuire, PhD[a]

[a]Center for OCD, Anxiety, and Related Disorders for Children, Division of Child and Adolescent Psychiatry, Department of Psychiatry & Behavioral Sciences, Johns Hopkins University School of Medicine, 1800 Orleans Street, Baltimore, MD 21287, USA; [b]Department of Mental Health, Bloomberg School of Public Health, Johns Hopkins University, Baltimore, MD, USA; [c]Department of Psychology, Towson University, Towson, MD, USA

KEYWORDS

- Psychotherapy • Cognitive behavior therapy • Behavioral therapy • Anxiety disorders
- Obsessive-compulsive disorder • Posttraumatic stress disorder • Virtual reality • Digital interventions

KEY POINTS

- The democratization of virtual reality (VR) devices with ergonomic controls can make VR therapeutic tools accessible and affordable to clinics and patients with limited resources.
- Research found VR therapeutic tools for psychiatric conditions generally more effective than inactive controls; at least as effective as in vivo tools; with mixed outcomes or no data for long-term efficacy.
- Team science approaches, such as software-sharing, interdisciplinary collaborations, and academic-industry partnerships, are essential to overcome the research to practice gap.
- Possible short-term approaches to bridge this gap include the following: experiments using VR devices practical for frontline clinicians, optimization of VR developed as therapeutics, and a team-science approach toward a unified tool.

INTRODUCTION

Virtual reality (VR) is broadly defined as digitally simulated environments that are 3-dimensional (3D), which can be immersive or nonimmersive, multisensory, or visual-only, and are interactive to various degrees (responsive to user inputs for navigation and/or manipulation of objects and/or characters). However, with the advances in consumer VR devices, the definition of VR is narrowing. The consensus is increasingly converging with the nomenclature of the technology sector and market space, where the term "virtual reality" is trending to exclusively refer to immersive, interactive VRs (eg, by the International Consortium of Extended Reality Safety Initiative [1]), which are generally multisensory (ie, at least with audio and visual simulation). Therefore, in the present discussion of the advances in psychotherapy with VR, this emerging consensus is observed whereby the term VR refers to immersive VRs unless otherwise specified. Furthermore, the name of specific products and companies are refrained from to avoid highlighting certain tools over others. Affordability is discussed in terms of costs in US dollars (low: \$0–\$300; medium: \$301–\$2000; high: >\$2000).

Benefiting from the advances of smartphone technology, low-cost, stand-alone, high-quality consumer VR devices have emerged, making VR dramatically

*Corresponding author, *E-mail address:* essoe@jhmi.edu

https://doi.org/10.1016/j.ypsc.2022.04.001
2667-3827/22/

more available, accessible, and affordable in the past 3 years. Sold for less than half the price of high-end smartphones, stand-alone VR devices are used in consumer entertainment (eg, video games and 3D movies or tours), fitness (eg, exercise-focused games), and relaxation (eg, relaxation training or exercises) with an ever-growing application marketplace (app stores).

For decades, the potential of VR as a tool to advance clinical care for psychiatric disorders has been widely recognized [2]. This body of literature has proliferated around this potential and this vision—especially in the past decade, with the advances of low-cost, high-capacity hardware, as well as easy-to-learn software for VR development. VR-based treatment for psychiatric disorders began in exposure therapy for phobias, which has developed a robust body of literature [2–5] and expanded into exposures for posttraumatic stress disorder (PTSD) [6,7], cue-based exposure for substance dependence [8,9] and eating disorders [10,11], social cognitive training for autism spectrum disorder (ASD) and attention-deficit/hyperactivity disorder (ADHD) [2,12], as well as for interventions for psychotic disorders [13,14], eating- and body-image-related disorders [10], and depression [15]. This body of literature is so expansive that more than 20 reviews and/or meta-analyses were published in the past 2 years, as well as some *reviews* of reviews/meta-analyses [16,17]. Literature reviews and meta-analyses agree that VR-therapeutics are more effective than nonactive controls (eg, waitlist), as effective as in vivo evidence-based treatments in the acute post-treatment phase, with mixed reports or insufficient research in terms of long-term benefit [2–4,6,8–29]. However, barriers remain for VR to fulfill its potential and become a commonplace therapeutic tool for psychiatric disorders.

Although effective treatments exist for psychiatric disorders, such as pharmacotherapy or psychotherapy, VR-based or VR-enhanced treatment has garnered much interest because it has potential beyond what is possible in real-world therapies. These promises broadly fall into 3 categories, that VR can do the following:

1. Enhance treatments that are already feasible in the clinic
2. Make feasible treatments that are not practical in the clinic
3. Make possible treatments that are otherwise impossible in the clinic

Despite these promises, hundreds of feasibility studies, and dozens of modest to large clinical trials, there remains a considerable research-to-practice gap. Namely, VR-based treatment tools are not available, accessible, and/or affordable to frontline clinicians.

Given the abundance of reviews of VR clinical research, this article aims to provide a future-focused examination of the foundational potentials or "promises" that VR brings to the treatment of individuals with psychiatric disorders. It begins with a discussion of each of these promises, the advances in research that have leveraged it, and practical examples of VR treatment tools that realize each promise using currently available technologies. This is followed by a discussion on research approaches that can close the research-to-practice gap—toward making VR treatment tools as available, accessible, and affordable as VR devices, to facilitate frontline clinicians' ability to implement this pivotal technology in everyday clinical practice.

THE PROMISES OF VIRTUAL REALITY

Promise 1. Enhance treatments already feasible in the clinic

Treatment guidelines for many psychiatric disorders recommend psychotherapies, either as a stand-alone treatment or in combination with pharmacotherapy. Many psychotherapeutic techniques are feasible and are widely practiced in frontline clinics worldwide. Building on evidence-based techniques such as exposure therapy, VR has the potential to enhance psychotherapies that are feasible in the real world—by making therapeutic stimuli more accessible, available, and controllable for clinicians (Box 1).

Current state-of-the-art

Specific phobia exposures. Clinical trials examining VR exposures for specific phobias [4,5] have generally found it to be at least as effective as real-world exposures [2,21]. Phobia exposure suites are available to clinicians but have a high cost. Although some use commercial VR devices driven by high-graphic capacity computers, others use proprietary VR hardware. Recent reviews [22,28] and meta-analysis [28] that specifically examined public speaking phobia suggest that VR exposures reduce fear. Specifically, VR public-speaking exposures-only conditions were more effective in symptom reduction than inactive control conditions (eg, waitlist), as effective as in vivo exposures-only conditions, and that cognitive behavioral therapy (CBT) with VR exposures was as effective as CBT with in vivo exposure [22,28]. VR public-speaking tools are commercially available, ranging from exposure-only public speaking practice, marketed

BOX 1
Practical example of using virtual reality in therapy: obsessive-compulsive disorder contamination exposures

Real world: When conducting exposures for OCD contamination fears related to rest rooms, a therapist and patient will have to leave the "the office setting" to a "contaminated bathroom setting" that the clinician may need to first create and then clean up.

VR enhancement: A well-designed VR software can present a virtual restroom at various levels of contamination to support different stages of the exposure hierarchy, which saves clinician and patient time and effort.

Current technological feasibility:

- Hardware: Low-cost, commercially available, stand-alone VR devices can readily support the required functionalities.
- Software: Development platforms/engines can readily support the required functionalities.
- Software availability: No clinical trial–tested therapeutic VR for OCD are available to clinicians.

Clinical evidence to date: Low. Generally, relevant VR stimuli trigger anxiety in patients with OCD and individuals with subclinical OCD symptoms [2]. Only 2 studies have reported that VR exposures reduced symptoms in individuals with contamination fears, with a collective sample size of 24 (21 with subclinical contamination fears [49] and 3 patients with OCD [50]).

Research-to-practice gap: Wide. Despite being technologically and theoretically feasible, the research-to-practice gap for VR-based OCD treatment tools remains wide because of the lack of translational research in adults and youth.

with digital coaching as self-help products, as well as therapeutic tools intended to be used to supplement clinician-led therapy such as CBT.

Social anxiety exposures. Reviews and meta-analyses on social anxiety exposures in general have found that VR exposures are as effective as in vivo exposures in the acute posttreatment phase [20,22,23,28,30] but may be inferior in long-term maintenance [20]. However, many of these randomized controlled trials (RCTs) included clinician-led CBT in both VR and in vivo exposure conditions [2,20], thus should only be considered to be evidence to support VR-therapeutics that are clinician-guided.

Posttraumatic stress disorder exposures. VR exposures for PTSD have been found to be more effective than nonactive controls (eg, waitlist), and as effective as active treatment conditions (eg, imaginal exposure) in acute posttreatment assessment. However, VR exposures for PTSD may serve some populations better than others [2,6]. The effects of combat-related, VR exposure sustain in follow-ups over some control conditions (waitlist, psychoeducation) [7], with mixed results when compared with prolonged imaginal exposure [31–34].

Cue exposures for substance dependence and eating disorders. Cue exposures for substance dependence disorders successfully trigger craving, but it remains unclear whether it is effective in reducing symptoms [8,9]. In cue exposure for bulimia nervosa and binge eating disorder, an RCT (n = 58) found that CBT non-responders who underwent nonimmersive VR food-related cue exposure reported greater reduction in binge episodes and food craving than participants who underwent additional CBT sessions at postacute treatment [35] and 6-month follow-up [36].

Psychotic disorders exposures and skill training. Examining individuals diagnosed with psychotic disorders with paranoid ideation, researchers found that exposure and behavioral exercises in nonimmersive VR social environments were found to reduce safety behavior and paranoid thoughts postacute treatment and at 6-month follow-up in an RCT (n = 116) comparing treatment as usual (TAU) + VR and TAU only [37]. A follow-up health care cost analysis found this specific VR therapeutic tool to be cost-effective [38]. Although there is promising evidence that VR-based exposures and behavioral exercises (ie, social skill training) can reduce social functioning impairments in individuals with psychosis, additional research is required in this growing field before it can be considered an evidence-based treatment [13,14,17].

Autism spectrum disorder skill training. For individuals with ASD, VR treatment tools are thought to increase patient motivation and engagement in skills training (eg, social skills, cognitive, or occupational training). A recent meta-analysis reported that VR-based skill trainings are promising, with moderate to large effect sizes, which vary depending on the skill of interest [12].

Attention-deficit/hyperactivity disorder assessment and cognitive training. "The Virtual Classroom" [39] is a VR classroom software with ecologically valid distractions that has been used in many studies [40] for assessment and cognitive training for ADHD. A recent small trial (n = 51) reported that cognitive training in this VR resulted in similar improvement in task-based assessment as pharmacotherapy, and greater improvement than psychotherapy; however, ADHD symptom improvement was only observed in the pharmacotherapy group [41].

Limitations and challenges

VR can make therapeutic stimuli accessible that are costly (eg, passenger flights [42], dental office [43]) and/or are unsafe (eg, combat scenario [6,7], social scenario during a pandemic). These, along with specific phobia stimuli, are the most researched area in this body of literature. VR can also deliver therapeutic stimuli that are not possible in a clinical setting (eg, sharks [44], lions, hellfire) or are more susceptible to refusal of in vivo exposure (eg, harm-related or religious obsessions). Interestingly, even though VR therapeutic stimuli that are not possible in real-world clinics would best showcase the potential of VR, they remained largely unexamined.

The promise of VR to enhance currently feasible treatments has mostly been tested in the arena of making therapeutic stimuli more accessible to clinicians and increasing clinician control, especially in exposure for phobias, social anxiety, and PTSD, as well as cue exposures. Theoretically, this would also contribute to disseminating treatment to patients.

Unfortunately, most of the software used in the aforementioned research is not yet available nor accessible to clinicians, with the notable exceptions of phobia and public speaking exposures as described above. Although supported by strong clinical evidence and wide availability, phobia exposure software is not yet affordable nor accessible. In addition to the cost of high graphic capacity computers, software costs may be beyond the budgets of most community clinicians. Accessibility can be increased by optimizing the software for stand-alone headsets, which require less physical space to operate and less technological skills for users to maintain. Public speaking exposures and training for adults experiencing social anxiety are generally supported by literature. These are commercially available at various levels of quality, functionality, and affordability (ranging from free to high cost). Functionality and quality range from noninteractive photo/video spheres via cardboard VR, to eye tracking and automated real-time feedback via head-mounted display.

However, even for the most widely available, accessible, and affordable VR-therapeutics, there remains a paucity of clinical evidence in children and adolescents. Although the lack of research in VR-therapeutic tools for youth is a fieldwide issue (except for ADHD and ASD), age-appropriateness is of particular importance in certain populations. For example, most public speaking and social anxiety VR-therapeutics have been developed for adults (eg, speaking in front of a large auditorium or board room to other adults). Meanwhile, youth might require adaptations in which presentations are conducted to same-aged peers in age-appropriate situations (eg, classrooms). Most VR public speaking studies were conducted in adults; none were in children under age 12, and only 3 studies were conducted with adolescents using mostly nonimmersive VRs (n = 20 [45], n = 47 [30], and a student study, n = 20 [46]). In youth (ages 12–18), VR public speaking exposures induced distress during presentation to an immersive video of an adult audience [30], in photosphere of a youth audience [46], and in a VR high-school classroom with an audience of adult-looking "bots" (3D characters operated by the VR software) wearing school uniforms [45]. Unfortunately, the use of child "bots" (3D child characters) in these exposures remains unexamined. The best effort to date is the student study already referenced, in which the experimenters recruited 20 youth to not only serve as participants but also serve as audience members for the 360° photospheres that are later used as exposure stimuli [46].

In addition, VR's potential to reduce treatment or exposure refusal is often discussed in the literature. The artificial nature of VR environments provides the clinician with total control over the therapeutic stimuli: the VR spider or dog may be rowdy, and the shopkeeper-bot may be rude—but only as far as they are programmed to be. Therefore, VR has the potential to overcome patients' reluctance in the early stages of therapy to build trust and therapeutic alliance between the patient and clinician. However, only one study directly compared the refusal rate of VR therapy to real-world therapy, reporting that the rates were similar [47]. The comparative refusal rates between VR and real-world therapy may best be examined via large-scale surveys of providers and patients, rather than clinical trials.

Areas of growth and considerations

Therapies such as exposures require specific stimuli. Most of these stimuli are available to the clinician but could be difficult to access because of limited resources, such as space, funding, personnel, or time. VR versions of these stimuli are reuseable once developed, and easier to maintain—but only if the software is well programmed and technically well supported. For example, although exposure therapy using real, live spiders is effective and feasible, virtual spiders are not perishable, nor do they require dedicated habitats or regular feeding. However, it is only beneficial and practical if the software is reliable and low maintenance, and if the clinician is well-trained to use it and can receive technical support when needed.

Another aspect of VR's promise to enhance feasible treatments, which remains largely unexamined, is its potential to increase treatment access to patients by enhancing dissemination, bridging the inequality in access to psychotherapy. In telehealth, for example, after psychoeducation and developing an exposure hierarchy via video conference, a multiuser VR can allow a clinician to guide a patient through exposures in real time. This is technologically feasible—a stand-alone headset can be preprogrammed and mailed to patients, along with mobile hotspots for those with limited Internet access. Although some studies have used preprogrammed virtual agents (bots, or so-called artificial intelligence characters) to serve as therapists [21,48] or exposure stimuli for social anxiety [20,23,49], multiuser VR for clinician-guided exposures remains largely unexamined. A notable exception is detailed in the next section, where patients with refractory auditory verbal hallucinations interacted with clinician-driven avatars that represent the voices they heard [50–53]. Despite technological feasibility, additional research is required to examine the effectiveness of other forms of psychotherapy using real-time, clinician-driven avatars in the context of multiuser VRs.

The advance of affordable VR technology allows high-quality VR therapeutic stimuli to be widely disseminated. The research-to-practice gap can be narrowed through creative research using low-cost, stand-alone, VR devices with well-built and well-supported therapeutic software that are not-for-profit or are subsidized such that its cost is based on the profit margin of each clinic. This can bridge inequality in mental health care access by improving care for patients served by community clinics with limited resources, reaching patients living in remote areas, or engaging patients with limited mobility or social impairments that could pose a barrier to psychotherapy.

Promise 2. Make feasible treatments that are not practical in the clinic

Most evidence-based, nonpharmacologic interventions for psychiatric disorders involve learning and memory. Associative learning processes, such as inhibitory learning, and/or nonassociative learning, such as habituation, have been proposed as mechanisms for CBT. In supportive psychotherapy, patients learn relaxation, communication, problem-solving skills, and strategies, through clinician guidance and social rewards.

As these interventions require patients to learn new skills and associations to cope with psychiatric disorders or to reduce symptoms, evidence-based learning/memory enhancement techniques can be incorporated to improve treatment outcomes. Although these techniques can be difficult or impractical in real-world clinical settings, VR can provide a feasible platform to implement and integrate learning enhancement techniques into evidence-based interventions—without modifying the interventions themselves, merely how they are implemented (Box 2).

Timely reinforcement ("gameful learning") in therapy

As a digital medium, VR can be programmed to provide time-locked feedback based on user input for reinforcement of therapeutic skills, which can, in turn, be optimized by evidence-based learning enhancement strategies. For example, a rewarding event can occur (eg, pleasant music, earning points) after the patient's gaze fixates on a therapeutic stimulus for a predetermined duration, or at the precise moment when a virtual hand comes into contact with feared stimuli. This can even incorporate other forms of user input for multimodal therapeutic learning. Examples of these inputs include physiologic signals, such as heart rate, skin conductance, and electroencephalography, as specialized measurement devices also become increasingly low-cost and portable.

Therapy in diverse contexts and with diverse stimuli. Based on learning and memory theories, therapeutic learning becomes more robust for retrieval when occurring in multiple contexts, and more generalizable through the use of diverse exposure stimuli (eg, various shapes, sizes, and ages of animals and humans). Although this is achievable in the real world, a diverse collection of these stimuli must be obtained and maintained by the clinician, which may strain the clinic's resources. VR can make accessible and affordable multiple

BOX 2
Practical example of using virtual reality in therapy: therapy in multiple contexts

Real world: Clinicians meet with patients within the clinic, usually within the same room across sessions. To implement therapy in multiple contexts would mean clinicians and patients move from location to location (eg, clinician's office, school/workplace, patient's home). Not only is this time consuming, but also some locations are not conducive for intense, private therapeutic conversations (eg, waiting room, crowded street, school cafeteria).

VR enhancement: VR provides diverse contexts that can be "traveled" to within moments, and public settings (eg, VR schools, amusement park, or supermarket populated with bots) within sandboxed VRs will allow for the privacy required for patient-clinician conversations. These VR paradigms can be single-user VR whereby only the patients are immersed, while clinicians could communicate directly or via a connected microphone, or it can be multiuser VR whereby clinicians and patient interact via avatars in the VR, which can also be used in a remote therapy setting.

Technological feasibility in 2022:

- Hardware: Low-cost, commercially available, stand-alone VR devices can readily support the required functionalities.
- Software: Development platforms/engines can readily support the required functionalities.
- Software availability: If only diverse and distinctive contexts are required, most commercial VR devices are sold with multiple VR environments out of the box, and many more are available in the application store, which vary in the level of interactivity. For treatment that requires specific functionality (eg, interactive bots, clinician driven-avatars, phobic stimuli), development platforms/engines can readily use a given set of treatment-related functionality in different VR environments.

Clinical evidence: See section entitled, "Phobia Exposure in Multiple Contexts" [56].

Research-to-practice gap: Theoretically narrow, see section entitled, "Evidence-Based Therapy, but in Multiple Contexts."

types of the feared stimuli (eg, spiders, dogs) programmed to present a diverse array of behavior.

Current state-of-the-art

Phobia exposure using diverse stimuli. As described in an earlier section, there is strong clinical evidence for phobia exposures in VR. Several available VR phobia exposure software have the functionality to provide multiple types of fear stimuli (eg, various breeds of dogs, bridges of varying heights); some include functionality for diverse animal behaviors (eg, stationary, moving, jumping).

Phobia exposure in multiple contexts. In individuals with spider phobia, spider exposure that occurred in multiple VR contexts was associated with lower fear renewal (ie, lower subjective ratings of distress when encountering a spider in a novel VR context, and less behavioral avoidance when encountering a real spider outside of the VR contexts), as compared with exposure in a single VR context [54]. Other research that used multiple VR contexts generally examined treatment or disorders in which context already plays a key role (eg, cue exposures [35,36], social avoidance exposures [37,55], acrophobia [5,15], fear of flying [42], and combat-related PTSD [6,7]). In these studies, multiple VR contexts are part of the treatment and were not examined as a factor.

Pharmacologic enhancement during virtual reality exposures. Pharmacotherapies suspected to enhance therapeutic learning (eg, D-cycloserine, dexamethasone) have been tested in combination with VR exposures with mixed results [2,56].

Inducing a relaxed state. VR has generally been found to be effective for leading to relaxation (distinct from formalized relaxation training) in the general population [29], for acute pain management [57], and for distraction or anxiety reduction during medical procedures [15,19,58], especially in children [25,27,59,60]. Most studies used noninteractive, relaxing sceneries (eg, beach, underwater scene, forests), and many have measured physiology (eg, heart rate/variability, skin conductance, electroencephalogram) as a measure of relaxation outcomes. However, most reviewers noted that this field of research varies widely in quality.

Biofeedback training. There is a growing body of research for VR biofeedback training (heart rate/variability, respiration, skin conductance). Studies have generally found VR biofeedback training to be as effective as traditional or nonimmersive biofeedback but may be more engaging [24,26]. Although most studies have been conducted in healthy adults or nonpsychiatric medical conditions, some have used VR and simultaneous physiology for skill-based relaxation training in adults with generalized anxiety disorder (GAD) [61,62], youth with ADHD or ASD [18], those with subclinical anxiety [63], and those with anxiety and externalizing problems [64].

Limitations and challenges

The integration of behavioral learning enhancement techniques in VR-therapeutics has remained largely unexamined, despite the strength of VR as a means to enhance therapeutic learning via gamefully designed therapeutic tools, beyond simply making treatment more engaging. Although promising early evidence suggests that VR exposure in multiple contexts and VR-biofeedback training is effective in healthy adults, more research is needed in psychiatric populations, especially for youth with psychiatric disorders.

Available VR treatment tools (eg, phobia suites) may contain diverse exposure stimuli, but the aforementioned barriers for accessibility and affordability remain. Some software also incorporates multiple contexts, but mostly for disorders whereby the external environments are entangled with the pathologic condition (eg, acrophobia, fear of flying). These use various subcontexts (eg, levels of height, areas in the airport) in the exposure hierarchy. Available VR therapeutic software for other phobias (eg, animal phobia) and other disorders (eg, obsessive-compulsive disorder [OCD], GAD, depression), whereby contexts are more incidental, either do not have multiple contexts or the diverse contexts are underdeveloped.

Although there is growing evidence for VR biofeedback relaxation training for psychiatric disorders, more research is needed—particularly in youth—to better integrate it into clinical care. However, *that* it is feasible is supported by the multitude of apps using consumer VR or augmented reality (AR) devices for relaxation training. Most of these apps are VR/AR only and low cost; some can be informed by physiology data from commercially available fitness devices (eg, fitness bands, rings, smart watches) or proprietary devices that are low to medium cost. These consumer relaxation training apps vary wildly in terms of empirical support and have yet to be systematically reviewed [65].

Areas of growth and considerations

Gameful reinforcement of therapeutic skill training. Behavior modification through reinforcement learning, as well as their associated enhancement strategies, often requires the minute manipulation of timely feedback, making it difficult to implement with precision in the real world. Although not strictly a psychiatric treatment, one small study examined approach-avoidance training (a type of cognitive bias modification paradigm) using VR to modify unhealthy food-choice bias in healthy adults. They found that as compared with the same training delivered via computer or smartphone, the VR group was more engaged and committed less errors during training [66].

Evidence-based therapy, but in multiple contexts. A low-barrier area to incorporate learning enhancement into therapy is to conduct therapy in multiple contexts as exemplified by the spider phobia exposure study described above [54]. Decades of research have found that human memory is context dependent [67–69]. That is, during learning, internal or environmental cues that seem irrelevant (ie, contexts) become bound to the information or association being learned. Therefore, if these cues are present during later recall, they can aid memory retrieval. Conversely, their absence can impair recall, a phenomenon referred to as *change-induced forgetting*. Meanwhile, the inverse of change-induced forgetting is *transfer*, the ability to recall information in one situation after having learned it in another.

These concepts are highly relevant to the treatment of psychiatric disorders. Most nonpharmacologic interventions occur in contexts (eg, clinician's office) that are different from where the learned information is to be retrieved (eg, school, home, work), reducing the probability of successful recall. It is possible for the clinician to conduct house-calls, such as meeting the patient at school for school phobia exposure sessions, or to return to a street corner where a traumatic event had occurred. However, this is costly for patients and clinicians alike.

Immersive VR can be used to increase transfer by allowing the therapy (ie, learning) to occur in multiple, diverse, and ecologically valid contexts. This enables the memory that is formed to be associated with a multitude of cues, increasing the probability of the retrieval cues being present during recall, leading to the formation of memory that is robust to context change [54,70,71].

There are exciting advances in realizing VR's potential to make feasible therapeutic techniques that are not practical in the real world. Although there is a paucity of research specifically examining the use of multiple VR contexts in psychotherapy [54], evidence-based therapy—especially those that rely mainly on therapeutic conversations—can be conducted in various

VR contexts with little or no change to treatment protocols, which is supported by established evidence. This may be an attainable area of rapid research development, as commercial VR becomes increasingly accepted into the consumer space, new-generation VR devices become less likely to induce simulator sickness [72], and distinctive contexts become readily accessible. If VR-therapeutics that incorporate evidence-based learning enhancement techniques can become available, accessible, and affordable to frontline clinicians, it can improve the efficacy, and thus cost-effectiveness, of psychotherapy.

Promise 3. Making possible treatments that are not possible in the clinic

VR has such wide-ranging potentials as a clinical tool because it can accomplish with fictional worlds what the real world simply cannot deliver. Everything in a VR world—time, space, characters, even physics—can be adjusted to suit the clinical needs of the condition or treatment at hand. Although this specific promise remains largely unexplored, it is well showcased by very creative work using VR to provide treatment that is not possible in the real world (Box 3).

Beyond therapeutic stimuli or treatment, VR offers opportunities for training providers, family, and caretakers as well. The subjective experiences of other human beings are generally only accessible to us via communication. However, perspective-taking VR [73] may serve as a clinician/family educational tool by allowing nonaffected individuals to experience the subjective reality of those with psychiatric conditions (eg, psychosis [74], schizophrenia [75], Asperger syndrome [76]), and this has been found to improve knowledge about the disorder and foster empathy toward those thus affected [74–76].

Current state-of-the-art

Body image disturbance. A VR training software was developed to confront body image disturbance in patients with eating disorders [77–79]. In one of these training stages, patients created avatars that were the sizes of their perceived weight and then adjusted the avatars until they conformed to the true sizes of the patients. When used in combination with CBT, it was found to be more effective in body image satisfaction than CBT alone [79,80], and effects were maintained when followed up in 6 [81] or 12 months [80]. When used in an inpatient setting for individuals with binge eating and obesity, the software + CBT was also more effective in maintaining weight loss than CBT alone or inpatient program alone in a 1-year follow-up [82].

Auditory verbal hallucination in psychosis. Although evidence for avatar therapy (ie, therapeutic interactions with an avatar operated by a person, or a bot operated by the VR software, serving as a coach, therapist, the patient, and similar) remains mixed [21,48], a specific form of avatar therapy that personifies the pathologic condition bears much promise. Three research groups have developed VR software in which patients with refractory auditory verbal hallucinations customize the faces and the voices of avatars to resemble the source of their auditory verbal hallucination [50,51,83]. Then the clinicians, presenting in VR as the customized avatars, engage in a conversation-based therapy with the patients. The VR-based treatments were more effective than TAU [50,84]; traditional CBT [53] effects were maintained in the 1-year follow-up [85], and another group reported that their software was rated as useable by providers [51].

Limitations and challenges

Although there is creative and on-going work [53] in using VR for treatments that are not possible in the real-world clinic, much remains unexplored in this area. To the best of the authors' knowledge, the body image disturbance training software is not yet publicly available to clinicians, but it seems newer software with similar purposes are being tested in healthy or subclinical samples and may become available in the near future [86]. On the other hand, the auditory verbal hallucination software is currently being tested in a blinded RCT [53] and may become available.

Areas of growth and considerations

It is understandable that VR-therapeutics begin with replicating real-world therapy, and as the field and VR technology mature, ventures into developing novel therapeutics. Some therapeutic stimuli are simply not accessible or available, separated by time, space, scale (eg, phobia of extraterrestrial life forms, fear of the planet losing its gravity and being flung into space), or perhaps, spiritual dimensions (eg, religions obsession about, or phobia of, angles, daemons, and hell). VR enables clinicians to access these "impossible" therapeutic stimuli that offer more control than imaginal therapy. Although more studies are needed, VR-therapeutic research in this area has been impressive and creative.

Not only is the research into avatar therapy for auditory verbal hallucination an exciting advance of VR-therapeutics but it also presents a potential roadmap for taking a VR-therapeutic software from the laboratory

BOX 3
Practical example of using virtual reality in therapy: germ exposures

Real world: A clinician treating a child with mysophobia first shows the patient images of microbes. As they move up the exposure hierarchy, the clinician asks the child to touch a door handle, and to imagine germs climbing up the hand, then up his arm. The child insists that he is imagining it as instructed and reports high subjective units of distress. The clinician is experienced with this patient and recognizes that the signs of distress he demonstrates during other exposures were absent. The clinician deduces that the child may not be able or willing to perform the imaginal exposure, and that an alternative exercise must be devised.

VR enhancement: VR can provide visual representation of the germs (eg, particles, clouds, sheets) that cling to the patient triggered when patient's virtual hand interacts with specific objects in the VR environment (eg, door handles, toilets, desks, mobile phones). The VR germs can come in different colors representing different types of microbes and can be programmed to express, digitally, the true form of the microbe in question when the patient's gaze lingers on it. These visual representations can disburse at the end of the exposure, or they can be paired with rewarding stimuli to reinforce the interaction with objects (eg, door handle) that triggered the germs. Although beyond the scope of this discussion, augmented reality may serve these types of exposure even better than VR.

Technological feasibility:

- Hardware: No special requirement. Commercial, stand-alone VR headsets can readily support required functionalities.
- Software: No special requirement. Development platforms/engines can readily support the required functionalities.
- Software availability: None, to the best of the authors' knowledge.

Clinical evidence to date: To the best of the authors' knowledge, no studies have examined this.

Research-to-practice gap: Wide, owing to the lack of clinical research.

toward day-to-day clinical usage. The research group led by Dr Dumais from the Université de Montréal first tested their therapeutic tool in a small pilot (n = 19) and found that it is more effective than TAU [50]. Then, a 1-year randomized trial was conducted, and it was found that the VR-therapeutic tool, as compared with traditional CBT, resulted in larger effect size in symptom reduction, greater improvement in quality of life, affective symptoms, and persecutory beliefs, and effects were maintained in the 1-year follow-up [85]. The group is now conducting a larger, blinded RCT [53]. To complete the roadmap, it may be beneficial to collect usability data during the trial—especially clinicians' and patients' feedback about using the software in treatment, and support staff's feedback in preparing the therapeutic stimuli with patients (ie, the process of creating the avatars for the persecutory voices)—followed by examining usability from an independent group of providers and support staff (eg, psychotherapists, nursing staff, and administrative staff) in a similar manner as Brander and colleagues [51]. Another promising aspect about this work is that in the clinical trial underway at Université de Montréal, the software requires head-mounted, smartphone-driven VR (as the treatment is conversation-based, navigation and high-fidelity movement tracking are not required), making the therapeutic tool more accessible than room-scale VR devices and more affordable than computer-driven VR devices.

DISCUSSION: BRIDGING THE RESEARCH-TO-PRACTICE GAP

As the practical examples illustrate, VR technological advances have outpaced advances in clinical research in that available, accessible, and affordable software are not generally well researched, and evidence-based software are generally not yet available, accessible, and affordable.

There are some issues or criticisms raised in past reviews about this field of research, some more fair than others. Some of these have seen progress and efforts to address them, including the need for larger sample sizes, large RCTs, the presence of effect size inflation owing to small sample sizes, and the use of inactive rather than active control conditions. Others are improving with efforts, such as open protocol and open data initiatives. Some criticisms remain valid and largely unaddressed. These include the heterogeneity of software and hardware used in research; the lack of integration with established research tools, such as psychophysiology, neurophysiology, and eye tracking; and some populations remain underexamined, namely, youth and OCD spectrum disorders. These criticisms, especially the first, factor into the gap between clinical research on VR therapeutic tools and their being implemented in day-to-day clinical care.

Although the democratization of VR makes this technology itself feasible in day-to-day clinical care, a barrier remains—a lack of well-researched, available, accessible/useable, affordable/low-cost VR therapeutic tools for frontline practicians. In this section, the authors propose some approaches to increase the quality of therapeutic tools while further facilitating the translation of laboratory findings into clinical practice, which consider the scalability of a VR therapeutic during the early stage.

Using portable consumer devices in research

The most direct way to shorten the distance between the laboratory and the clinic is to forego using VR systems that are expensive to operate, such as those requiring large empty spaces (eg, CAVES), technical expertise (eg, accelerometers), or even high-graphic capacity computer systems. Instead, new-generation, consumer VR devices with ergonomic interaction should be used, ideally stand-alone, head-mounted devices. A recent meta-analysis of cognitive neuroscience studies found that these devices resulted in no adverse effects (eg, motion sickness) and attrition that were traditionally associated with VR studies [72]. Therefore, not only are these devices now affordable and more accessible for day-to-day clinical use, but also they are safer for participants and patients than other devices tested in research.

When stand-alone VR devices with ergonomic interactions—interactions that resemble real-world movements, such as virtual hands rather than joysticks or keypress controls—became available in 2019, it was affordable enough to open a wide window of possibilities for use in clinical care, especially for the clinic with limited space, funding, and human resources. As of the time of this writing, the following technology are widely available in the consumer space.

Virtual reality devices

Stand-alone VR headsets with ergonomic interactions are sold for low cost. Many, including the most affordable product, have Bluetooth and wi-fi capacity, as well as tracking, visual, and positional audio that are more than adequate. Moreover, these stand-alone devices tend to cost less and require less space to operate than computer-driven models. Although it is beyond the scope of the current discussion, some of the stand-alone headsets, including the lowest-cost product, can also implement AR software, which could be particularly useful for contamination fears and cue exposures.

Internet connectivity. Although single-player therapeutic software can operate independently of the Internet, multiuser VR may require an Internet connection. To serve patients living in remote regions with poor Internet connection, a stand-alone headset can be preconfigured to access the Internet via a mobile hotspot, and both can be sent together to the patients. At least one mobile plan exists with the speed and data required for $50 USD per month at the time of writing.

Psychophysiology devices. For VR biofeedback, research quality Bluetooth and audio-port devices measuring heart rate and skin conductance are available for low cost, and neurofeedback devices are also available but less affordable. Commercially available fitness devices can measure some physiologic responses, but the software development kits may be proprietary.

Using technology in research that is also practical for frontline clinicians, especially for modestly funded community clinics, will shorten the distance between the laboratory and clinics, as well as further decreasing inequality in treatment access.

Design and optimization of virtual reality therapeutic tools

One potential barrier for researchers to use stand-alone VR systems is that it requires front-end optimization and design. These front-end investments help to narrow the research-to-practice gap in the long term and also make multisite, large-scale clinical trial more manageable. For example, shipping 5 commercial devices preloaded with the therapeutic software is much less burdensome than shipping 5 high-graphic capacity PCs, connection cables, and VR system that requires 5 large rooms to operate.

Optimization. Without the luxury of a high-capacity PC system, optimization can conserve resources and prevent system lag—which can lead to motion sickness. For example, certain assets (eg, a 3D model of a dog) can be designed to render at different levels of details so that less polygons are rendered when the camera is far away, or custom scripts can save data to disk every 10 seconds instead of every frame.

Design. One advantage of the PC-driven system is that the clinician can monitor the patients and manage the VR outside of the VR—sitting at a computer desk, monitoring patients' view on one computer screen, while adjusting the behavior of the therapeutic stimuli (eg, a virtual spider) on another computer screen. However, the clinician can do the same in-game with either a well-designed multiuser VR or a VR that communicates with a mobile app.

Team science approach to research and development of virtual reality-therapeutics

As advances in VR technology outpace research evidence for VR-therapeutics, it is beneficial to reconsider certain structural barriers within academic and institutional practices. Although policies and laws are beyond the scope of this discussion, some barriers are more surmountable than others, in some institutions more than others. Here, the authors focus on the barriers that can be addressed by drawing upon precedents of published studies and those used in multisite clinical trials.

Interdisciplinary collaboration. Although optimization and game design can be self-taught, interdisciplinary collaboration, or industry-academic partnership, would greatly benefit from the advancement of VR-therapeutics for psychiatric disorders. Colleagues in game development, digital animation, and visual arts and design have much to contribute. Moreover, as one does not receive psychotherapy from a game designer, why should one expect a VR therapeutic tool to be everything that it can be without the input of experts in VR development?

An example of this interdisciplinary collaboration was described in the aforementioned game-based VR approach-avoidance training study [66]. Following the codesign principle [87], a team of designers, psychologists, human-computer interface researchers, and VR game developers collaboratively designed the game, consulting with potential future treatment recipients. The game is then developed in an iterative process with a focus group for usability and user understanding.

Intradisciplinary collaboration. Another barrier to bringing VR-therapeutics into the clinic is that much of the research, even for highly similar tools, were conducted using entirely custom software, often developed by the researchers themselves—including the authors' own ongoing work. This results in the lack of a consensus-based, widely available VR therapeutic tool even for well-researched disorders in this field.

There are many reasons making software sharing between universities difficult. It is hopeful that this barrier is becoming increasingly surmountable, including the growing advocacy for open protocols and open data by funding agencies and journals, and the funding opportunities for industry-academic collaboration. Thus, a concerted effort should begin to organize an interinstitutional, interdisciplinary, international consortium toward the development of a unified, comprehensive VR therapeutic tool for multisite testing, with the understanding that the end-product will remain open source and affordable to the clinician serving patients across the economic spectrum. This will enable clinical scientists to pool resources and talents across industry and borders, build upon one another's work, iteratively improve the therapeutic tool, and afford high-quality clinician training.

SUMMARY

VR bears much promise to improve clinical care for patients with psychiatric conditions: (1) enhancing treatments that are currently feasible in the clinic, (2) making feasible treatments that are impractical in the clinic, and (3) making possible what is impossible in the clinic. The field has excelled in the first promise; much progress has been made on the second promise, and the last, although showcased by creative and important work, remains largely unexplored.

Research to date has found that VR-based treatment tools are generally more effective in symptom reduction than inactive control conditions, at least as effective as in vivo therapy or standard of care, with mixed results or a lack of data in terms of long-term efficacy. Nevertheless, VR has the added potential of being more accessible, especially to clinicians and patients with limited resources.

The field of research using VR as a therapeutic tool for psychiatric conditions is still maturing, and there has been progress in addressing the decades-long issues plaguing this work. However, there remains a research-to-practice gap. With the democratization of VR and as it becomes increasingly acceptable into the consumer space, the burden to close the research-to-practice gap leans firmly on the clinical research aspect, rather than on the technological aspects. Some small changes to and investment in clinical research approach can help bridge the gap, but concerted effort across institutions and industry may be required to develop a comprehensive, consensus-based VR therapeutic tool for multisite testing. Despite the mammoth effort this would require, the resulting gold-standard, low-cost, comprehensive VR therapeutic can benefit patients across the globe and the economic spectrum.

CLINICS CARE POINTS

- Virtual reality has the potential to enhance clinical care but requires careful consideration of how to best incorporate it into treatment. Some disorders and software are better supported by research evidence than others, and some devices are more suitable for certain treatment than others.
- When using virtual reality in treatment, consider the level of interactivity necessary for treatment. Some patients may require minimal activity and/or motion tracking. Meanwhile, other patients might require greater interactivity and/or immersion to achieve therapeutic goals.
- When navigable or interactive virtual reality is required, whenever possible, select devices and software with new-generation tracking and ergonomic interactions. These are safer and less likely to lead to adverse reactions (eg, motion sickness) compared with older devices and those with nonergonomic controls (eg, remote control or joystick).

DISCLOSURE

This work was supported in part by Tourette Association of America (to Drs. J. K.-Y. Essoe, K. A. Ramsey), Misophonia Research Fund (Dr. J. F. McGuire), and the Hilda and Preston Davis Foundation (Dr. J. F. McGuire). Declarations of interest: None.

REFERENCES

[1] Extended reality safety initiative (XRSI). The XRSI definitions of extended reality (XR). 2022. Available at. https://xrsi.org/publication/the-xrsi-definitions-of-extended-reality-xr. Accessed February 10, 2022.

[2] Emmelkamp PMG, Meyerbröker K. Virtual reality therapy in mental health. Annu Rev Clin Psychol 2021;17: 495–519.

[3] Chou PH, Tseng PT, Wu YC, et al. Efficacy and acceptability of different interventions for acrophobia: a network meta-analysis of randomised controlled trials. J Affective Disord 2021;282:786–94.

[4] Thng CEW, Lim-Ashworth NSJ, Poh BZQ, et al. Recent developments in the intervention of specific phobia among adults: a rapid review. F1000Res 2020;9:F1000.

[5] Wechsler TF, Kümpers F, Mühlberger A. Inferiority or even superiority of virtual reality exposure therapy in phobias? -A systematic review and quantitative meta-analysis on randomized controlled trials specifically comparing the efficacy of virtual reality exposure to gold standard in vivo exposure in agoraphobia, specific phobia, and social phobia. Front Psychol 2019;10:1758.

[6] Eshuis LV, van Gelderen MJ, van Zuiden M, et al. Efficacy of immersive PTSD treatments: A systematic review of virtual and augmented reality exposure therapy and a meta-analysis of virtual reality exposure therapy. J Psychiatr Res 2021;143:516–27.

[7] Deng W, Hu D, Xu S, et al. The efficacy of virtual reality exposure therapy for PTSD symptoms: a systematic review and meta-analysis. J Affect Disord 2019;257: 698–709.

[8] Ghiţă A, Gutiérrez-Maldonado J. Applications of virtual reality in individuals with alcohol misuse: a systematic review. Addict Behav 2018;81:1–11.

[9] Segawa T, Baudry T, Bourla A, et al. Virtual reality (VR) in assessment and treatment of addictive disorders: a systematic review. Front Neurosci 2020;13. Available at. https://www.frontiersin.org/article/10.3389/fnins.2019.01409. Accessed February 23, 2022.

[10] Clus D, Larsen ME, Lemey C, et al. The use of virtual reality in patients with eating disorders: systematic review. J Med Internet Res 2018;20(4):e157.

[11] Low TL, Ho R, Ho C, et al. The efficacy of virtual reality in the treatment of binge-purging eating disorders: a meta-analysis. Eur Eat Disord Rev 2021;29(1):52–9.

[12] Karami B, Koushki R, Arabgol F, et al. Effectiveness of virtual/augmented reality-based therapeutic interventions on individuals with autism spectrum disorder: a comprehensive meta-analysis. Front Psychiatry 2021;12:887.

[13] Bisso E, Signorelli MS, Milazzo M, et al. Immersive virtual reality applications in schizophrenia spectrum therapy: a systematic review. Int J Environ Res Public Health 2020;17(17):6111.

[14] Riches S, Pisani S, Bird L, et al. Virtual reality-based assessment and treatment of social functioning impairments in psychosis: a systematic review. Int Rev Psychiatry 2021;33(3):337–62.

[15] Ioannou A, Papastavrou E, Avraamides MN, et al. Virtual reality and symptoms management of anxiety, depression, fatigue, and pain: a systematic review. SAGE Open Nurs 2020;6:2377960820936163.

[16] Cieślik B, Mazurek J, Rutkowski S, et al. Virtual reality in psychiatric disorders: a systematic review of reviews. Complement Ther Med 2020;52:102480.

[17] Dellazizzo L, Potvin S, Luigi M, et al. Evidence on virtual reality–based therapies for psychiatric disorders: meta-review of meta-analyses. J Med Internet Res 2020; 22(8):e20889.

[18] Bossenbroek R, Wols A, Weerdmeester J, et al. Efficacy of a virtual reality biofeedback game (deep) to reduce anxiety and disruptive classroom behavior: single-case study. JMIR Ment Health 2020;7(3):e16066.

[19] Czech O, Wrzeciono A, Rutkowska A, et al. Virtual reality interventions for needle-related procedural pain, fear and anxiety—a systematic review and meta-analysis. J Clin Med 2021;10(15):3248.

[20] Emmelkamp PMG, Meyerbröker K, Morina N. Virtual reality therapy in social anxiety disorder. Curr Psychiatry Rep 2020;22(7):32.

[21] Franco M, Monfort C, Piñas-Mesa A, et al. Could avatar therapy enhance mental health in chronic patients? a systematic review. Electronics 2021;10(18):2212.

[22] Hinojo-Lucena FJ, Aznar-Díaz I, Cáceres-Reche MP, et al. Virtual reality treatment for public speaking anxiety in students. Advancements and results in personalized medicine. J Pers Med 2020;10(1):E14.

[23] Horigome T, Kurokawa S, Sawada K, et al. Virtual reality exposure therapy for social anxiety disorder: a systematic review and meta-analysis. Psychol Med 2020;50(15): 2487–97.

[24] Kothgassner OD, Goreis A, Bauda I, et al. Virtual reality biofeedback interventions for treating anxiety : A systematic review, meta-analysis and future perspective. Wien Klin Wochenschr 2022;134(Suppl 1):49–59.

[25] Lambert V, Boylan P, Boran L, et al. Virtual reality distraction for acute pain in children. Cochrane Database Syst Rev 2020;10:CD010686.

[26] Lüddecke R, Felnhofer A. Virtual reality biofeedback in health: a scoping review. Appl Psychophysiol Biofeedback 2022;47(1):1–15.

[27] Nordgård R, Låg T. The Effects of Virtual Reality on Procedural Pain and Anxiety in Pediatrics: A Systematic Review and Meta-Analysis. Frontiers in Virtual Reality 2, 2021. Available at: https://www.frontiersin.org/article/10.3389/frvir.2021.699383.

[28] Reeves R, Curran D, Gleeson A, et al. A meta-analysis of the efficacy of virtual reality and in vivo exposure therapy as psychological interventions for public speaking anxiety. Behav Modif 2021;3:145445521991102.

[29] Riches S, Azevedo L, Bird L, et al. Virtual reality relaxation for the general population: a systematic review. Soc Psychiatry Psychiatr Epidemiol 2021;56(10):1707–27.

[30] Parrish DE, Oxhandler HK, Duron JF, et al. Feasibility of virtual reality environments for adolescent social anxiety disorder. Res Social Work Pract 2016;26(7):825–35.

[31] Reger GM, Koenen-Woods P, Zetocha K, et al. Randomized controlled trial of prolonged exposure using imaginal exposure vs. virtual reality exposure in active duty soldiers with deployment-related posttraumatic stress disorder (PTSD). J Consulting Clin Psychol 2016; 84(11):946–59.

[32] McLay RN, Wood DP, Webb-Murphy JA, et al. A randomized, controlled trial of virtual reality-graded exposure therapy for post-traumatic stress disorder in active duty service members with combat-related post-traumatic stress disorder. Cyberpsychology, Behav Social Networking 2011;14(4):223–9.

[33] McLay RN, Baird A, Webb-Murphy J, et al. A randomized, head-to-head study of virtual reality exposure therapy for posttraumatic stress disorder. Cyberpsychology, Behav Social Networking 2017;20(4):218–24.

[34] Ready DJ, Gerardi RJ, Backscheider AG, et al. Comparing virtual reality exposure therapy to present-centered therapy with 11 U.S. Vietnam veterans with PTSD. Cyberpsychology, Behav Social Networking 2010;13(1):49–54.

[35] Ferrer-García M, Gutiérrez-Maldonado J, Pla-Sanjuanelo J, et al. A Randomised controlled comparison of second-level treatment approaches for treatment-resistant adults with bulimia nervosa and binge eating disorder: assessing the benefits of virtual reality cue exposure therapy. Eur Eat Disord Rev 2017; 25(6):479–90.

[36] Ferrer-Garcia M, Pla-Sanjuanelo J, Dakanalis A, et al. A randomized trial of virtual reality-based cue exposure second-level therapy and cognitive behavior second-level therapy for bulimia nervosa and binge-eating disorder: outcome at six-month followup. Cyberpsychol Behav Soc Netw 2019;22(1):60–8.

[37] Pot-Kolder RMCA, Geraets CNW, Veling W, et al. Virtual-reality-based cognitive behavioural therapy versus waiting list control for paranoid ideation and social avoidance in patients with psychotic disorders: a single-blind randomised controlled trial. Lancet Psychiatry 2018;5(3):217–26.

[38] Pot-Kolder R, Veling W, Geraets C, et al. Cost-effectiveness of virtual reality cognitive behavioral therapy for psychosis: health-economic evaluation within a randomized controlled trial. J Med Internet Res 2020;22(5): e17098.

[39] Rizzo AA, Bowerly T, Buckwalter JG, et al. A virtual reality scenario for all seasons: the virtual classroom. CNS Spectr 2006;11(1):35–44.

[40] Parsons TD, Rizzo A. "Skip." A review of virtual classroom environments for neuropsychological assessment. In: Rizzo A, Bouchard S, editors. *Virtual Reality for Psychological and neurocognitive interventions.* Virtual reality technologies for health and clinical applications. Springer New York; 2019. p. 247–65. https://doi.org/10.1007/978-1-4939-9482-3_11.

[41] Bioulac S, Micoulaud-Franchi JA, Maire J, et al. Virtual remediation versus methylphenidate to improve distractibility in children with ADHD: a controlled randomized clinical trial study. J Atten Disord 2020;24(2):326–35.

[42] Price M, Anderson P, Rothbaum BO. Virtual reality as treatment for fear of flying: a review of recent research. Int J Behav Consultation Ther 2008;4(4):340.

[43] Gujjar KR, van Wijk A, Kumar R, et al. Are technology-based interventions effective in reducing dental anxiety in children and adults? a systematic review. J Evid Based Dent Pract 2019;19(2):140–55.

[44] Malbos E, Burgess GH, Lançon C. Virtual reality and fear of shark attack: a case study for the treatment of squalophobia. 2020. Available at. https://journals.sagepub.com/doi/full/10.1177/1534650120940014. Accessed January 10, 2022.

[45] Kahlon S, Lindner P, Nordgreen T. Virtual reality exposure therapy for adolescents with fear of public speaking: a non-randomized feasibility and pilot study. Child Adolesc Psychiatry Ment Health 2019;13:47.

[46] Frantz A, Grosenbacher K. A mixed method study on the effectiveness of using virtual reality to improve adolescent public speaking. J Stud Res 2021;10(4). https://doi.org/10.47611/jsrhs.v10i4.2098.

[47] Garcia-Palacios A, Botella C, Hoffman H, et al. Comparing acceptance and refusal rates of virtual reality exposure vs. in vivo exposure by patients with specific phobias. Cyberpsychology Behav 2007;10(5):722–4.
[48] Aali G, Kariotis T, Shokraneh F. Avatar therapy for people with schizophrenia or related disorders. Cochrane Database Syst Rev 2020;5:CD011898.
[49] Chesham RK, Malouff JM, Schutte NS. Meta-analysis of the efficacy of virtual reality exposure therapy for social anxiety. Behav Change 2018;35(3):152–66.
[50] du Sert OP, Potvin S, Lipp O, et al. Virtual reality therapy for refractory auditory verbal hallucinations in schizophrenia: a pilot clinical trial. Schizophrenia Res 2018; 197:176–81.
[51] Brander M, Egger ST, Hürlimann N, et al. Virtual reality human-human interface to deliver psychotherapy to people experiencing auditory verbal hallucinations: development and usability study. JMIR Serious Games 2021; 9(2):e26820.
[52] Dellazizzo L, Potvin S, Phraxayavong K, et al. L'amélioration de la qualité de vie chez les patients atteints d'une schizophrénie réfractaire ayant suivi la Thérapie assistée par la Réalité Virtuelle : une analyse de contenu. smq 2021;46(1):157–74.
[53] Dumais A. A randomized controlled trial comparing avatar therapy to cognitive behavioral therapy in schizophrenia with treatment refractory hallucinations. clinicaltrials.gov. 2021. Available at. https://clinicaltrials.gov/ct2/show/NCT04054778. Accessed February 17, 2022.
[54] Shiban Y, Pauli P, Mühlberger A. Effect of multiple context exposure on renewal in spider phobia. Behav Res Ther 2013;51(2):68–74.
[55] Kampmann IL, Emmelkamp PMG, Hartanto D, et al. Exposure to virtual social interactions in the treatment of social anxiety disorder: A randomized controlled trial. Behav Res Ther 2016;77:147–56.
[56] Maples-Keller JL, Rauch SAM, Jovanovic T, et al. Changes in trauma-potentiated startle, skin conductance, and heart rate within prolonged exposure therapy for PTSD in high and low treatment responders. J Anxiety Disord 2019;68:102147.
[57] Mallari B, Spaeth EK, Goh H, et al. Virtual reality as an analgesic for acute and chronic pain in adults: a systematic review and meta-analysis. J Pain Res 2019;12: 2053–85.
[58] Pourmand A, Davis S, Marchak A, et al. Virtual reality as a clinical tool for pain management. Curr Pain Headache Rep 2018;22(8):53.
[59] Eijlers R, Utens EMWJ, Staals LM, et al. Systematic review and meta-analysis of virtual reality in pediatrics: effects on pain and anxiety. Anesth Analg 2019;129(5): 1344–53.
[60] Canares T, Parrish C, Santos C, et al. Pediatric coping during venipuncture with virtual reality: pilot randomized controlled trial. JMIR Pediatr Parenting 2021;4(3): e26040.
[61] Repetto C, Gaggioli A, Pallavicini F, et al. Virtual reality and mobile phones in the treatment of generalized anxiety disorders: a phase-2 clinical trial. Pers Ubiquit Comput 2013;17(2):253–60.
[62] Gorini A, Pallavicini F, Algeri D, et al. Virtual reality in the treatment of generalized anxiety disorders. Stud Health Technol Inform 2010;154:39–43.
[63] van Rooij M, Lobel A, Harris O, et al. DEEP: a biofeedback virtual reality game for children at-risk for anxiety. In: Proceedings of the 2016 CHI conference extended abstracts on human factors in computing systems. CHI EA '16. Association for Computing Machinery; 2016. p. 1989–97. https://doi.org/10.1145/2851581.2892452.
[64] Schuurmans AAT, Nijhof KS, Engels RCME, et al. Using a videogame intervention to reduce anxiety and externalizing problems among youths in residential care: an initial randomized controlled trial. J Psychopathol Behav Assess 2018;40(2):344–54.
[65] Pallavicini F, Pepe A, Mantovani F, et al. Commercial off-the-shelf video games for reducing stress and anxiety: systematic review. JMIR Ment Health 2021;8(8):e28150.
[66] Kakoschke N, Page R, de Courten B, et al. Brain training with the body in mind: towards gamified approach-avoidance training using virtual reality. Int J Human-Computer Stud 2021;151:102626.
[67] Smith SM, Vela E. Environmental context-dependent memory: a review and meta-analysis. Psychon Bull Rev 2001;8(2):203–20.
[68] Smith SM. Effects of environmental context on human memory. The SAGE Handbook Appl Mem 2013;162.
[69] Rosas JM, Todd TP, Bouton ME. Context change and associative learning. Wires Cogn Sci 2013;4(3):237–44. https://doi.org/10.1002/wcs.1225.
[70] Dunsmoor JE, Ahs F, Zielinski DJ, et al. Extinction in multiple virtual reality contexts diminishes fear reinstatement in humans. Neurobiol Learn Mem 2014;113: 157–64.
[71] de Jong R, Lommen MJJ, de Jong PJ, et al. Using multiple contexts and retrieval cues in exposure-based therapy to prevent relapse in anxiety disorders. Cogn Behav Pract 2019;26(1):154–65.
[72] Kourtesis P, Collina S, Doumas LAA, et al. Technological competence is a precondition for effective implementation of virtual reality head mounted displays in human neuroscience: a technological review and meta-analysis. Published online January 14, 2021. doi:10.31234/osf.io/6vxe3
[73] Estrada Villalba É, San Martín Azócar AL, Jacques-García FA. State of the art on immersive virtual reality and its use in developing meaningful empathy. Comput Electr Eng 2021;93:107272.
[74] Formosa NJ, Morrison BW, Hill G, et al. Testing the efficacy of a virtual reality-based simulation in enhancing users' knowledge, attitudes, and empathy relating to psychosis. Aust J Psychol 2018;70(1):57–65.
[75] Kalyanaraman SS, Penn DL, Ivory JD, et al. The virtual doppelganger: effects of a virtual reality simulator on

perceptions of schizophrenia. J Nerv Ment Dis 2010; 198(6):437–43.

[76] Hadjipanayi C, Michael-Grigoriou D. Conceptual knowledge and sensitization on Asperger's syndrome based on the constructivist approach through virtual reality. Heliyon 2020;6(6).

[77] Perpiñá C, Botella C, Baños RM. Virtual reality in eating disorders. Eur Eat Disord Rev 2003;11(3):261–78. https://doi.org/10.1002/erv.520.

[78] Riva G, Bacchetta M, Cesa G, et al. Is severe obesity a form of addiction?: rationale, clinical approach, and controlled clinical trial. CyberPsychology Behav 2006; 9(4):457–79.

[79] Riva G, Bacchetta M, Cesa G, et al. The use of VR in the treatment of eating disorders. Cybertherapy 2004; 121–63.

[80] Marco JH, Perpiñá C, Botella C. Effectiveness of cognitive behavioral therapy supported by virtual reality in the treatment of body image in eating disorders: one year follow-up. Psychiatry Res 2013;209(3):619–25.

[81] Riva G, Bacchetta M, Cesa G, et al. Six-month follow-up of in-patient experiential cognitive therapy for binge eating disorders. CyberPsychology Behav 2003;6(3): 251–8.

[82] Cesa GL, Manzoni GM, Bacchetta M, et al. Virtual reality for enhancing the cognitive behavioral treatment of obesity with binge eating disorder: randomized controlled study with one-year follow-up. J Med Internet Res 2013;15(6):e2441.

[83] Leff J, Williams G, Huckvale M, et al. Avatar therapy for persecutory auditory hallucinations: what is it and how does it work. Psychosis 2014;6(2):166–76.

[84] Leff J, Williams G, Huckvale MA, et al. Computer-assisted therapy for medication-resistant auditory hallucinations: proof-of-concept study. Br J Psychiatry 2013;202(6): 428–33.

[85] Dellazizzo L, Potvin S, Phraxayavong K, et al. One-year randomized trial comparing virtual reality-assisted therapy to cognitive–behavioral therapy for patients with treatment-resistant schizophrenia. NPJ Schizophr 2021; 7:9.

[86] Turbyne C, Goedhart A, de Koning P, et al. Systematic review and meta-analysis of virtual reality in mental healthcare: effects of full body illusions on body image disturbance. Front Virtual Reality 2021;2. Available at. https://www.frontiersin.org/article/10.3389/frvir.2021.657638. Accessed March 9, 2022.

[87] Sanders EBN, Stappers PJ. Co-creation and the new landscapes of design. CoDesign 2008;4(1):5–18.

Advances in Psychiatry and Behavioral Health 2 (2022) 95–105

ADVANCES IN PSYCHIATRY AND BEHAVIORAL HEALTH

Affective Computing in Psychotherapy

Rahul Khanna, MBBS, FRANZCP[a,*], Nicole Robinson, PhD[b], Meaghan O'Donnell, PhD[a], Harris Eyre, MBBS, PhD[c], Erin Smith[d]

[a]Phoenix Australia, Department of Psychiatry, University of Melbourne, 161 Barry Street, Carlton, VIC 3053, Australia; [b]Electrical and Computer Systems Engineering and Turner Institute for Brain and Mental Health, Monash University, 18 Alliance Lane, Clayton Campus, Victoria 3800, Australia; [c]Brain Capital Alliance, San Francisco, CA, USA; [d]Atlantic Fellow for Equity in Brain Health at the Global Brain Health Institute at University of California, 548 E Crescent Drive, Palo Alto, CA 94301, USA

KEYWORDS

- Digital mental health • Affective computing • Telehealth • Artificial intelligence • Machine learning
- Digital psychotherapy

KEY POINTS

- Psychotherapy is evolving away from its roots as an individual, face-to-face interaction to cope with workforce shortages in the face of overwhelming demand and a destabilizing pandemic.
- Affective computing is the branch of computer science focused on detecting, interpreting, processing, and simulating human emotion. It has the potential to overcome the limitations of contemporary approaches to digital therapy.
- Advances in affective computing and adjacent technologies can enhance our understanding and delivery of psychotherapy, though several practical and ethical barriers remain.
- Effective partnerships between system developers and mental health clinicians and consumers will be crucial to widespread clinical adoption.

BACKGROUND

Emerging Trends in Psychotherapy

Psychotherapy, colloquially called the *talking cure*, is an approach to mental health treatment that traditionally used the relationship between a therapist and a client to impart skills or insight to relieve suffering. Psychotherapeutic approaches differ on several dimensions, including by (individual, family, or group), intended aim (personal insight vs direct behavioral change), the centrality of relational elements, duration, and more. Common themes, however, include attention to emotion, thoughts, and behavior. Although formative concepts of psychotherapy trace their roots much further in human history, the psychoanalytic approach pioneered by Freud in the early twentieth century is commonly accepted as the birth of modern psychotherapy [1]. Contemporary approaches represent an evolution or reaction to analysis.

Despite this divergence in foci and content, for most of its history, psychotherapy has primarily been carried out as a face-to-face interaction between a client and a professional mental health care provider. Increasingly, however, the talking cure has evolved into a *communication cure*, representing a broadening of the definition of therapist interaction and the notion of the "therapeutic space." The modality of communication has become increasingly diverse, ranging from face-to-face to telehealth and even text messaging or live chat. The COVID-19 pandemic also has resulted in a global surge in telehealth and other psychotherapy innovations by both increasing demand and breaking prior service models

*Corresponding author, *E-mail address:* Rahul.khanna@unimelb.edu.au

https://doi.org/10.1016/j.ypsc.2022.05.006
2667-3827/22/

in the interest of infection control [2]. Emerging technology-first providers such as Ginger.io, which recently merged with Headspace, use a stepped-care model, whereby a spectrum of modalities is offered based on the need. These evolving modalities have also made it possible for therapy to occur asynchronously. In this approach, the interaction with the therapist can occur asynchronously. The client may communicate their thoughts to a clinician via text, email, or video at any hour, and the therapist would respond when available. Although much less widely used than synchronous telehealth, adoption is growing [3]. Although these approaches bring new advantages to the treatment process, they have been principally motivated by a shortage of qualified therapists. For instance, in the United States, in March 2021, 37% of the population lived in an area experiencing mental health professional shortages. This rises to over 94% in more sparsely populated states [4].

These new modalities increase flexibility and, therefore, access to psychotherapy but have limitations. One aspect of traditional psychotherapy and mental health clinical practice more broadly is the mental state examination (MSE), which is used alongside other clinical assessments and therapeutic modalities during psychotherapy. This examination reflects the clinicians' systematic observation of a client's presentation, including their overt behavior, therapeutic engagement, speech and language use, the coherence and goal-directedness of their thought process, reported mood, visible effect, insight, and judgment. However, an inexact skill, the ability to conduct an MSE is considered a core clinical competency that informs diagnoses and treatment planning. As practice moves further from its face-to-face individual treatment roots, conducting a thorough MSE becomes increasingly challenging as it depends greatly on nonverbal cues lost in videoconferencing. This is one of several spaces where affective computing is demonstrating early promise.

Introducing Affective Computing

Rosalind Picard, widely credited with founding affective computing, defined *affective computing* as "computing that relates to, arises from, and deliberately influences emotion" [5]. Today, it is the discipline of computer science focused on detecting, interpreting, processing, and simulating human emotions (Fig. 1).

The field has several motivations, ranging from improved computer decision-making to enhancing human–computer interactions. As Picard later summarized, emotion "...kept coming up as essential in perception. Emotion biased what we saw and heard. Emotion played major roles not only in perception but also in many other aspects of intelligence that artificial intelligence (AI) researchers had been trying to solve from a cortical-centric perspective. Emotion was vital in forming memory and attention and in rational decision-making. And, of course, emotional communication was vital in human–machine interaction. Emotions influence action selection, language, and whether or not you decide to double-check your mathematical derivations, comment your computer code [or] initiate a conversation." Pertinently for the topic of psychotherapy, Picard reiterates that emotion is a principal "motivating and guiding force in perception and attention" [6].

These diverse aims of affective computing are usually enabled through the combination of data and machine learning. Traditionally, the field focused on interpreting visual and audio data. Examples include using computer vision to interpret facial expressions or audio recordings to infer emotional valence through features such as vocal tone, speed, pitch, prosody, and so forth. Such data points are captured, and a machine learning algorithm is used to "train" software to estimate the probability of a given emotion based on an initial set of previously human-labeled data.

Although speech and facial expressions were the most common data sources of algorithmic training in the early decades of affective computing, in principle any computationally measurable manifestation of an emotional state can be used (see Fig. 1). For example, a clinical bot titled SimSensei uses psychophysiological measures such as heart rate and galvanic skin response to augment vocal features, speech content, and facial expression [7].

Psychophysiological signals have been a mainstay of psychology research since the 1950s but previously had considerable limitations. Chief among them has been the inconvenience, expense, and biasing nature of contact sensors required to capture such data. Once strapped onto a participant's body, they could collect several parameters of the autonomic nervous system, such as temperature, heart rate, and vascular tone. Recent advances in signal processing, however, have led to the emergence of computational psychophysiology techniques. These involve the use of imaging, such as those collected from standard video and thermal cameras, to deduce psychophysiological status through machine learning [8]. Such methods add a rich array of features that can support affective computing.

Affective computing has been improved by the increasing capability of mobile devices, which now

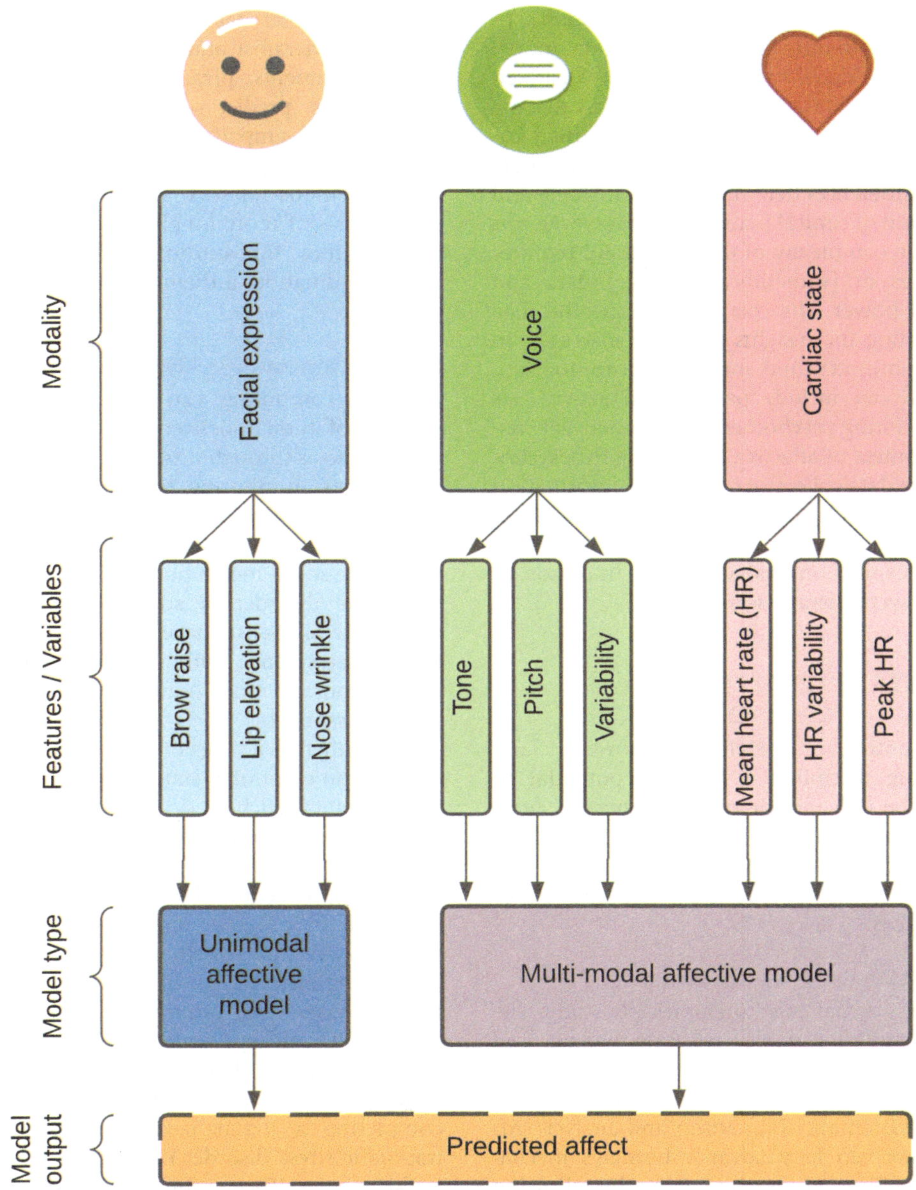

FIG. 1 Affective computing systems commonly consist of affective modalities, derived features, and machine learning models that predict affect.

accompany billions of people throughout the day. Now nearly ubiquitous, smartphones unobtrusively collect rich sensor data spanning multiple modalities, including location, proximity to other devices (and therefore those who carry them), communication behavior, and more. Mobile devices are also capable of increasingly complex computing on their own, reducing the inconvenience and privacy issues associated with the cloud computing previously necessary. Politou and *colleagues* (2017) identified 131 research papers using mobile devices to infer effect [9]. These ranged from unidimensional models like stress levels to more nuanced classifiers capable of distinguishing more distinctive affective states.

Modality, in this context, refers to the data stream(s) used to create the affective computing machine learning software. A unimodal model uses a single source of data, such as voice, to infer effect. A multimodal model can leverage several signal streams at once, as illustrated in Fig. 1. Individual data inputs from a modality that are used by the machine learning algorithm are termed *features*. This approach may make the model more accurate and robust to differences between the training data and the messier world of clinical practice [10]. However, this also adds to the complexity of the model and requires greater volumes of (sometimes intrusive) data and computational power. The cost of acquiring the data and implementing the insights therefore increases. In addition, for unimodal and multimodal approaches, data collection can include passive and active tests that can occur during psychotherapy or in-between sessions. In the context of affective computing for psychotherapy, passive data collective can include information collected from smartphone usage or social media activity, whereas active data collection may involve specific vocal or facial expression analyses during in-person or telemedicine psychotherapy sessions.

CURRENT STATE OF AFFECTIVE COMPUTING APPLIED TO THERAPY

Affective computing is, therefore, a powerful and rapidly evolving discipline. It has the potential to contribute to the full lifecycle of psychotherapy, from advancing our mechanistic understanding of therapy to training clinicians and supporting human-led psychotherapy through autonomous care. A selection of such work follows.

Exploring Underlying Mechanisms

Psychotherapy is a challenge to empirically study. The number of potential variables affecting process and outcome, the complexity of each therapy session, and the subjectivity of human assessors are some of the challenges for systematic comparison and analysis. Affective computer can help advance human's mechanistic understanding of psychotherapy by allowing them to measure affective states more systematically. Such studies featured prominently in Wilshire's (2020) systematic review [11] on interpersonal coordination dynamics in psychotherapy. They note evidence indicating that the affective states of clinicians and their clients covary within a psychotherapeutic interaction. Theoretic constructs, such as the common factors model and polyvagal theory, suggest such covariance may moderate effectiveness. Although some included studies used human-coded data, affective computing is used in an increasing number of studies reviewed. Reviewed studies demonstrated that coordination between the therapist and the client in features such as body movements, physiology, language, and speech patterns can predict outcomes, including symptom improvement, empathy, and therapeutic alliance.

As the investigators note [11], the use of computational methods for such analyses not only allows for the analysis of more longitudinal data but also opens opportunities for automated feedback to improve such coordination, a theme discussed in the following section.

Supporting Human-Delivered Therapy

Affective computing can also support the client's journey of human-delivered therapy, from screening and diagnosis through actual therapeutic content delivery, progress monitoring, and more. These systems have been used to try to screen people who may benefit from therapy (eg, through the affective computing methods to analyze social media posts for the evidence of major depressive disorder or suicide risk [12,13]). Virtual agents like SimSensei have been used to conduct diagnostic assessments, with some suggestions that they may encourage more honest self-disclosure than human assessors [14].

Then, there is a range of work seeking to map digital behavior to emotional states, particularly those of clinical relevance, such as depression and mania. Signals used for such affective systems range from vocal features, as previously described, to more abstract ones like typing behavior. These systems could be used for diagnosis or progress monitoring. Such approaches could enhance measurement-based care (MBC) that is developing an evidence base for enhancing rates and time to recovery in multiple disorders [15]. In traditional MBC, self-report scales are completed on a regular basis to guide therapy. For example, in a protocol developed by Nixon and Elizabeth [16], participants completing a manualized psychotherapy for post-traumatic stress disorder complete a weekly symptom questionnaire. Those who are not showing decreases in questionnaire scores by the fifth session have a reformulation session, whereby the biopsychosocial barriers to recovery are collaboratively reconsidered. Based on this reformulation, the therapist will deviate from the manualized treatment to address barriers (such as substance use) before returning to the core therapy. Replacing or augmenting self-reported measures with affective computing would add a more objective layer to this. Another advantage of such an approach is that it can occur within a client's own environment rather than in the artificial setting of a clinic. This allows for a more naturalistic understanding of the individual's experiential rather than reporting self, which the authors know do not always align [17]. Fig. 2 illustrates an affective computing-based dashboard.

An example of work in this vein comes from Ieso, an online cognitive behavioral therapy (CBT) provider in the United Kingdom. As a large provider of text-based therapy, they were able to leverage a deep learning algorithm to analyze over 90,000 psychotherapy session transcripts to understand the relationship between patient language, therapy content, and outcomes [18,19]. These insights were then distilled into a decision support tool that provides live feedback on the therapist's work within a session, nudging them toward techniques shown to improve outcomes [20]. Using these systems, Ieso was able to achieve recovery rates of 12% and 15% more than the national average in 2021 for depression and generalized anxiety disorder, respectively [21].

Although Ieso's model was limited to text data, the broader concept of live therapist guidance has enormous potential when paired with the latest in affective computing. Although in its infancy, the expansion of teletherapy prompted by the COVID-19 pandemic presents another opportunity to collect the large volumes of data required to build similar models using a broader range of affective signals. Recordings of video therapy sessions could yield not just transcripts but vocal features, facial expressions, and computationally derived physiologic data as well.

Such affective systems could also aid in the training of future psychotherapists. For example, Wilcocks and colleagues demonstrated a psychotherapy simulator to facilitate training in intensive short-term dynamic psychotherapy, helping to train clinicians in a cost-effective way using simulated interactions with the clients. This virtual patient was able to respond to dialogue and display affects to allow trainees to begin practicing skills in a safe environment [22]. Such tools could be paired with Ieso-like clinical guidance systems to present unparalleled training opportunities. Innovative digital training experiences like this would be particularly important in low-income and middle-income countries, where they can help nonspecialists rapidly develop basic psychotherapeutic skills [23].

Delivering Autonomous Therapy

Autonomous therapy systems are stand-alone interventions like chatbots that aim to deliver care without human interaction. They typically use text, audio, and video to teach self-management skills and encourage healthy thought patterns based on CBT principles. By allowing more organic interaction, they present an improvement on online course-like approaches, which linearly deliver therapeutic content. Contemporary systems like *Wysa* or *Woebot* store some persistent information about the user, allowing more tailored therapy delivery and facilitating a sense of connection. In fact, a recent analysis of *Woebot* data showed scores on a therapeutic alliance inventory equal to that of human therapists [24].

Till recently, studies on such tools consistently show that outcomes are enhanced when such programs and paired with a human, even a lay coach or peer, without

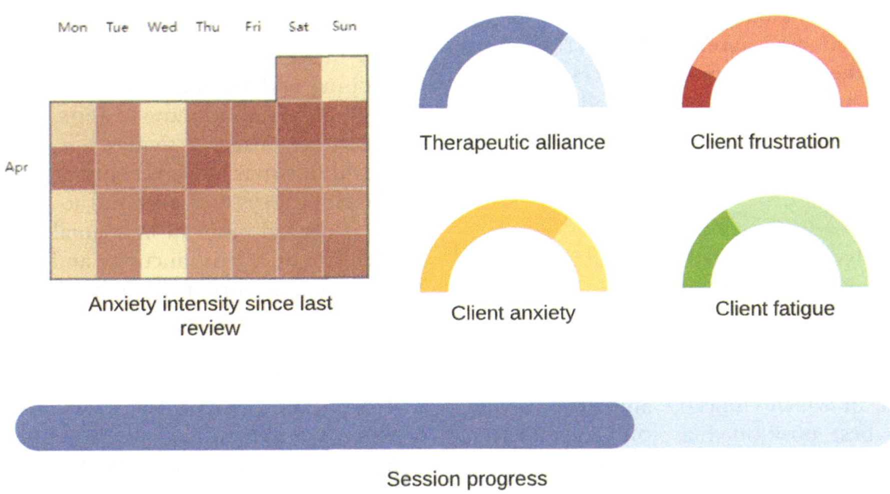

FIG. 2 An affective computing-based dashboard that could support human-delivered therapy.

which both engagement and efficacy markedly drop. Successful therapy depends on a process of learning, which is inherently an emotional process. *Feelings* of curiosity that often trigger learning are reenforced by the pleasure of mastery and sometimes are inhibited by feelings of frustration. A human therapist, coach, or peer can detect such shifts and respond appropriately to keep the client engaged. More mature use of affective computing has the potential to detect and use this nuance to narrow the gap between human-aided and autonomous therapy.

CLINICAL INTEGRATION

Despite the exciting emerging evidence discussed to date, truly clinically integrated solutions such as Ieso's are rare. The strong demand for mental health services and the volume of research and investment activities, however, suggests that they will transform care in the next decade. Ieso themselves raised $53 million in their latest funding round, and Forbes estimated that venture capital funding for United States-based mental health start-ups in 2020 alone exceeded $1.5 billion [25].

Therapists as Key Partners

Ultimately, the successful integration of affective computing into psychotherapy practice will depend on effective partnerships between clinicians and technologists. Most importantly, therapists are best placed to understand and identify improvement opportunities in clinical workflows. This is crucial for an appropriate prioritization of research and investment. Fig. 3 shows an example of workflows that may benefit from affective computing-based applications. Although such outlines seem basic, there will be many nuances between disciplines and therapy types that need broader engagement. Beyond this, there are several roles clinical experts can play in the future of this technology.

High-Quality Data and Expert Evaluation

Another key enabler is the labeled data that forms the backbone of any affective computing system. Such systems perform best when able to "learn" from a large corpus of diverse, high-quality data sets. For clinical applications, this ideally means sensitive recordings of therapy content, of which clinicians and their clients themselves are best positioned as joint custodians. Although clients should be the final arbiter of the data they are comfortable with sharing for system training, this is the best done in dialogue with a clinician who is able to convey the value of their data for improving care.

Further, the existing corpus of data used to train current systems has mostly been coded by the laypeople. That is, nonexperts have provided the human labels for what affect an individual was displaying at the time of data collection. A study that is an exception to this theme illustrates how problematic this can be. Liu and *colleagues* built a robot-assisted rehabilitation therapy for children with autism spectrum disorder [26]. The system was trained to recognize anxiety, engagement, and liking using a mixture of self-reports by children and labeling of videos by parents and clinicians. Interestingly, depending on the pairing (parent, clinician vs child-participant) and the emotional target, the agreement between reporters (measured by kappa score) ranged from 0.15 to 0.63. Given that 1 represents perfect agreement and 0 is the level expected by chance, the study is a reminder that the views of clinically trained and lay observers in effect may differ widely.

It would be impractical to have all such data sets labeled by expert clinicians, but it is important for systems to be able to learn "on the job." That is, systems must be designed to receive and improve based on expert feedback on performance. In this way, affective clinical systems can continuously improve alongside the clinicians that use them.

Appropriate Incentives

The above points around clinician input and improved data will be difficult to achieve without rethinking incentives. Models with the maturity of Ieso's remain rare, and as such early-adopting clinicians of other affective systems may experience inconveniences not immediately offset by benefits. Researchers and enterprises developing and leveraging such tools must, therefore, think creatively about how to appropriately incentivize and remunerate such activities.

Health insurers, governments, and developers of affective clinical systems all stand to gain from scalable, effective clinical innovation. Mental ill-health is associated with reduced productivity and increased physical health costs, on top of the individual human toll and direct health care expenses. All three parties should consider ways to encourage clinicians and patients to adopt novel affective tools, financially and otherwise.

The question of data ownership, and the role of the patients themselves, also needs active thought. Huag wrote a poignant reminder that the clients' perspectives have often been neglected in debates about clinical data ownership, which generally occur between and among

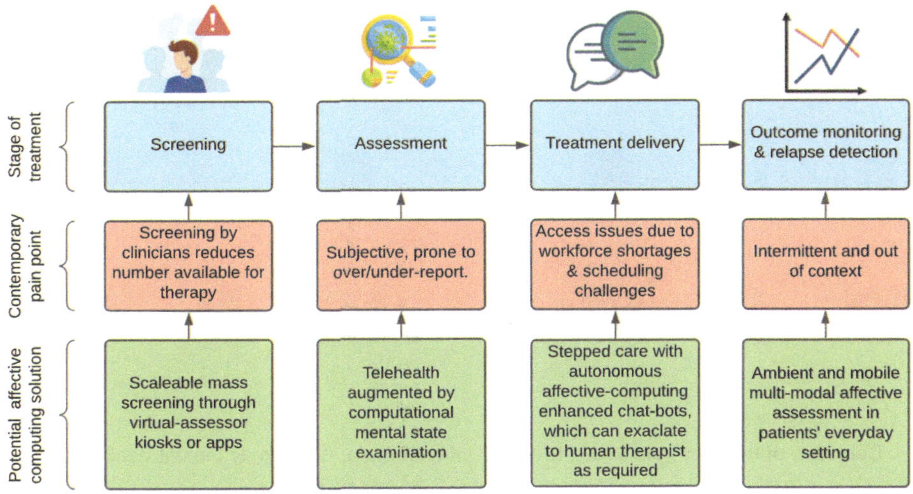

FIG. 3 Example therapy workflows that may benefit from affective computing-based applications.

clinicians, researchers, regulators, and other health enterprise stakeholders. Consumers need to be brought into that data-sharing discussion [27]. Consumers of digital health care products are increasingly skeptical around data privacy and control, including for medically sensitive data. As Huag stresses, however, they can also be savvy about its value, and many are altruistically motivated to share in the interests of other sufferers. Ignoring consumer views can lead to overly permissive and overly restrictive policies and regulations, depending on the level of the paternalism of regulators in a given setting. Both can be a detriment to ethical innovation.

One technology-first path forward may be the use of blockchain-based systems, increasingly termed "Web3." Unlike contemporary "Web2" infrastructure, where data typically reside on institutionally owned servers that are accessed and authored by clients (devices owned by individuals or organizations), Web3 relies on peer-to-peer computing. The technical detail is outside the scope of this article, but the principal distinction between the two for health purposes is data residence and ownership. In a peer-to-peer framework, data remain individually owned. Ownership is tracked on distributed ledgers ("the blockchain"), and protocols enable *smart contracts*. This means that instead of relying on a central authority to manage data and govern use, such requirements are coded directly into the system collecting and sharing the data. Fig. 4 summarizes the structural shift from Web2 to Web3. Odyssey Decentralised Autonomous Organisation (DAO) and other resources are readily available to better understand Web3 principles [28].

Precision Psychology

Affective computing biomarkers may assist in a precision medicine approach to certain psychotherapy modalities. As there are many different types of psychotherapy, affective computing biomarkers may be used to monitor response to psychotherapy and determine which type of therapy a patient is most likely to respond to. Affective computing can be combined with other modalities, such as functional neuroimaging for this decision support [29].

Managing Errors

Another aspect that clinicians, regulators and, other stakeholders must resolve is how to deal with inaccuracies. Affective computing is by no means infallible, and the further a model strays from the context of its training data set and the lower the quality of that data, the less accurate it is likely to be. Particularly problematic are cross-cultural differences in emotional expressions, such as differences in the meaning behind facial expressions, hand gestures, levels of eye contact, physical proximity, and dozens of other variables.

One possible way of managing this is mandating transparency of training data sets for affective computing systems. Much like food labeling, this might necessitate the disclosure of the demographics and context of that data set. It may enumerate which countries the model was trained in and the demographic profiles of participants, including age, gender, ethnicity,

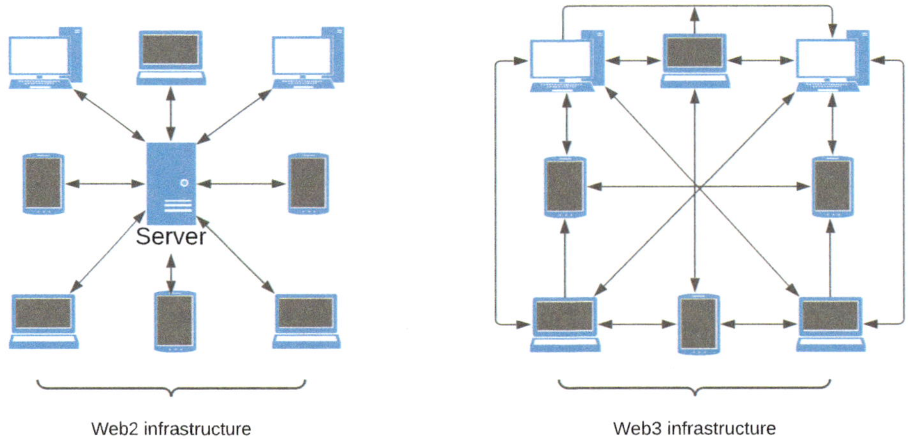

FIG. 4 Depiction of the shift from Web2 to Web3 infrastructure, which may benefit health applications.

and any other dimensions that may influence affective expression. Certain medical conditions or medication may also alter some of the features used in typical models, such as facial scarring for systems relying on expression recognition.

Although there is a formidable challenge, it is important to remember that humans share similar limitations. As Liu's study above reminds us, humans frequently disagree about affective expression. Like our digital counterparts, cultural differences pose particular challenges. Humans, however, have clearer legal standing and greater flexibility to recognize, reflect on, and address their limitations.

THE PATH FORWARD FOR CLINICAL AFFECTIVE COMPUTING

In addition to the above clinical integration questions, the technology has several other challenges that must be considered when developing systems for therapeutic use. Many such issues are considered in the 2021 International Institute of Electrical and Electronics Engineers (IEEE), Global Initiative on Ethics of Autonomous, and Intelligent Systems, which include an article on affective computing [30].

One interesting point posed in this document is the bidirectional relationship between humans and technology. Specifically, just as people shape the systems that accompany them, they are in turn shaped by those they engage with. Tellingly, it seems children as young as 7 months old can assign agency to an autonomous robot [31]. It is uncertain then how generations raised alongside such systems will have their affective experience and expression shaped by such interaction. Even adults may not be immune to the bidirectional influence of affective computing. At a minimum, there may be a shift toward the affective behaviors of the cultural context of the affective system's creators, akin to the impact of colonialism. This is not to say that societal changes are inherently negative, societies are always in a state of evolution. Rather, it highlights the need for cautious implementation and broad investment, where possible, in "home grown" (or at least "home trained") affective systems.

Earlier, the importance of designing systems that clinicians can improve post-implementation was discussed. Similar considerations are important for the therapists' clients who are being analyzed via affective computing. It is ideal for them to also know the outputs of the system. This may serve not only a therapeutic purpose in terms of developing personal insight and reflection but also an ethical duty in terms of transparency and the ability to correct errors. The exact implementation of such feedback, however, must be subject to empirical investigation to detect and address unintended consequences. For example, research suggests the phenomenon of *Zoom fatigue* (fatigue associated with videoconferencing) may partially result from "mirror anxiety" [32]; that is, users having to look at themselves for protracted periods during online interactions.

From a developmental context, we know that children look to carers as a source of truth to learn to understand and regulate their internal emotional states. The accuracy of the carers' regard and the interpretation of the child's effect is, therefore, thought to be a developmental predictor of future psychopathology [33]. It is possible that similar issues may arise with affective systems. The bottom line, as the IEEE concludes, is that stakeholders must be attuned to these risks and seek to mitigate and proactively assess them. As the issue of errors, human actors are not immune to such issues, so it is important to be measured such risks.

In addition, the 2021 "Ethics and governance of artificial intelligence for health: World Health Organization (WHO) guidance" report by the WHO highlights key ethical principles for the use of artificial intelligence in health care, which include protecting autonomy; promoting human well-being, human safety, and the public interest; ensuring transparency, explainability, and intelligibility; fostering responsibility and accountability; ensuring inclusiveness and equity; and promoting artificial intelligence that is responsive and sustainable [34]. These ethical principles must guide the development of affective computing applications for psychotherapy to ensure human rights are upheld and that patient and community interests do not become subordinate to the powerful commercial interest of technology companies or the interests of governments in surveillance and social control [35].

Finally, it is important to start thinking of such systems, as clinical products, and applying similar expectations to those preceding them. This includes publicly acknowledging side effects and somewhat uniquely for more autonomous systems, highlighting their status as *designed and deliberately built* rather than entities in their own right [30]. The IEEE guidelines also suggest that more autonomous systems need to be capable of detecting their use case and modifying accordingly. For example, they should recognize and deal differently with a minor who may not be able to judge the risks and benefits of an affective therapeutic system and give appropriate consent.

SUMMARY

Traditional psychotherapy is inaccessible to many who need it, and the lack of innovative approaches such as affective computing in psychotherapy remains largely absent. The psychotherapy field has begun to innovate to meet this challenge in several ways, including an embrace of telehealth, asynchronous care, and the inclusion of new disciplines like coaches. There have also been attempts at digitizing therapy more comprehensively, such as the use of online treatment companions and chatbots.

In parallel, strides have been made in affective computing. These systems have increased in speed and sophistication, using a range of modalities to interpret, express, and influence emotion. Although there are few such systems already deployed in clinical workflows, many others are demonstrating promise in research and development settings. The billions invested annually speak volumes of the need for such novel techniques in clinical practice.

Work to date demonstrates potential in deepening our mechanistic understanding of psychotherapy, training future therapists, screening those requiring help, assisting in diagnostic assessments, and participating directly in care delivery. This can take the form of supporting human-delivered therapy through clinical decision support and outcome monitoring or delivering sophisticated autonomous treatment.

Maximizing the potential of this emerging technology will depend on effective partnerships with clinicians and consumers. Therapists can contribute by helping prioritize technology to match important clinical challenges and workflows and providing expert feedback on algorithm outputs. They are also key stakeholders in the broader discussion about data ownership. Although Web3 frameworks may facilitate new ways of securing data, consensus and transparency remain important. Consensus is even more crucial when systems fail, and the technology will require the broader health ecosystem, including regulators and insurers, to adapt. The key publications by the WHO and IEEE can help guide the next stages in the broader development and dissemination affective computing systems for psychotherapy.

CLINICS CARE POINTS

- Clinical affective computing systems are beginning to reach clinical application and are attracting substantial consumer, investment, and research interest.
- They have the potential to increase access and quality of psychotherapy, both by supporting human-delivered therapy and supplementing it with autonomous care on a stepped-care model.
- Clinicians should be encouraged to explore adoption into clinical practice while demanding adherence to published guidelines on autonomous systems published by the International Institute of Electrical and Electronics Engineers and World Health Organization from developers.

DISCLOSURE

R. Khanna volunteers as an advisor to Flintworks and More Good Days. He is supported by an Australian

Government Research Training Program (RTP) Scholarship. H. Eyre is an employee of PRODEO LLC. E. Smith has nothing to disclose. N. Robinson is a company director and shareholder with LYRO Robotics.

REFERENCES

[1] Porter R. Madness: a brief history. Oxford University Press; 2021. p. 183–215.

[2] Khanna R, Forbes M. Telepsychiatry as a public health imperative: slowing COVID-19. Aust N Z J Psychiatry 2020;54(7):758.

[3] Chan S, Li L, Torous J, et al. Review of use of asynchronous technologies incorporated in mental health care. Curr Psychiatry Rep 2018;20(10). https://doi.org/10.1007/s11920-018-0954-3.

[4] Hubbard K. Many states face shortage of mental health providers. U.S News World Rep 2021. Available at: https://www.usnews.com/news/best-states/articles/2021-06-10/northeastern-states-have-fewest-mental-health-provider-shortages.

[5] Picard RW. Affective Computing 1995. doi:10.1007/bf01238028.

[6] Calvo R, D'Mello S, Gratch J, et al. The promise of affective computing. Oxford Handb Affect Comput; 2014. p. 1–11. https://doi.org/10.1093/oxfordhb/9780199942237.013.013.

[7] DeVault D, Artstein R, Benn G, et al. SimSensei Kiosk: a virtual human interviewer for healthcare decision support. In: *Proceedings of the 2014 international Conference on autonomous Agents and multi-agent systems*. AAMAS '14. International Foundation for Autonomous Agents and Multiagent Systems; 2014. p. 1061–8.

[8] Cardone D, Pinti P, Merla A. Thermal infrared imaging-based computational psychophysiology for psychometrics. Comput Math Methods Med 2015;2015:1–8.

[9] Politou E, Alepis E, Patsakis C. A survey on mobile affective computing. Comput Sci Rev 2017;25:79–100.

[10] Poria S, Cambria E, Bajpai R, et al. A review of affective computing: from unimodal analysis to multimodal fusion. Inf Fusion 2017;37:98–125.

[11] Wiltshire TJ, Philipsen JS, Trasmundi SB, et al. Interpersonal coordination dynamics in psychotherapy: a systematic review. Cognit Ther Res 2020;44(4):752–73.

[12] Coppersmith G, Leary R, Crutchley P, et al. Natural language processing of social media as screening for suicide risk. Biomed Inform Insights 2018;10:117822261879286.

[13] Chen L, Magdy W, Whalley H, et al. Examining the role of mood patterns in predicting self-reported depressive symptoms. In: 12th ACM conference on web science. WebSci '20. Association for Computing Machinery; 2020. p. 164–73. https://doi.org/10.1145/3394231.3397906.

[14] Lucas GM, Gratch J, King A, et al. It's only a computer: virtual humans increase willingness to disclose. Comput Hum Behav 2014;37:94–100.

[15] Guo T, Xiang Y-T, Xiao L, et al. Measurement-based care versus standard care for major depression: a randomized controlled trial with blind raters. Am J Psychiatry 2015;172(10):1004–13.

[16] Nixon R, Elizabeth M. Does case formulation improve outcomes in cognitive processing therapy for PTSD? a randomized controlled trial. In: ; 2020:151.

[17] Kahneman D, Riis J. Living, and thinking about it: two perspectives on life. Sci Well-being 2005;285–304.

[18] Ewbank MP, Cummins R, Tablan V, et al. Understanding the relationship between patient language and outcomes in internet-enabled cognitive behavioural therapy: a deep learning approach to automatic coding of session transcripts. Psychother Res 2020;31(3):326–38.

[19] Ewbank MP, Cummins R, Tablan V, et al. Quantifying the association between psychotherapy content and clinical outcomes using deep learning. JAMA Psychiatry 2020;77(1):35–43.

[20] Cummins R, Tablan V, Ewbank MP, et al. A tool for gaining insights into psychotherapy. Proc Int World Wide Web 2019;3503–6. https://doi.org/10.1145/3308558.3314128x.

[21] Jee C, Douglas Heaven W. The therapists using AI to make therapy better. MIT Technol Rev 2021. Available at: https://www.technologyreview.com/2021/12/06/1041345/ai-nlp-mental-health-better-therapists-psychology-cbt/.

[22] Wilcocks K, Kapralos B, Kalpin A, et al. A dialogue intervention simulation framework to facilitate psychotherapy training. IEEE 23rd Int Symp Consum Technol 2019;74–5. https://doi.org/10.1109/ISCE.2019.8900976.

[23] Naslund JA, Shidhaye R, Patel V. Digital technology for building capacity of nonspecialist health workers for task sharing and scaling up mental health care globally. Harv Rev Psychiatry 2019;27(3):181–92.

[24] Darcy A, Daniels J, Salinger D, et al. Evidence of human-level bonds established with a digital conversational agent: cross-sectional, retrospective observational study. JMIR Form Res 2021;5(5):1–7.

[25] Jennings K. Venture funding for mental health startups hits record high as anxiety, depression skyrocket. Forbes 2021. Available at: https://www.forbes.com/sites/katiejennings/2021/06/07/venture-funding-for-mental-health-startups-hits-record-high-as-anxiety-depression-skyrocket/?sh=15f1e99e1116.

[26] Liu C, Conn K, Sarkar N, et al. Affect recognition in robot assisted rehabilitation of children with autism spectrum disorder. Proc IEEE Int Conf Robot Autom 2007;1755–60. https://doi.org/10.1109/ROBOT.2007.363576.

[27] Haug CJ. Whose data are they anyway? can a patient perspective advance the data-sharing debate? N Engl J Med 2017;376(23):2203–5.

[28] Odyssey DAO. Intro to Web3. 2022. Available at: https://www.odysseydao.com. Accessed January 29, 2021.

[29] Beam E, Potts C, Poldrack RA, et al. A data-driven framework for mapping domains of human neurobiology. Nat Neurosci 2021;24(12):1733–44.

[30] The IEEE global initiative on ethics of autonomous and intelligent systems. Affective Computing; 2021.

[31] Kamewari K, Kato M, Kanda T, et al. Six-and-a-half-month-old children positively attribute goals to human action and to humanoid-robot motion. Cogn Dev 2005;20(2):303–20.

[32] Fauville G, Luo M, Queiroz ACM, et al. Nonverbal mechanisms predict zoom fatigue and explain why women experience higher levels than men. SSRN Electron J 2021;1–18. https://doi.org/10.2139/ssrn.3820035.

[33] Fonagy P, Gergely G, Target M. The parent-infant dyad and the construction of the subjective self. J Child Psychol Psychiatry 2007;48(3–4):288–328.

[34] World Health Organization. Ethics and governance of artificial intelligence for health. WHO Guidance; 2021.

[35] Buolamwini J, Timnit G. Gender shades: intersectional accuracy disparities in commercial gender classification. Proc Mach Learn Res 2018;81:1–15.

Women's Mental Health

Advances in Psychiatry and Behavioral Health 2 (2022) 107–118

ADVANCES IN PSYCHIATRY AND BEHAVIORAL HEALTH

Perimenopause and Mental Health

Implications for the Assessment and Treatment of Women at Midlife

Nicole Leistikow, MD[a,*], Milena H. Smith, MD, PhD[b]

[a]Department of Psychiatry, University of Maryland School of Medicine, Baltimore, MD, USA; [b]Department of Psychiatry & Behavioral Sciences, Johns Hopkins University School of Medicine, Baltimore, MD, USA

KEYWORDS

- Mental illness in perimenopause
- Perimenopausal depression
- Evaluation of midlife women

KEY POINTS

- The perimenopausal transition, or the 4 to 9 years leading up to menopause (average age 51 years), is a window of increased risk for new onset or recurrence of depression that should trigger universal depression screening of midlife women in primary care settings.
- Assessment for perimenopausal depression should include screening for vasomotor symptoms, sleep disturbance, cognitive complaints, urogenital symptoms, and joint pain and assessment of perimenopausal symptoms should rule out depression as an exacerbating or underlying factor.
- Severe or concerning perimenopausal symptoms should be further investigated and alternative causes ruled out.
- Perimenopausal depression treatment should be guided by medications that have been effective in the past for a particular individual or medications that might also treat concomitant problems, such as vasomotor symptoms or chronic pain.
- Menopausal hormone therapy (MHT) may have benefit for treatment or prevention of perimenopausal depression, but extant research is not definitive. MHT is an adjunctive option in women who have moderate to severe vasomotor symptoms, and who are younger than 60 or within 10 years of menopause with no contraindications.

CLINICAL VIGNETTE

A 47-year-old married mother of 2 teens reports worsening irritability and anxiety, difficulty sleeping, trouble concentrating at work, loss of pleasure in her regular activities, daily dread, and feeling overwhelmed for the last 2 months and has gradually increased her alcohol use to 2 glasses of wine each evening. She has a history of mild premenstrual irritability and experienced an episode of postpartum depression 1 month after her first delivery, successfully treated with an antidepressant and therapy. She has not received any psychiatric treatment since. How would you proceed?

Introduction

Perimenopause is defined as the years leading up to the cessation of menstruation. This window of time—which typically starts in a woman's mid-40s, lasts 4 to 9 years, and ends on average at age 51 years— is marked by myriad potential symptoms. These symptoms include, but are not limited to: irregular menses; hot flashes; sleep disturbance; cognitive complaints; sexual, vaginal, and urinary problems; and joint pain [1–3]. These hormonally driven physical changes may be related to or simply concomitant with additional changes in mood and well-being. The effects of

*Corresponding author, *E-mail address:* nleistikow@som.umaryland.edu

https://doi.org/10.1016/j.ypsc.2022.05.004

2667-3827/22/

perimenopause on mental health are greatly underappreciated.

The lack of attention given to perimenopause contrasts with the relatively recent acceptance of the perinatal period—another stage of hormonal fluctuation—as a window of vulnerability for, and opportunity to address, threats to women's mental health. Postpartum depression (PPD) is now understood by the medical establishment, media, and general public to be a serious psychiatric illness that can be treated and potentially prevented. Resources allotted to address PPD are rightly seen as an investment yielding dividends to women, their families, and society. Strikingly, the same women who experience PPD will also be at increased risk for depression later in life, when they begin the perimenopausal transition.

Building on our knowledge of the peripartum, it is time to extend our appreciation of the brain's sensitivity to reproductive stages and to recognize perimenopause as a similar window of both risk and opportunity in women's mental health. Given the growing body of research and clinical expertise, it is expected that perimenopause will soon gain recognition, both within and beyond psychiatry, as an important phase of physiologic changes and health sequelae. Recognizing and sufficiently treating perimenopausal mental illness and its associated symptoms could significantly improve the health of women at midlife.

This article describes the effects of perimenopause on mood, sleep, and cognition and elucidates how an understanding of perimenopause informs the assessment of mental illness in midlife women and guides evidence-based treatment.

The role of perimenopause in women's mental health

Much of our current understanding of how perimenopause affects women's mental health comes from 4 longitudinal prospective studies that were started in the United States in the 1990s: the Harvard Study of Moods and Cycles, the Penn Ovarian Aging Study (POAS), the Seattle Midlife Women's Health Study (SMWHS), and the Study of Women's Health Across the Nation (SWAN).

These studies demonstrated an increased incidence of both depressive symptoms and major depressive disorder during the perimenopausal transition, when compared with women not yet in the transition to menopause. SWAN found that the prevalence of dysphoric mood increased from 9% to 15% as women went from premenopause to perimenopause, and that women were 2 to 4 times more likely to have a major depressive episode in perimenopause or early postmenopause than when premenopausal [4]. The percentage of women experiencing a major depressive episode during the 13-year SWAN study period was high: 39% of all women, broken down into 28% of those with no history of a prior episode and 59% of those with a past history of depression [5]. POAS found that, whether or not they had a history of depression, women were at increased risk of clinically significant depressive symptoms in the 10 years leading up to the last menstrual period and at decreased risk afterward. However, similar to SWAN, women in POAS with a history of depressive episodes were 13 times more likely to experience severe depressive symptoms during perimenopause than those without a prior history [6]. Although 10% to 30% of women without a history of depression had significant depressive symptoms during perimenopause, this incidence dropped to 0% to 15% by the second year after their last menstrual period, a sharp decrease underlining the likely role of perimenopause [6]. Likewise, the Harvard Study of Moods and Cycles found that women with no history of depression were twice as likely to have depressive symptoms after entering perimenopause than those who remained premenopausal [7]. In summary, perimenopause confers an increased risk of depression for all women, particularly those with a prior history of the disease. Given that a significant percentage of women will experience either depressive symptoms or major depression during this window of time, all medical professionals who treat midlife women should consider screening for depression.

Although less well established than the data on perimenopausal depression, there is evidence that the perimenopausal window is also a time of increased risk for onset or recurrence of other mental illnesses, including bipolar disorder and schizophrenia [8–11]. For bipolar disorder in particular, studies suggest that depressive symptoms increase in perimenopause, but conclusions have been limited by the lack of prospective design and standardized menopausal staging [11,12]. There is also evidence for increased anxiety symptoms, although not necessarily anxiety disorders, during the perimenopausal window, with a link between vasomotor symptoms (VMS) (hot flashes and night sweats) and both anxiety and panic attacks [13–15]. Given that estrogen has demonstrated neuroprotective effects, promoting synaptic plasticity and decreasing inflammation [16], one theory as to why exacerbation occurs in this window is that the loss of neuroprotection can put perimenopausal women with a history of serious mental illness at risk for increased symptoms [17,18].

Fluctuations in other reproductive hormones, such as progesterone and its neuroactive steroid derivative, allopregnanolone, are also hypothesized to play a role [19].

An increased risk of substance use disorders may also exist during the perimenopausal transition. Theories as to the cause of this include the loss of the neuroprotective effects of estrogen cited earlier , as well as the lost benefit of estrogen in reducing impulsivity [18]. Women may also become more vulnerable to the effects of alcohol at lower levels of consumption as they age, with data suggesting that a subset of women may be at risk of transitioning to excessive drinking during the menopausal transition [20,21]. In addition, an increasing number of midlife women are using cannabis to alleviate symptoms of perimenopause, despite a lack of data showing efficacy for this purpose [22]. In one study of women with chronic pain, menopausal symptoms were associated with increased long-term opioid prescriptions, potentially conferring a risk of opioid dependence and opioid use disorder [23]. There may also be an increased risk of disorders of eating and body image during this window, but few studies have investigated this connection thus far [24,25].

Finally, in addition to representing a window of risk for the development or exacerbation of depressive and other psychiatric disorders in women, the menopausal transition is also notable for an increased incidence of a diverse array of other symptoms. As stated earlier, these include hot flashes and night sweats, difficulty falling asleep and staying asleep, cognitive challenges including memory problems and difficulty concentrating, sexual dysfunction, vaginal dryness, urinary incontinence, and joint pain [3]. As described in later sections, it is important to ask about such symptoms, which can overlap with the symptoms of depression, to properly diagnose and treat women at midlife and also to rule out more concerning causes, topics explored in the following section.

How perimenopause affects the assessment of women at midlife

Given that the menopausal transition is a time of increased risk for women experiencing new onset or recurrent major depression, universal screening for depression should be adopted by all providers treating women at midlife, similar to steps that have recently been taken to screen pregnant and postpartum women [26]. The United States Preventive Services Task Force began recommending universal depression screening for all adults in 2016. These recommendations give special attention to the risk of depression for women during pregnancy and postpartum, but fail to note perimenopause as an additional period of increased risk [27]. One recent survey of obstetricians/gynecologists found that 34% of respondents did not screen perimenopausal patients for depression and 44% did not feel confident in treating depression at this time of life [28].

Despite the need for depression screening during perimenopause, there is no consensus on exactly when to screen or which instrument to use [29]. Whether a woman has entered perimenopause is established clinically, by enquiring whether periods have become persistently irregular, defined by a greater than 7-day difference in the length of at least 2 cycles over the course of 10 months [30]. Because levels of sex hormones vary significantly throughout the day and month, checking them is not standard practice for establishing perimenopause [19,30,31]. The Meno-D, a perimenopause-specific brief screening instrument, was recently developed and validated, but is not yet in widespread use [32]. The Patient Health Questionnaire (PHQ-9), which has been validated for use in primary care settings, is appropriate for this population, although it does not ask about some of the somatic symptoms that can overlap with and complicate the diagnosis of major depression in perimenopause [33,34].

The physical symptoms of perimenopause may present independently of, exacerbate, or be worsened by depression. As described earlier, common complaints are hot flashes and night sweats, which are referred to collectively as VMS; sleep disturbances; cognitive symptoms; sexual, vaginal, or urinary symptoms; and joint pain [3,35]. When patients present to primary care providers with these complaints, it is important that co-occurrence of depression be considered. When midlife women present with depressed mood as their primary complaint, it is important that clinicians include in their review of systems questions about common perimenopausal symptoms (Box 1). Clinicians should also be prepared to counsel patients about the potential interconnection of mood and perimenopausal symptoms and to plan appropriate overlapping interventions. Three general instruments that can be used to elicit perimenopausal symptoms across different domains are the Menopause Rating Scale (11 items that focus on the domains listed previously) [36], the Menopause-Specific Quality of Life (23 items that cover broader topics such as feelings about home and work) [37], and the Greene Climacteric Scale (21 items that focus on specific physical symptoms) [38].

VMS are the most common perimenopausal symptoms, experienced by up to 80% of women during

Box 1
Questions to Include When Evaluating Midlife Women

How to Ask Patients About Specific Topics	
Onset of perimenopause	1. Have you noticed any changes in your menstrual cycle? Heavier, lighter, more irregular?
Vasomotor symptoms	2. Have you noticed any sudden sweating during the day? Do you ever wake at night hot and sweaty? Is your nightwear or bedding ever wet?
Sleep complaints	3. Have you been having any trouble sleeping?
Cognitive complaints	4. Are you having any trouble with forgetfulness or concentration?
Genitourinary complaints	5. Are you experiencing any bladder problems (frequency or incontinence), vaginal dryness, or pain with sex?
Somatic complaints	6. Are you noticing any changes in your body such as new weight gain or joint pain?

These topics can be remembered with the mnemonic: please make very good midlife suggestions (PMVGMS) = pain, memory, VMS, genitourinary, menstrual, sleep.

perimenopause [39]. VMS are closely related to the second most common perimenopausal symptom: sleep disturbance, experienced by 39% to 47% of women during perimenopause [40]. Research into the relationship between VMS and sleep disturbance suggests a more complex interplay than VMS simply causing sleep disturbance, and sleep problems can also exist independently of VMS [41]. The Hot Flash-Related Daily Interference Scale is one detailed instrument for measuring VMS [42], and the Insomnia Severity Index is an instrument for assessing sleep disturbance [43]. In practice, however, asking about the number, duration, and severity of hot flashes will reveal the extent to which VMS may be interfering with sleep or other activities. As discussed in the section "Treatment of Perimenopausal Depression," there is compelling evidence that several antidepressants can reduce the severity of VMS. For sleep, asking what time the patient fell asleep, what time they awoke, and the causes, number, and duration of middle-of-the-night interruptions will start to reveal problematic patterns and additional relevant information and provide the basis for recommending behavioral interventions or further investigation (Fig. 1). Of note, obstructive sleep apnea and restless leg syndrome are 2 of the more common causes of sleep disturbance in this population [44]. Assessing whether perimenopausal depression is accompanied by VMS with or without sleep disturbance can clarify contributors to low mood and guide treatment.

Another common perimenopausal symptom is cognitive change. Women most frequently report subjective problems with verbal memory, such as losing objects, forgetting names or words, or forgetting whether information has been shared or received from others. These symptoms were experienced by 50% or more of the women in SWAN [3,45,46]. SWAN also found a transient decrease in expected learning during perimenopause using an objective measure, while also noting that the presence of anxiety and depression symptoms negatively affected cognitive performance across different domains [47]. Problems with subjective executive functioning have also been investigated [48,49]. However, extant studies demonstrate cognitive complaints during perimenopause to be primarily subjective, not severe, and transient. If cognitive complaints are severe or advancing noticeably, further investigation using standard tools such as the Montreal Cognitive Assessment and additional workup is important to accurately identify the cause (Fig. 2) [50].

If severe or advancing cognitive complaints have been ruled out, one question to explore is that of worsening or previously undiagnosed attention-deficit disorder/hyperactivity disorder (ADHD), given the underdiagnosis of women with this condition [51]. No studies have thus far been published characterizing the effects of perimenopause on the symptoms or treatment of patients with ADHD, including any potential effects of menopausal hormone therapy (MHT) [52].

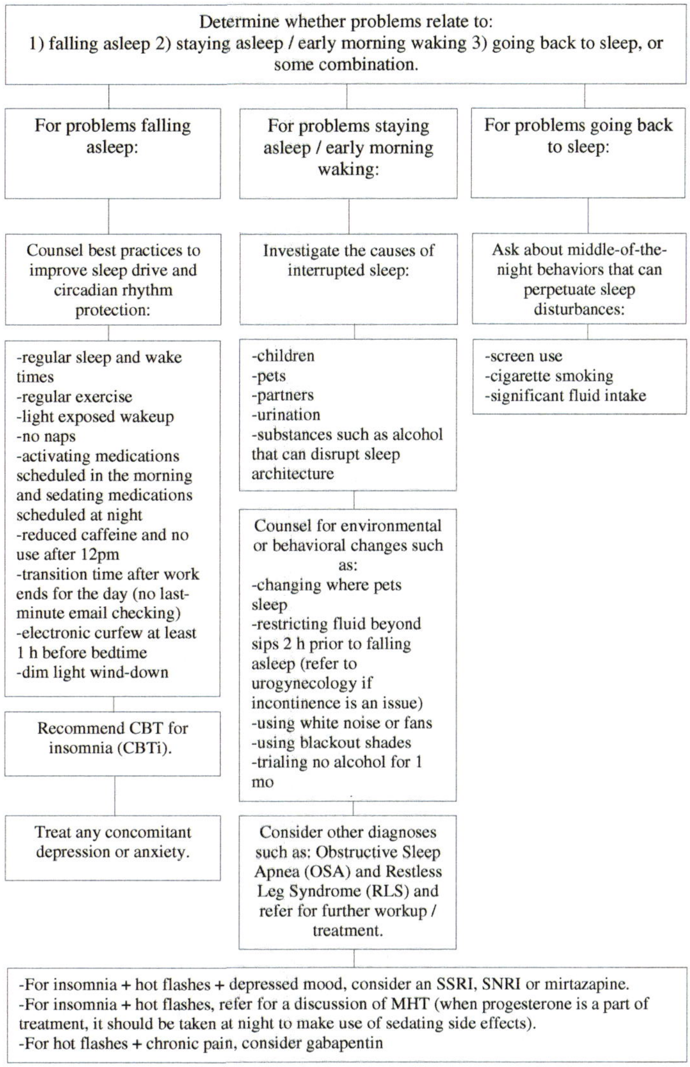

FIG. 1 Steps for addressing sleep problems. CBTi, CBT for insomnia; OSA, obstructive sleep apnea; RLS, restless leg syndrome.

Two studies, however, have looked at the efficacy of lisdexamfetamine in women with new-onset executive function difficulties during the menopausal transition, without a formal diagnosis of ADHD. Both trials found benefit for cognitive symptoms [48,49].

Additional common symptoms of perimenopause include pain with sex, vaginal dryness, and urinary frequency and incontinence. These symptoms may be either directly related to the impact of estrogen withdrawal on tissue health or influenced by factors such as: mechanical problems caused by childbearing; social and relationship stressors; past experiences of trauma; or exacerbations of depression and anxiety [3,53,54]. Although problems in these domains may significantly affect a woman's quality of life, she may neither volunteer these complaints unless asked nor be aware that treatment exists. Identifying issues in these domains and referring patients to appropriate providers such as urogynecologists or pelvic floor physical therapists, or to treatment options such as vaginal estrogen cream or over-the-counter lubricants, may form an important component of the treatment of depression. Finally, providers may want to ask about joint pain or other episodic or chronic pain, which can present at midlife

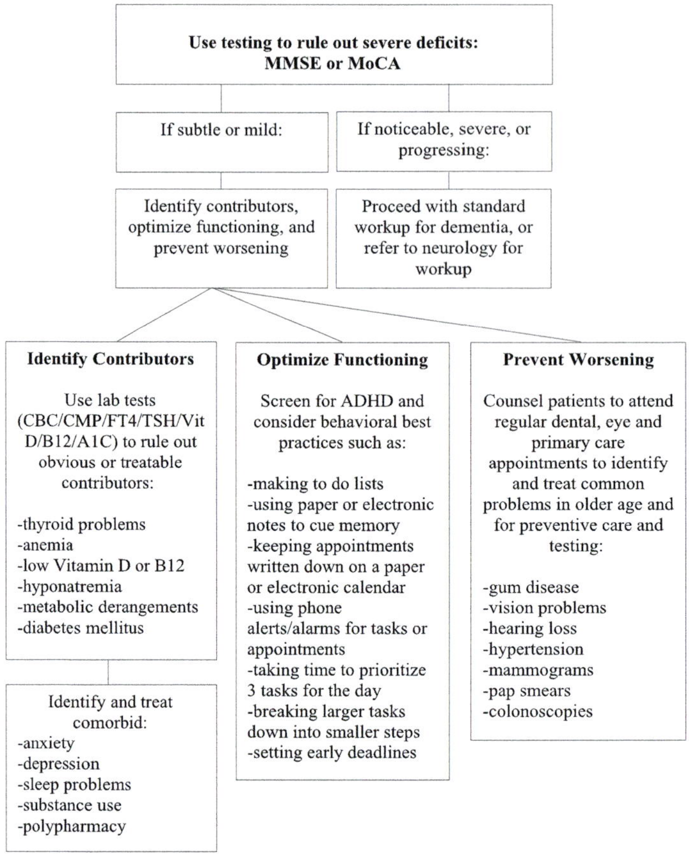

FIG. 2 Steps for addressing cognitive complaints. ADHD, attention-deficit/hyperactivity disorder; CBC, complete blood cell count; HBA$_{1c}$, glycated haemoglobin A$_{1c}$; MoCA, Montreal Cognitive Assessment; TSH, thyrotropin.

and may affect sleep, depression, capacity to engage in physical activity, or make patients more at risk of opioid dependence. Such comorbidities may also guide treatment recommendations of specific agents, as discussed in the section "Treatment of Perimenopausal Depression."

In addition to screening for depression and asking about perimenopausal symptoms, the treatment of women's mental health at midlife should include assessing factors that could contribute to or worsen symptoms, such as inadequate nutrition or unhealthy eating habits, tobacco use, excessive caffeine intake, and the misuse of alcohol, cannabis, or illegal substances. Women in this age group are at greater risk of thyroid disorders, which can also mimic perimenopausal symptoms in their presentation, thus thyroid function should be regularly assessed [55]. Checking a complete blood cell count, comprehensive metabolic panel, and vitamin B$_{12}$ and vitamin D levels may be appropriate, similar to psychiatric evaluation at other times of life.

Treatment of perimenopausal depression

As described earlier, the first step in treating women at midlife is a thorough assessment, identifying not only symptoms of depression but also symptoms of perimenopause that may be co-occurring and require treatment.

For mild to moderate depression, psychotherapy may be sufficient, as at other times of life, along with educating patients about lifestyle and behavioral modifications. Important behaviors to address are improving sleep hygiene and reducing caffeine, alcohol, cannabis, and the use of other substances that can negatively affect sleep, cognition, and mood. Increasing exercise, particularly strength training, may help regulate sleep, improve

Box 2
Medications to Consider in Perimenopause

Agents with evidence supporting use for both depression and VMS[a]	
SSRIs	Citalopram, escitalopram, fluoxetine, paroxetine
SNRIs	Duloxetine, venlafaxine, desvenlafaxine
Other	Mirtazapine and vortioxetine
Other agents to consider	
MHT	• Clear evidence of benefit for VMS, less clear whether evidence shows benefit for depression when combined with progesterone (required to prevent increased risk of endometrial cancer in women with a uterus) • Indicated for women with bothersome VMS who are younger than 60 y or within 10 y of menopause and have no contraindications • Some evidence of benefit for women with schizophrenia
Gabapentin/pregabalin	May be helpful in treating VMS in women who cannot take MHT or who also have chronic nerve pain
Antipsychotics (neuroleptics)	Efficacy and bioavailability can be reduced by low-estrogen states; therefore, midlife women reliant on them may need an increase in dose or change to depot formulation

[a]Therapeutic doses of antidepressants for treating VMS alone without depression are typically much lower, for example, venlafaxine 37.5 mg for VMS versus 150 mg for depression.

energy, and mitigate the loss of muscle mass and bone density that occurs in perimenopause [56].

For moderate to severe perimenopausal depression, antidepressants are indicated and remain the gold standard, in addition to therapy and behavioral modifications. The only randomized controlled double-blind studies of antidepressants in the perimenopausal population have been of desvenlafaxine [34,57]. Given the lack of clinical trials in this population, clinicians should use medications that have worked previously for patients with a history of benefit from specific antidepressants. For patients who have not taken antidepressants in the past, there is evidence that many SSRIs and SNRIs also have efficacy for VMS, so one of these can be initiated. Agents with specific evidence of benefit for both depression and VMS include several SSRIs (citalopram, escitalopram, fluoxetine, paroxetine), the SNRIs (duloxetine, venlafaxine, desvenlafaxine), and mirtazapine and vortioxetine (Box 2) [34,58,59]. For patients with chronic pain as part of their presentation, SNRIs appeal as potentially offering the triple benefit of treating pain, VMS, and depression. In addition, for those patients who may benefit from the use of gabapentin/pregabalin (eg, for neuropathic pain or other indications) or clonidine, there is also some evidence of these agents' efficacy for VMS [58,59].

Women may ask about supplements or alternative treatments for perimenopausal depression or VMS, and it is important for clinicians to be familiar with the evidence and risks surrounding these [60]. The 2015 Position Statement of the North American Menopause Society provides a useful summary of the current data on nonhormonal treatments for VMS [58]. In particular, the popular supplements evening primrose oil (*Oenothera biennis*) and dong quai (*Angelica sinensis*) have been found to have no benefit over placebo and may confer significant risks, such as anticoagulation [58,61]. There is some evidence that regulated extracts of black cohosh may reduce VMS; however, most black cohosh products are sold as unregulated food supplements that have been found to be ineffective when compared with placebo and may contain adulterated ingredients with risk of harm [62,63]. There is a small study showing that chasteberry (*Vitex agnus-castus*) may help with VMS, with possible safety concerns for women with hormone-sensitive cancers [64].

For women with both depression and VMS for whom antidepressants do not sufficiently treat hot flashes or night sweats, estrogen remains the gold standard for treating VMS. MHT was widely used before the Women's Health Initiative (WHI) study, which was stopped early due to data suggesting overall increased risk of cardiovascular disease in postmenopausal women [65]. Subsequent analyses of the WHI data revealed minimal risk in younger women, and the current recommendation is to consider MHT for women with bothersome VMS who are younger than 60 or within 10 years of menopause and have no contraindications (such as a history of breast cancer, venous thromboembolism, or myocardial infarction) [66].

The question of whether MHT can treat or prevent perimenopausal depression remains unsettled. Multiple studies of estrogen alone have suggested benefits for mood, but the effects when combined with progesterone (required in women with a uterus to prevent increased risk of endometrial cancer) are less clear, and differences in study design, lack of studies specific to the perimenopausal population, and the paucity of studies comparing MHT to antidepressants have hampered clear conclusions and make this an ongoing area of research [34,67,68]. Current guidelines suggest considering MHT for treatment of perimenopausal depression with caution or when there are other indications for its use such as VMS [34]. If MHT is desired, referral is typically made to a primary care provider or gynecologist with competence in this area.

Treatment of other mental illnesses during perimenopause

Estrogen increases the efficacy and bioavailability of the antipsychotic/neuroleptic class of medications, thus waning estrogen in perimenopause may make these medications less effective [18]. Women who rely on neuroleptics, whether for bipolar disorder, schizophrenia, delusional disorder, obsessive-compulsive disorder, or treatment-resistant depression, may be at risk of recurrence of symptoms during perimenopause simply because the physiologic changes of perimenopause may cause their dose to become ineffective [18,69,70]. In women for whom an antipsychotic has efficacy that wanes in perimenopause, increasing the dose is an obvious first step. If a higher dose is ineffective or intolerable, switching to a depot formulation, which avoids first-pass metabolism and thus may be less affected by estrogen's influence on hepatic enzymes, is an alternative [17,71].

In addition, midlife women with schizophrenia often benefit psychiatrically from adjunctive MHT, which has been shown to decrease psychotic and cognitive symptoms in this population, and also to improve negative symptoms [17]. Depression, which burdens the large majority of people with schizophrenia, may also be improved in women with schizophrenia treated with MHT through the menopausal transition and beyond [17].

For women with treatment-resistant schizophrenia for whom adjunctive MHT is contraindicated, the selective estrogen receptor modulator raloxifene hydrochloride may be an option to treat both the positive and negative symptoms of schizophrenia [72]. Raloxifene has been associated with reduced cognitive impairment in both healthy women after menopause and women with schizophrenia [72,73]. Although it has not been directly studied in this population, raloxifene may also prove useful for women with treatment-resistant bipolar disorder who are unable to take MHT [74].

Perimenopause as a window of risk and opportunity

In conclusion, perimenopause, like the perinatal period, confers an increased risk of mood symptoms for women who are vulnerable to hormonal fluctuations, as well as multiple other potentially overlapping problems. Given the high incidence of depressive episodes during perimenopause, primary care providers who treat women in their 40s and 50s should implement universal screening for depression, and psychiatric clinicians should be aware of and screen for concomitant symptoms of VMS, sleep disturbance, cognitive complaints, genitourinary problems, and joint pain. As at other stages of life, screening laboratory tests, including a thyroid panel, may be indicated. For problems such as cognitive changes that are severe or rapidly advancing, further evaluation, workup, and referral is warranted.

Treating perimenopausal depression successfully will involve attention to those agents that have worked well for patients in the past, as well as a knowledge of which agents might treat overlapping symptoms such as VMS, sleep disturbance, or pain. Assessing, treating, and making appropriate referrals for additional perimenopausal symptoms that affect quality of life should not be overlooked.

CLINICAL VIGNETTE POSTSCRIPT

Returning to the case of the 47-year-old woman presenting with 2 months of depressive symptoms, her history suggests sensitivity to hormonal fluctuations, a prior episode of depression, and daily alcohol use, all of which may increase her risk for perimenopausal depression. You gather further history and ask targeted questions about the domains often affected by perimenopause (see Box 1); this reveals irregular periods over the past year, sleep interrupted 3 to 4 times a night by hot flashes, diminished attention and motivation at work, vaginal dryness causing pain with sex, and a 4.5-kg weight gain over the past 6 months. You assess her as experiencing a recurrence of depression. Given that she responded well in the past to an antidepressant that also has efficacy for hot flashes, you recommend that she restart this medication with the goal of treating depression, VMS, and interrupted sleep. If this trial is helpful for low mood but insufficient for VMS, MHT can be considered to treat VMS and may also improve vaginal dryness. In the meantime, you advise her to try an over-the-counter lubricant before sex. You also ask her to consider a trial of no alcohol for 1 month to see if this helps with sleep, concentration, irritability, and weight loss. Additional behavior changes that could help include improved sleep hygiene, regular exercise, and exploring whether work/life boundaries need to be asserted or whether more social support can be sought. You recommend a course of psychotherapy to work on these and other potential goals. Given her full recovery from her previous episode of depression, her prognosis is excellent.

CLINICS CARE POINTS

- When evaluating midlife women, determine perimenopausal status by asking whether periods have become irregular.
- For women in perimenopause with somatic complaints, screen for depression, which can contribute to or exacerbate physical perimenopausal symptoms.
- For women in perimenopause with depression or flares of mental illness, screen for somatic symptoms, especially sleep disturbance and VMS, which can contribute to or exacerbate depression.
- A useful mnemonic for perimenopausal symptoms is: please make very good midlife suggestions (PMVGMS): pain, memory, VMS (hot flashes and night sweats), genitourinary problems, menstruation, sleep.
- Screen midlife woman for substance use disorders, which can contribute to or exacerbate depression or somatic symptoms.
- For women with both depression and VMS, consider antidepressants that can treat both.
- For woman with only VMS, MHT is the gold standard for women within 10 years of menopause or younger than 60 without contraindications.
- For women reliant on neuroleptics, watch for loss of efficacy due to waning estrogen reducing bioavailability; a dose increase or a change to depot formulation may be required.

ACKNOWLEDGMENTS

The authors would like to acknowledge Katherine E. Williams, MD, and C. Neill Epperson, MD, whose involvement in our prior writing on perimenopause has helped shape our ideas.

DISCLOSURE

Neither author has any commercial or financial conflicts of interest. Dr N. Leistikow receives support from NIMH grant 5R37MH121564-03.

REFERENCES

[1] Gold EB, Bromberger J, Crawford S, et al. Factors associated with age at natural menopause in a multiethnic sample of midlife women. Am J Epidemiol 2001;153(9):865–74.

[2] Paramsothy P, Harlow SD, Nan B, et al. Duration of the menopausal transition is longer in women with young age at onset: the multi-ethnic Study of Women's Health Across the Nation. Menopause N Y N 2017;24(2):142–9.

[3] Woods NF, Mitchell ES. The Seattle Midlife Women's Health Study: a longitudinal prospective study of women during the menopausal transition and early postmenopause. Womens Midlife Health 2016;2(1):6.

[4] Bromberger JT, Kravitz HM, Chang YF, Cyranowski JM, Brown C, Matthews KA. Major depression during and after the menopausal transition: study of women's health across the nation (SWAN). Psychol Med 2011;41(9):1879–88.

[5] Bromberger JT, Schott L, Kravitz HM, Joffe H. Risk factors for major depression during midlife among a community sample of women with and without prior major depression: Are they the same or different? Psychol Med 2015. https://doi.org/10.1017/S0033291714002773.

[6] Freeman EW, Sammel MD, Boorman DW, Zhang R. Longitudinal pattern of depressive symptoms around natural menopause. JAMA Psychiatry 2014;71(1):36–43.

[7] Cohen LS, Soares CN, Vitonis AF, Otto MW, Harlow BL. Risk for new onset of depression during the menopausal transition: the harvard study of moods and cycles. Arch Gen Psychiatry 2006;63(4):385–90.

[8] Crow E, Jasberg S, Crow EA. Schizophrenia during Menopausal Transition. Ment Health Fam Med 2016;12(02). https://doi.org/10.25149/1756-8358.1202005.

[9] Gupta R, Assalman I, Bottlender R. Menopause and schizophrenia. Menopause Int 2012;18(1):10–4.
[10] Hu LY, Shen CC, Hung JH, et al. Risk of psychiatric disorders following symptomatic menopausal transition. Medicine (Baltimore) 2016;95(6):e2800.
[11] Perich T, Ussher J, Meade T. Menopause and illness course in bipolar disorder: a systematic review. Bipolar Disord 2017;19(6):434–43.
[12] Truong D, Marsh W. Bipolar disorder in the menopausal transition. Curr Psychiatry Rep 2019;21(12):130.
[13] Bromberger JT, Kravitz HM, Chang Y, et al. Does risk for anxiety increase during the menopausal transition? Study of Women's Health Across the Nation. Menopause 2013; 20(5):488–95.
[14] Hantsoo L, Epperson CN. Anxiety disorders among women: a female lifespan approach. FOCUS 2017; 15(2):162–72.
[15] Freeman EW, Sammel MD. Anxiety as a risk factor for menopausal hot flashes: evidence from the penn ovarian aging cohort. Menopause 2016;23(9):942–9.
[16] Yilmaz C, Karali K, Fodelianaki G, et al. Neurosteroids as regulators of neuroinflammation. Front Neuroendocrinol 2019;55. https://doi.org/10.1016/j.yfrne.2019.100788.
[17] Brzezinski A, Brzezinski-Sinai NA, Seeman MV. Treating schizophrenia during menopause. Menopause 2017; 24(5):582–8.
[18] Brand BA, de Boer JN, Sommer IEC. Estrogens in schizophrenia: progress, current challenges and opportunities. Curr Opin Psychiatry 2021;34(3):228–37.
[19] Gordon JL, Girdler SS, Meltzer-Brody SE, et al. Ovarian hormone fluctuation, neurosteroids, and HPA axis dysregulation in perimenopausal depression: a novel heuristic model. Am J Psychiatry 2015;172(3):227–36.
[20] Milic J, Glisic M, Voortman T, et al. Menopause, ageing, and alcohol use disorders in women. Maturitas 2018; 111:100–9.
[21] Peltier MR, Verplaetse TL, Roberts W, et al. Changes in excessive alcohol use among older women across the menopausal transition: a longitudinal analysis of the Study of Women's Health Across the Nation. Biol Sex Differ 2020;11:37.
[22] Mejia-Gomez J, Phung N, Philippopoulos E, Murphy KE, Wolfman W. The impact of cannabis use on vasomotor symptoms, mood, insomnia and sexuality in perimenopausal and postmenopausal women: a systematic review. Climacteric J Int Menopause Soc 2021;24(6):572–6.
[23] Gibson CJ, Li Y, Huang AJ, Rife T, Seal KH. Menopausal symptoms and higher risk opioid prescribing in a national sample of women veterans with chronic pain. J Gen Intern Med 2019;34(10):2159–66.
[24] Baker JH, Runfola CD. Eating disorders in midlife women: a perimenopausal eating disorder? Maturitas 2016;85:112–6.
[25] Mangweth-Matzek B, Rupp CI, Vedova S, et al. Disorders of eating and body image during the menopausal transition: associations with menopausal stage and with menopausal symptomatology. Eat Weight Disord EWD 2021. https://doi.org/10.1007/s40519-021-01141-4.
[26] Kendig S, Keats JP, Hoffman MC, et al. Consensus bundle on maternal mental health. Obstet Gynecol 2017;129(3):422–30.
[27] Siu AL, the US Preventive Services Task Force (USPSTF). Screening for depression in adults: US preventive services task force recommendation statement. JAMA 2016; 315(4):380–7.
[28] Raglan GB, Schulkin J, Juliano LM, Micks EA. Obstetrician-gynecologists' screening and management of depression during perimenopause. Menopause 2020;27(4): 393–7.
[29] Willi J, Ehlert U. Assessment of perimenopausal depression: a review. J Affect Disord 2019;249:216–22.
[30] Harlow SD, Gass M, Hall JE, et al. Executive summary of the stages of reproductive aging workshop + 10: Addressing the unfinished agenda of staging reproductive aging. J Clin Endocrinol Metab 2012. https://doi.org/10.1210/jc.2011-3362.
[31] American College of Obstetricians and Gynecologists Committee on Gynecologic Practice, American Society for Reproductive Medicine Practice Committee. Compounded bioidentical menopausal hormone therapy. Fertil Steril 2012;98(2):308–12.
[32] Kulkarni J, Gavrilidis E, Hudaib AR, Bleeker C, Worsley R, Gurvich C. Development and validation of a new rating scale for perimenopausal depression—the Meno-D. Transl Psychiatry 2018;8:123.
[33] Arroll B, Goodyear-Smith F, Crengle S, et al. Validation of PHQ-2 and PHQ-9 to screen for major depression in the primary care population. Ann Fam Med 2010; 8(4):348–53.
[34] Maki PM, Kornstein SG, Joffe H, et al. Guidelines for the evaluation and treatment of perimenopausal depression: summary and recommendations. J Womens Health 2019;28(2):117–34.
[35] Woods NF, Mitchell ES. Symptoms during the perimenopause: Prevalence, severity, trajectory, and significance in women's lives. Am J Med 2005;118:14–24. https://doi.org/10.1016/j.amjmed.2005.09.031, Elsevier Inc.;.
[36] Heinemann K, Ruebig A, Potthoff P, et al. The Menopause Rating Scale (MRS) scale: a methodological review. Health Qual Life Outcomes 2004;2:45.
[37] Hilditch JR, Lewis J, Peter A, et al. A menopause-specific quality of life questionnaire: development and psychometric properties. Maturitas 1996;24(6):161–75.
[38] Greene JG. A factor analytic study of climacteric symptoms. J Psychosom Res 1976;20(5):425–30.
[39] Avis NE, Crawford SL, Green R. Vasomotor symptoms across the menopause transition differences among women. Obstet Gynecol Clin North Am 2018;45: 629–40.
[40] Kravitz HM, Zhao X, Bromberger J, et al. Sleep disturbance during the menopausal transition in a multiethnic community sample of women. Sleep 2008; 31(7):979–90.

[41] Thurston RC, Chang Y, Buysse DJ, Hall MH, Matthews KA. Hot flashes and awakenings among midlife women. Sleep 2019;42(9). https://doi.org/10.1093/sleep/zsz131.
[42] Carpenter JS. The Hot Flash Related Daily Interference Scale: a tool for assessing the impact of hot flashes on quality of life following breast cancer. J Pain Symptom Manage 2001;22(6):979–89.
[43] Morin CM, Belleville G, Bélanger L, Ivers H. The insomnia severity index: psychometric indicators to detect insomnia cases and evaluate treatment response. Sleep 2011;34(5):601–8.
[44] Joffe H, Massler A, Sharkey KM. Evaluation and management of sleep disturbance during the menopause transition. Semin Reprod Med 2010. https://doi.org/10.1055/s-0030-1262900.
[45] Epperson CN, Sammel MD, Freeman EW. Menopause effects on verbal memory: findings from a longitudinal community cohort. J Clin Endocrinol Metab 2013;98(9):3829–38.
[46] Woods NF, Mitchell ES, Adams C. Memory functioning among midlife women: observations from the seattle midlife women's health study. Menopause 2000;7(4):257–65.
[47] Greendale GA, Wight RG, Huang MH, et al. Menopause-associated symptoms and cognitive performance: results from the study of women's health across the nation. Am J Epidemiol 2010;171(11):1214–24.
[48] Epperson CN, Shanmugan S, Kim DR, et al. New onset executive function difficulties at menopause: a possible role for lisdexamfetamine. Psychopharmacology (Berl) 2015;232(16):3091–100.
[49] Shanmugan S, Loughead J, Nanga RPR, et al. Lisdexamfetamine effects on executive activation and neurochemistry in menopausal women with executive function difficulties. Neuropsychopharmacol 2017;42(2):437–45.
[50] Nasreddine ZS, Phillips NA, Bédirian V, et al. The Montreal Cognitive Assessment, MoCA: a brief screening tool for mild cognitive impairment. J Am Geriatr Soc 2005;53(4):695–9.
[51] Quinn PO, Madhoo M. A review of attention-deficit/hyperactivity disorder in women and girls: uncovering this hidden diagnosis. Prim Care Companion CNS Disord 2014;16(3). https://doi.org/10.4088/PCC.13r01596.
[52] Camara B, Padoin C, Bolea B. Relationship between sex hormones, reproductive stages and ADHD: a systematic review. Arch Womens Ment Health 2021. https://doi.org/10.1007/s00737-021-01181-w.
[53] Avis NE, Colvin A, Karlamangla AS, et al. Change in sexual functioning over the menopausal transition: results from the Study of Women's Health Across the Nation. Menopause 2017;24(4):379–90.
[54] Waetjen LE, Crawford SL, Chang PY, et al. Factors associated with developing vaginal dryness symptoms in women transitioning through menopause: a longitudinal study. Menopause 2018;25(10):1094–104.
[55] Stuenkel CA. Thyroid disease in women at midlife. NEJM J Watch 2014;2014. https://doi.org/10.1056/nejm-jw.NA34807.
[56] Sipilä S, Törmäkangas T, Sillanpää E, et al. Muscle and bone mass in middle-aged women: role of menopausal status and physical activity. J Cachexia Sarcopenia Muscle 2020;11(3):698–709.
[57] Clayton AH, Kornstein SG, Dunlop BW, et al. Efficacy and safety of desvenlafaxine 50 mg/d in a randomized, placebo-controlled study of perimenopausal and postmenopausal women with major depressive disorder. J Clin Psychiatry 2013;74(10):1010–7.
[58] Carpenter J, Gass MLS, Maki PM, et al. Nonhormonal management of menopause-Associated vasomotor symptoms: 2015 position statement of the North American Menopause Society. Menopause 2015;22(11):1155–74.
[59] Joffe H, Soares CN, Cohen LS. Assessment and treatment of hot flushes and menopausal mood disturbance. Psychiatr Clin North Am 2003;26(3):563–80.
[60] Hutner LA, Catapano L, Nagle-Yang SM, et al, editors. Textbook of women's reproductive mental health. 1st edition. American Psychiatric Association Publishing; 2021.
[61] Kronenberg F, Fugh-Berman A. Complementary and alternative medicine for menopausal symptoms: a review of randomized, controlled trials. Ann Intern Med 2002;137(10):805–13.
[62] Leach MJ, Moore V. Black cohosh (Cimicifuga spp.) for menopausal symptoms. Cochrane Database Syst Rev 2012;9:CD007244.
[63] Castelo-Branco C, Gambacciani M, Cano A, et al. Review & meta-analysis: isopropanolic black cohosh extract iCR for menopausal symptoms – an update on the evidence. Climacteric 2021;24(2):109–19.
[64] Naseri R, Farnia V, Yazdchi K, Alikhani M, Basanj B, Salemi S. Comparison of vitex agnus-castus extracts with placebo in reducing menopausal symptoms: a randomized double-blind study. Korean J Fam Med 2019;40(6):362–7.
[65] Chester RC, Kling JM, Manson JAE. What the Women's Health Initiative has taught us about menopausal hormone therapy. Clin Cardiol 2018;41(2):247–52.
[66] Pinkerton JAV, Aguirre FS, Blake J, et al. The 2017 hormone therapy position statement of the North American Menopause Society. Menopause 2017;24(7):728–53.
[67] Gordon JL, Eisenlohr-Moul TA, Rubinow DR, Girdler SS, Xia K, Schmidt PJ. Efficacy of transdermal estradiol and micronized progesterone in the prevention of depressive symptoms in the menopause transition. JAMA Psychiatry 2018. https://doi.org/10.1001/jamapsychiatry.2017.3998.
[68] Rubinow DR, Johnson SL, Schmidt PJ, Girdler S, Gaynes B. Efficacy of estradiol in perimenopausal depression: so much promise and so few answers. Depress Anxiety 2015;32(8):539–49.

[69] González-Rodríguez A, Catalán R, Penadés R, et al. Antipsychotic response worsens with postmenopausal duration in women with schizophrenia. J Clin Psychopharmacol 2016;36(6):580–7.

[70] González-Rodríguez A, Guàrdia A, Palao DJ, Labad J, Seeman MV. Moderators and mediators of antipsychotic response in delusional disorder: Further steps are needed. World J Psychiatry 2020;10(4):34–45.

[71] Seeman MV. Treating schizophrenia at the time of menopause. Maturitas 2012;72(2):117–20.

[72] Kulkarni J, Gurvich C, Lee SJ, et al. Piloting the effective therapeutic dose of adjunctive selective estrogen receptor modulator treatment in postmenopausal women with schizophrenia. Psychoneuroendocrinology 2010;35(8):1142–7.

[73] Yang ZD, Yu J, Zhang Q. Effects of raloxifene on cognition, mental health, sleep and sexual function in menopausal women: a systematic review of randomized controlled trials. Maturitas 2013;75(4):341–8.

[74] Torrey EF, Davis JM. Adjunct treatments for schizophrenia and bipolar disorder: what to try when you are out of ideas. Clin Schizophr Relat Psychoses 2012;5(4):208–16.

Advances in Psychiatry and Behavioral Health 2 (2022) 119–132

ADVANCES IN PSYCHIATRY AND BEHAVIORAL HEALTH

Infertility and Its Association with Depression, Anxiety, and Emotional Distress: A Current Review

Neha Shroff Hudepohl, MD[a,*], Kelsey Smith, MD[b]

[a]Department of Psychiatry, University of South Carolina School of Medicine Greenville/Prisma Health, 701 Grove Road, Greenville, SC 29605, USA; [b]Prisma Health/University of South Carolina School of Medicine Greenville – Psychiatry Residency Program (Greenville), 701 Grove Road, Greenville, SC 29605, USA

KEYWORDS

• Infertility • Mental health • Assisted reproductive technology • Depression • Stress • Anxiety

KEY POINTS

- Depression, anxiety, and emotional distress have higher rates in infertility than in the general population, and quality of life is often negatively affected.
- Depression, anxiety, and emotional distress may affect assisted reproductive technology (ART) outcomes, but this is controversial.
- ART and associated medications can worsen psychiatric outcomes and symptoms in susceptible individuals.
- Psychotherapy is considered first-line treatment of depression and anxiety in infertility, with multiple effective treatment modalities.
- Certain psychotropic medications may cause or exacerbate infertility through their effect on the HPG axis and other biological risk factors.

INTRODUCTION

Infertility is a complex medical phenomenon with potential for profound impact on mental health (MH). Infertility is defined as the failure to establish a clinical pregnancy after 12 months (before age 35 years), 6 months (after age 35 years), or anytime (after age 40 years) of regular, unprotected sexual intercourse [1,2]. The relationship between infertility and MH is bidirectional; infertility is known to increase the risk of stress, depression, and anxiety, and is affected by the same [3]. Various biological factors contribute to the cause of infertility (Table 1), as well as age and medical, menstrual, and sexual history [2,4]. Medications used in assisted reproductive technology (ART) have neuropsychiatric impact and may exacerbate underlying MH conditions (Table 2). MH care in infertility is a critical aspect of treatment and is more commonly provided in fertility clinics using evidence-based approaches than by primary psychiatric providers [5].

*Corresponding author, *E-mail address:* neha.hudepohl@prismahealth.org

https://doi.org/10.1016/j.ypsc.2022.05.005

TABLE 1
Common Male and Female Factors Related to Infertility

Male factors	Sperm	Oligospermia or azoospermia Decreased sperm motility Abnormal sperm morphology Varicocele Retrograde ejaculation
	Testicular	Unilateral or bilateral cryptorchidism Hypogonadism
Female factors	Ovulatory dysfunction	Maternal age Amenorrhea Polycystic ovarian syndrome HPG axis dysfunction Eating disorders Medication-induced (eg, antidepressants, antipsychotics, corticosteroids)
	Uterine or tubal	Fallopian tube obstruction Pelvic adhesions Pelvic inflammatory disease Structural uterine anomalies (eg, bicornuate uterus) Uterine leiomyoma Endometriosis
	Endocrine	Thyroid dysfunction Pituitary adenoma/hyperprolactinemia

Data from Zegers-Hochschild FG, Adamson D, Dyer S, et al. The international glossary on infertility and fertility care. Hum Reprod 2017;23(9):1786-1801; and Cunningham J. Infertility: A primer for primary care providers. JAAPA 2017;30(9):19-25.

PREVALENCE, CAUSE, AND EVALUATION OF INFERTILITY

Prevalence/Incidence

Infertility affects 15% of reproductive-aged couples in the United States [2], with wide ranges in global prevalence due to inconsistency in definitions [6–8]. Approximately 12% of women of reproductive age undergo infertility evaluation annually [4]. Approximately 37% of infertility cases are attributed to female factors, 8% to male factors, and 35% to combined factors; the remaining 20% are unexplained [2,4]. ART interventions (Table 3) grow in prevalence each year [9]. Between 42% and 76% of women with infertility seek treatment [4,10].

Causes of Infertility

Many causes of infertility are conditions associated with psychiatric illness or symptoms. Polycystic ovarian syndrome (PCOS) is a common cause of infertility that affects 6% to 10% of women of reproductive age. One study reported a prevalence of infertility as high as 73% in women who report PCOS compared with those who do not [11,12]. PCOS is also associated with higher rates of anxiety and depression, as well as eating disorders, particularly binge-eating disorder [13,14]. Endometriosis also has high rates of infertility, and a 2021 retrospective matched-cohort study revealed higher rates of depression, anxiety, and self-directed violence in women with endometriosis compared with those without [15]. Pelvic pain in endometriosis has also been associated with higher levels of depression [16,17]. Autoimmune thyroid disorders are associated with infertility and higher rates of pregnancy loss. Thyroid disorders are known to contribute to changes in mood, energy, anxiety, and depression [18–21]. Common pathways may link many of these illnesses to both infertility and psychiatric symptoms and are discussed later.

Evaluation

Initial evaluation for infertility is conducted after 12 months of frequent, unprotected intercourse when the female partner is younger than 35 years without known risk factors, after 6 months from 35 to 40 years,

TABLE 2
Assisted Reproductive Technology Medications and Potential Neuropsychiatric Impact in Infertility

ART Medication	Use in ART	Potential Neuropsychiatric Impact in Infertility
COCPs	Suppression of HPG axis and ovulation	Mood destabilization in women with history of sensitivity to COCPs
CC	SERM leading to ovarian stimulation and follicular development	Mood lability Insomnia Decreased libido Case reports of transient psychosis [75,76,78]
Gonadotropins	Increase ovarian follicular stimulation Associated with high serum estradiol levels [99]	Mood lability Increased depressive symptoms while moving from follicular phase to luteal phase of menstrual cycle (with changes in estrogen levels), particularly in women with previous history of anxiety or depression [76,77,100]
AI: letrozole	Decrease peripheral conversion of androgens to estrogen creating a low estrogen state, increasing FSH and LH levels leading to ovarian follicular stimulation [100]	No studies in women undergoing fertility treatment Reports of depression, anxiety, memory, and concentration issues when used for cancer treatment [101]
GnRH agonists and antagonists	Used in IVF to prevent premature ovulation leading to temporary hypogonadal state [102]	With long-term exposure: hot flashes, sleep disturbance, irritability, depressed mood and mood lability, memory/concentration difficulties Short-term exposure: not associated with significant mood changes in some studies [103]; in others, increased mood lability with elevated baseline mood lability and/or neuroticism [103,104]
Progesterone	Endometrial support of implantation and embryo development	Synthetic progestins associated with depression and anxiety in some women [105,106]
Metformin	Oral insulin-sensitizing medication used in PCOS to decrease insulin resistance at ovulation induction	Potential improvement in depression and anxiety symptoms [107]
Bromocriptine and cabergoline	Ergot-derived D2 agonists used in patients with hyperprolactinemia	Hypomania or psychosis, especially in patients with preexisting mood or psychotic disorders [78,79] Increased risk of impulse-control disorders [108]
Corticosteroids	Enhance uterine receptivity especially with history of recurrent pregnancy loss or failed IVF cycles	Insomnia, irritability, anxiety, new-onset mania or psychosis, depression, suicidality [80]

Abbreviations: AI, aromatase inhibitors; CC, clomiphene citrate; COCP, combination oral contraceptives; GnRH, gonadotropin-releasing hormone; HPG, hypothalamic-pituitary-gonadal; IVF, in vitro fertilization; PCOS, polycystic ovarian syndrome; SERM, selective estrogen receptor modulator.

TABLE 3
Assisted Reproductive Technology: Description of Selected Procedures

ART Procedure	Description
OI	Female patient is given medication to stimulate development of more than 1 follicle, combined with timed intercourse or IUI
IUI	Ovulation stimulation with clomiphene citrate or aromatase inhibitor, followed by ovulation induction triggered by HCG injection. Sperm is injected into uterine cavity for fertilization Entails serial ultrasonographies to track follicular development
IVF	HPG axis suppression, followed by ovarian stimulation and induction via gonadotropin injection and HCG injection to trigger ovulation. Progesterone and/or estrogen is added for luteal phase support. Retrieval of oocytes following ovarian stimulation, and combination with sperm to achieve fertilization. One or more embryos are transferred to uterine cavity for implantation Requires frequent, sometimes daily, visits to monitor hormone levels and follicular development
ICSI	Technique in which an individual sperm is introduced to an oocyte for purposes of fertilization
Oocyte cryopreservation	Preserve oocytes via freezing and storage for later use in fertilization and transfer to uterus. Often used in the setting of female patients with cancer before chemotherapy or radiotherapy.
Gestational surrogacy	Use of a healthy person with a uterus to carry a pregnancy for an individual or couple. The gestational carrier does not provide the egg used in conception

Abbreviations: HCG, human chorionic gonadotropin; ICSI, intracytoplasmic sperm injection; IUI, intrauterine insemination; IVF, in vitro fertilization; OI, ovulation induction.

Data from Zegers-Hochschild FG, Adamson D, Dyer S, et al. The international glossary on infertility and fertility care. Hum Reprod 2017;23(9):1786-1801; and Cunningham J. Infertility: A primer for primary care providers. JAAPA 2017;30(9):19-25.

or sooner for those older than 40 years or with risk factors, such as history of abnormal menstrual cycles, endometriosis, past groin or testicular surgery, adult mumps, chemotherapy, or radiation therapy, among others [2,4]. A thorough history and physical examination with detailed menstrual and sexual history, medications, supplements, and substance use history is vital for the woman seeking pregnancy. Targeted laboratory testing for women with infertility includes serum progesterone, luteinizing hormone (LH), follicle-stimulating hormone (FSH), human chorionic gonadotropin, testosterone, prolactin, estradiol, and thyroid-stimulating hormone; for male partners it includes semen analysis [2,4]. Imaging is necessary to fully assess uterine and tubal anatomy for potential anomalies and is done via transvaginal/pelvic ultrasonography or hysterosalpingogram. Those with identified risk factors or complications may need more invasive exploratory procedures [2].

MENTAL HEALTH AND INFERTILITY

Screening

Because infertility is considered a chronic stressor and ART involves treatments with potential neuropsychiatric effects, thorough psychiatric screening is important for all individuals with infertility, with a particular focus on the presence of symptoms at times of hormone fluctuation, including the premenstrual and peripartum periods, and with exogenous hormone use. Common screening tools for depression and anxiety have shown to be reliable and valid in those with infertility; these include the Patient Health Questionnaire (PHQ-9 and PHQ-2) [22] and PHQ-4, a tool composed of the PHQ-2 and Generalized Anxiety Disorder-2 [23]. Although brief, they allow for rapid assessment of new or underlying MH concerns that may be exacerbated with infertility. Studies show that women are more likely to report depression and anxiety symptoms during screening than are their partners [22,24], likely because of the relative direct involvement with ART [9]. This observation further supports the need for not only comprehensive initial screening but also routine ongoing assessment of MH in both partners.

Early detection of distress aids in treatment outcomes by allowing providers to offer preventive services early in ART [3]. SCREENIVF is a scale used to identify emotional distress and maladjustment before and during treatment by assessing depression, anxiety, helplessness, acceptance of infertility, and social support [3,25]. Appropriate MH screening, as well as assessment of personal, marital, and physical stress, may allow patients greater ability to cope with the rigors of ART and potential pregnancy failure [26,27].

Clinical Course

Infertility, emotional distress, and quality of life

Emotional distress is a common consequence of infertility and ART [10,28]. Women undergoing infertility evaluation experience profound psychological impact [29], and the variability in ART outcomes leads to variability in emotional distress [30]. Treatment failure increases the risk of emotional distress in both men and women, particularly guilt, anger, and a sense of isolation in women [3,31,32]. The unfulfilled desire to have a child is clearly linked to emotional distress and poorer quality of life [3,33–35]. The identification with the role of parent and the potential inability to achieve parenthood can lead to a sense of defeat and entrapment [30], and individuals may experience a grief reaction over the lost hope of parenthood [36]. Many couples report ART as the most distressing experience of their lives [28,36]. Infertility may cause strain on both a personal sense of identity and partnership conflicts, but some studies also show positive benefit to marital relationships, particularly with in vitro fertilization (IVF) [31,35]. Stress levels are associated with medical intervention type, outcome uncertainty, communication with medication professionals, and financial burden [34]. High perceived stress levels are associated with depression relapse [7]. Women attribute emotional distress to childlessness and depression, whereas partners attribute distress to dissatisfaction with relationship and sexuality [37]. Patients cite high levels of psychological distress as a primary reason for treatment dropout [28]. A 2019 study identified an association between high levels of physical, personal, and marital stress in women undergoing ART and later antidepressant prescription redemption, which was strongest in women who did not deliver a child [26]. Coping skills can affect emotional and psychological response; avoidant coping styles are associated with negative emotions, whereas active coping is associated with positive adjustment [36].

Quality of life in infertility focuses on psychosocial well-being, relationship fulfillment, and sexual satisfaction and is typically measured by self-report scales that are detailed in Table 4 [5,26,38]. Quality-of-life measures are often worse in ART, particularly with prolonged duration [33]. Multiple studies suggest that quality-of-life measures for the female partner are lower [37–39]. A 2013 study examining quality of life in infertile females reports higher scores in anxiety, depression, helplessness, and acceptance subscales on SCREENIVF questionnaires in 63.8% of women compared with 45.6% of their partners [38]. These higher scores may be related to differences in coping styles [40], as well as differences in reported areas of distress. A 2020 Austrian study examining variables including self-reported stress, negative affect, worry, partnership quality, and perceived social support showed that overall life satisfaction scores were lower than those of age-matched controls in both male and female partners. Additional findings pointed to lower social support, high stress levels, and reduced self-value as contributors to poor quality of life [34].

Depression and infertility

Women with infertility have higher depression prevalence compared with other women of reproductive age, with rates ranging from 20% to 40% [29]. In a study of couples in an infertility clinic, 56% of women and 32% of men reported significant symptoms of depression [41]. Premorbid major depressive disorder (MDD) is a risk factor for depression relapse during ART [42], and prevalence estimates are as high as 39.5% in one study [9]. Women frequently discontinue psychiatric medication with ART in advance of pregnancy, leading to higher relapse rates, although this is inconsistently reported in the infertility population [7]. Increased relapse rates in the female partner are attributed to the chronic stress of treatment and occur despite psychopharmacologic intervention [7,33]. Heightened perceived stress may affect medication efficacy and lead to reemergence of mood symptoms [7].

Personality traits, including neuroticism and avoidance, are associated with increased risk of depression in infertility [43]. A 2010 study examining this relationship shows significant association of depression with somatic trait anxiety, psychic trait anxiety, stress susceptibility, lack of assertiveness, and embitteredness [43]. Cognitive distortions around helplessness and lack of control are often present. A sense of failure, perception of defeat, or feelings of entrapment can affect the risk of

TABLE 4
Quality-of-Life Measures in Infertility

Measure	Description
FertiQoL [5,49,109]	Multidimensional instrument that is the gold standard for assessment of QoL in patients with infertility. Composed of 2 forms, the Core FertiQoL and Treatment module (which assessed QoL during ART, including treatment environment and tolerability) Core FertiQoL measures 4 domains: • Emotional • Mind-body • Relational • Social
SCREENIVF [110]	Designed for use at the start of infertility treatment to identify women or men at risk of emotional maladjustment after treatment. Has better concurrent validity than predictive validity and should not be used as a predictive tool. Scale has 34 items on a 4-point Likert scale divided into the following domains: • State and trait anxiety (derived from Spielberger state and trait anxiety inventory) • Depression (derived from the short Beck Depression Inventory) • Social support (derived from the Inventory of Social Involvement) • Helplessness and acceptance (derived from the Illness Cognition Questionnaire for Infertility)
FPI [5]	Specific measure of infertility-related stress in men and women. Assesses the following domains: • Need for parenthood • Relationship concern • Sexual concern • Social concern • Rejection of child-free lifestyle • Global stress
FPS [5]	Assess infertility-related stress via 3 domains: • Martial stress • Social stress • Personal stress
IFQ [5]	Simple method of assessing the emotional impairment that accompanies infertility via the following domains: • Guilt-blame • Sexuality • Self-image Does not assess treatment satisfaction and has not been widely used in research
ICQ-I [5]	Adaptation from the Illness Cognition Questionnaire that relates to helplessness and acceptance

Abbreviations: FertiQol, fertility quality of life; FPI, fertility problem inventory; FPS, fertility problem stress; ICQ-I, illness cognition questionnaire adapted for infertility; IFQ, infertility questionnaire; QoL, quality of life.

Data from Kitchen H, Aldhouse N, Trigg A, et al. A review of patient-reported outcome measures to assess female infertility-related quality of life. Health and Quality of Life Outcomes 2017;15(1):86.

depression, more so than the lack of achievement of parenthood alone [30].

ART failure is associated with increased risk of depression and anxiety. A 2018 meta-analysis demonstrated that depression and anxiety are present even 6 months after a failed procedure [31]. Another systematic review showed that failed ART and unsuccessful achievement of parenthood increases the risk of depression [44], and this risk may persist 20 years or more following IVF [45]. A prospective study showed increased depression in couples after multiple ART cycles compared with those at initial phases of treatment [46]. An increased risk of postpartum depression has not been demonstrated in women undergoing IVF [45], but multiple unsuccessful ART cycles can increase the risk of depressive symptoms in a subsequent perinatal period [47]. A recent cohort study comparing women with a live birth found a significant difference in antidepressant initiation rate during the postpartum period in those requiring ART, raising concern for ongoing psychological impact of fertility treatment [48].

Anxiety disorders and infertility

Prevalence of anxiety disorders in infertility is high, ranging from 15% to 40% in women undergoing ART [24,29]. A study looking at anxiety, depression, and quality of life in women undergoing IVF showed higher anxiety levels and distress in women with female factor infertility, correlated with a sense of guilt [33]. Other factors, such as uncertainty of cause, treatment outcomes, and financial considerations, can also increase the risk of anxiety [49,50].

Although ART has been linked to elevated anxiety, the timing of symptom peak is inconsistent. A 2015 study looking at the Hospital Anxiety and Depression Scale in patients with infertility found higher anxiety scores in women compared with men, as well as with number of treatment failures, but no association with overall length of infertility diagnosis [50]. A 2018 meta-analysis confirmed that failed ART was associated with increased anxiety and depression in both men and women, but showed no improvement in anxiety after successful ART treatment [31]. Studies examining the psychological impact of ART find that couples initiating treatment experienced higher anxiety states compared with those who had completed multiple cycles and continued treatment [46]. Other studies demonstrate that women with infertility experience increased levels of anxiety compared with their partners, with a positive correlation between anxiety symptoms and treatment duration [9].

Suicide and infertility

Few studies have examined suicide rates in infertility. A 2011 Danish study showed that women with primary infertility who were unable to conceive had a suicide rate 2 times higher than women who conceived following fertility evaluation [51]. A 2019 Swedish study demonstrated that men with infertility-related diagnoses had higher suicide rates [52]. The psychological distress that accompanies infertility may increase the risk of self-harm in vulnerable populations. More research is needed in this important area.

Psychiatric illness as a risk factor for infertility

The role of psychiatric illness as a primary risk factor for infertility is unclear, because the 2 conditions may have similar underlying biological processes. Studies that report depression, anxiety, or stress in patients with infertility do not always control for confounding variables or specify the directionality of the impact between infertility and the psychiatric condition [29,53]. MH also affects nutrition, overall health, substance and tobacco use, and engagement with health care, which can in turn affect fertility or ART outcome [4].

Depression may affect fertility through alterations in physiology, including via hypothalamic-pituitary-thyroid axis, hypothalamic-pituitary-adrenal axis, or hypothalamic-pituitary-gonadal dysfunction. Women with MDD may have alterations in LH pulsatility, leading to changes in menstruation and subsequent infertility [54]. Cortisol is a biomarker for both depression in infertility and ART [55]. Depression in women undergoing ART is associated with higher inflammatory biomarkers, including C-reactive protein, but not with elevations in interleukin-6 or cortisol [7]. Elevations in cytokine levels may also affect biological systems implicated in both infertility and ART outcome, although this is a nonspecific finding [56]. A subset of female patients may have higher levels of inflammation associated with depression and be responsive to certain types of anti-inflammatory treatments, such as omega-3-fatty acids [7,57]. Just as depression can be associated with chronic inflammation, so can obesity. Obese women were more than twice as likely to have 4 to 5 biomarkers of inflammation compared with obese men, and those individuals with higher biomarker levels were more likely to respond to the omega-3 fatty acid than the placebo as evidenced by improvement in HAM-D-17 scores. These findings suggest that there is a relationship between these processes; however, further research is needed in this area [57].

Women who screen positive for depression are less likely to initiate fertility treatment [58,59] and are more likely to stop future fertility treatment [60]. A 2010 study examining the relationship between women with depression and the likelihood of seeking medical advice for infertility finds that women who report symptoms or a diagnosis of depression or other mental illness are less likely to seek medical advice or intervention, thus conceptualizing depression as a barrier to care [59]. Depressed women may initiate fewer ART cycles and have fewer live births compared with those without depression [61], although this is a controversial finding.

MH and emotional distress do not always have a negative impact on ART outcomes [3]. Studies examining the impact of depression, anxiety, and stress on ART outcome are mixed and lacking in clarity. One systematic review and meta-analysis showed nonsignificant effect sizes of depression, anxiety, and distress on ART outcome [62], whereas another meta-analysis showed a small negative effect size of depression and anxiety on ART outcome and more profound effect from emotional distress [63,64]. The birth rate in nonclinical populations of self-reported infertile women with emotional distress is not associated with depression and anxiety [65]. Lack of consistency among studies has created controversy over the impact of depression, anxiety, and emotional distress on ART outcomes and pregnancy rates [53]. Studies do not always control for the complexity in variables associated with emotional distress, such as medical and behavioral factors or the presence of social support, which may explain the variability seen across methodologies [3].

Therapeutic Options

Impact of psychotropic medications on infertility

There is concern that psychotropic medication may increase the risk of infertility through downstream effects on prolactin levels, weight gain, insulin resistance, and thyroid function. Antipsychotics, notably first-generation and risperidone/paliperidone, can increase prolactin levels via dopaminergic effect on the tuberoinfundibular pathway [66], which results in suppression of LH and FSH via negative feedback and inhibition of gonadotrophin-releasing hormone, and finally inhibition of ovulation. Hyperprolactinemia can also cause oligomenorrhea, amenorrhea, and sexual dysfunction, in addition to other short- and long-term side effects [66]. Although not as common, studies show that selective serotonin reuptake inhibitors (SSRIs) can also lead to elevated prolactin levels [67]. More common potential side effects of SSRIs, including decreased libido, erectile dysfunction, delayed ejaculation, and anorgasmia, can inherently negatively affect the frequency of conception events [68]. A 2020 prospective study looking at the impact of SSRIs on fecundability and pregnancy loss showed that SSRIs may lower the probability of conception; however, there was no significant association between overall SSRI use and pregnancy loss. Risk may differ among specific SSRIs [69]. Antipsychotics, lithium, and, to a lesser extent, SSRIs, can lead to weight gain and insulin resistance, which are associated with infertility. Lithium can also lead to hypothyroidism; thyroid levels should be monitored carefully because thyroid dysfunction is a known risk factor for infertility [70].

Impact of psychotropic medications on assisted reproductive technology

Studies examining the impact of psychotropic medication on ART show inadequate evidence of a negative impact of SSRIs on ART outcomes [71]. A systematic review focusing on the effects of antidepressants during ART found no impact on gamete quality or pregnancy outcomes, including number of oocytes retrieved, embryos transferred, and implantation rates [72]. A 2018 study investigating non-IVF ART showed that women treated with antidepressants had higher miscarriage rates compared with women not taking any antidepressants, and male partners with active depression had lower conception rates compared with men without currently active depression [73]. A 2016 study examining the relationship among depression, anxiety, antidepressant use, and IVF outcome including pregnancy, live birth, and miscarriage showed no change in outcome in pregnancy or live birth after IVF cycle for those treated with an SSRI when compared with women without a history of depression or anxiety; however, women who received an SSRI prescription within 3 months following the IVF start date had decreased odds for pregnancy and live birth. In addition, those requiring non-SSRI antidepressants (tricyclic antidepressants, serotonin-norepinephrine reuptake inhibitors [SNRIs], mirtazapine, bupropion) had higher risk of miscarriage and the lowest odds for pregnancy and live birth. Similar findings are noted in those with depression and anxiety without antidepressant exposure, pointing to illness severity and associated factors as increasing risk, rather than use of medication [74]. Although future research is needed, it is important to note that inadequate treatment of mental illness increases the risk of illness severity, poor initiation of infertility evaluation and ART, negative pregnancy outcomes after embryo transfer [74], and negative impact of maternal depression and anxiety on subsequent pregnancy and postpartum health.

Assisted reproductive technology and psychiatric symptoms

Pharmacologic treatment options in ART may cause or exacerbate psychiatric symptoms, as detailed in Table 2. Many medications used in ART can affect mood and associated symptoms, including sleep patterns, anxiety, memory, and concentration. Medications that affect hormone concentrations systemically, such as clomiphene citrate, gonadotropins, and aromatase inhibitors, have been linked to mood lability, depressed symptoms, and memory and concentration changes in various studies [75–77]. Case reports of transient psychosis associated with clomiphene citrate are also in the literature [75,76,78]. Nonhormonal treatments may also exacerbate psychiatric symptoms in some patients, particularly D2 agonists such as bromocriptine and cabergoline, which are used in patients with hyperprolactinemia and can lead to hypomania or psychosis [78,79], and corticosteroids, which are associated with irritability, anxiety, mania, and psychosis [80]. Women with premorbid psychiatric illness should be carefully monitored for worsening symptoms on initiation of these treatments.

Psychotherapy and infertility

Psychotherapy is the first-line treatment of patients with infertility with mild-to-moderate symptoms of depression and anxiety, including cognitive-behavioral therapy (CBT), mind/body interventions (MBI), psychodynamic psychotherapy, interpersonal and brief supportive therapy, music therapy, and coping therapy [81–83]. Mindfulness-based CBT groups have been adapted for patients with infertility [84]. A meta-analysis including randomized controlled trials of psychotherapy modalities showed that interventions including CBT and MBI have positive effects on anxiety, pregnancy rates, and marital function. A reduction in anxiety levels during embryo transfer was noted with music therapy and hypnosis; however, there was no significant positive effect for those awaiting pregnancy outcome, a time considered to be the most distressing [82]. A 2018 study noted that mind/body therapy, a group model incorporating the patient's partner for several sessions, and implementing a variety of skills including CBT, relaxation techniques, and lifestyle changes, was helpful in relieving stress and increasing pregnancy rates [53]. Unfortunately, the literature is inconsistent in terms of intervention efficacy [53,82], likely due to variability in duration of therapy, patient willingness and motivation, and therapy compliance [85]. A cross-sectional, prospective study looking at cognitive coping strategies showed that rumination/catastrophizing had a positive significant association with self-reported symptoms of depression and anxiety, whereas positive refocusing had a negative significant association [86]. Finally, mindfulness-based CBT and relaxation techniques have been examined in depressed and anxious women with infertility, and in one randomized controlled trial, shown to reduce infertility-related stress scores more than either fluoxetine or control [87].

Special Populations

LGBTQIA+ population, infertility, and mental health

Studies on the MH and emotional impact of infertility treatment center on cisgender heterosexual couples. For those in the LGBTQIA+ community, as well as single individuals who are interested in family planning, referral to reproductive endocrinology for counseling on fertility options should occur early [88]. Continued stigmatization of this population may pose a barrier to accessing appropriate care [89].

Transgender men, who are typically born with reproductive organs that allow for pregnancy, should discuss the impact of transition on fertility before initiation of the process. Testosterone therapy is often the first treatment in transition and leads to masculine physical appearance, anovulation, and amenorrhea [4]. An Australian study examining the experiences of transgender men with a gestational pregnancy found that initiation of testosterone was a validating experience, with overall improvement in depression and anxiety symptoms. Subsequent discontinuation of testosterone in advance of pregnancy leads to the return of feminine physical characteristics, and can lead to heightened stress levels, poor energy, mood fluctuations, and depressed mood [90].

Although pursuing similar interventions to their cisgender, heterosexual counterparts, members of the LGBTQIA+ community seeking ART often do not have an infertility diagnosis [89]. Qualitative focus groups in lesbian and bisexual women initiating ART show that those with an infertility diagnosis face a unique set of challenges during a stressful time, including the potential for the partner to take on the role of childbearing mother or the need to find alternative sperm donors. Treatment recommendations include offering specialized infertility groups unique to the population, involving all parties who plan to parent in the process, and creating a welcoming environment in an effort to lessen the fear of discrimination based on sexual orientation [91].

Infertility and male mental health

Male factors are causative in 8% of infertility cases and contributory in 35% [2,4]. The literature focuses primarily on the MH impact of infertility in women or heterosexual couples, with comparisons between male and female partners; few studies focus on male MH alone. Heightened stress in the male partner is a contributing factor to infertility and unsuccessful ART outcomes, although to a lesser degree than for the female partner [92]. Infertile men experience low self-esteem and feelings of inadequacy [93]. Men use different coping mechanisms, including distancing and self-controlling, and have unique problem-solving strategies compared with women [40]. In quality-of-life studies, men tend to report lower relationship and sexual satisfaction compared with their female partners [37]. As for women, high neuroticism in men correlates with higher rates of depression [43].

Men with infertility score significantly higher on depression and anxiety screening compared with their fertile counterparts. A 2017 study showed that higher scores on the Beck Depression Inventory correlated with significantly lower testosterone levels, higher prolactin and cortisol levels, and lower sperm count and ejaculate volume. Higher scores on the State-Trait Anxiety Inventory correlated with higher prolactin and cortisol levels and lower sperm count and ejaculatory volume. Neither depression nor anxiety seemed to affect FSH or LH, and both showed an inverse relationship with sex hormone-binding globulin (SHBG) and dehydroepiandrosterone sulfate (DHEA-S) levels [94]. This study shows clear impact of mood and anxiety on hormone levels and sperm quality, whereas others present conflicting data. A 2019 study examining MH symptoms in men at initial infertility assessment showed a significant, albeit small, correlation between depression scores and infertility duration, but no association with anxiety scores, suggesting that anxiety symptoms may develop during treatment itself. This study did not show a correlation between depression and anxiety symptoms and sperm count, motility, and morphology [93].

Studies demonstrate decreased sperm concentration, increased DNA fragmentation, and lower sperm motility with SSRI use compared with male infertility patients not taking an SSRI [71,95]. Results are not consistent across studies, and further research is prudent.

Surrogacy

There is a paucity of literature examining MH outcomes of gestational surrogacy, despite its use increasing 4-fold since 1999 [96]. Surrogacy offers high birth rates compared with ART in infertility, particularly in women older than 42 years [97]. A 2021 systematic review of literature on MH outcomes in surrogacy, focusing primarily on the MH of the gestational carrier (GC) and the child of surrogacy, finds that most studies focus on the GC's coping mechanisms, including the experience of joy, accomplishment, pride, and satisfaction, but these outcomes are strongly influenced by geographic, cultural, and socioeconomic context [96]. Another systematic review finds no difference in MH outcomes for children of surrogacy versus children of ART or natural pregnancy [98]. The American Society of Reproductive Medicine and other international organizations recommend MH screening for GCs and counseling for the GC and intended family.

SUMMARY

Infertility and MH have a complex, bidirectional relationship, and the impact of emotional distress in patients undergoing infertility evaluation and ART can be profound. Fertility treatment affects psychiatric stability in women, and MH may also have an impact on fertility and ART outcomes, although this is controversial. Individuals and couples struggling with infertility should be screened for MH and emotional distress, and early referrals for support and intervention provided to ensure the best outcomes.

CLINICS CARE POINTS

- MH screening is recommended for all patients with infertility, and common tools including the PHQ-2, PHQ-9, and PHQ-4 have been validated in this population.
- Many pharmacologic treatments used in ART can affect preexisting MH conditions, and it is prudent to monitor and treat symptoms appropriately.
- Depression, anxiety, and emotional distress may not affect the outcome of ART in infertility; the evidence is contradictory across studies.
- Irrespective of the aforementioned facts, depression, anxiety, and emotional distress are common in the infertility population, and evidence-based treatment options should be offered.
- Psychotherapy is the first-line treatment of depression and anxiety in infertility, with multiple effective modalities including CBT, MBI, mindfulness, and others.

- The LGBTQIA+ community seeking fertility intervention may or may not have a diagnosis of infertility; those that do should be provided specific resources for this unique struggle. Transgender males who are transitioning should discuss their reproductive plans with their providers before and during the transition process.

DISCLOSURE

The authors have nothing to disclose.

REFERENCES

[1] Zegers-Hochschild FG, Adamson D, Dyer S, et al. The international glossary on infertility and fertility care. Hum Reprod 2017;23(9):1786–801.

[2] Committee on Gynecologic Practice, American Society for Reproductive Medicine. ACOG committee opinion: infertility workup for the women's health specialist. Obstet Gynecol 2019;133(6):e377–84.

[3] Boivin J. How does stress, depression and anxiety affect patients undergoing treatment? Curr Opin Obstet Gynecol 2019;31:195–9.

[4] Cunningham J. Infertility: a primer for primary care providers. JAAPA 2017;30(9):19–25.

[5] Kitchen H, Aldhouse N, Trigg A, et al. A review of patient-reported outcome measures to assess female infertility-related quality of life. Health Qual Life Outcomes 2017;15(1):86.

[6] Mascarenhas MN, Flaxman SR, Boerma T, et al. National, regional, and global trends in infertility prevalence since 1990: a systematic analysis of 277 health surveys. PLoS Med 2012;9(12):e1001356.

[7] Freeman MP, Lee H, Savella GM, et al. Predictors of depressive relapse in women undergoing infertility treatment. J Womens Health (Larchmt) 2018;27(11):1408–14.

[8] Gurunath S, Pandian Z, Anderson RA, et al. Defining infertility - a systematic review of prevalence studies. Hum Reprod Update 2011;17(5):575–88.

[9] Gdańska P, Drozdowicz-Jastrzębska E, Grzechocińska B, et al. Anxiety and depression in women undergoing infertility treatment. Ginekol Pol 2017;88(2):109–12.

[10] Boivin J, Bunting L, Collins JA, et al. International estimates of infertility prevalence and treatment-seeking: potential need and demand for infertility medical care. Hum Reprod 2007;22:1506–12.

[11] Bozdag G, Mumusoglu S, Zengin D, et al. The prevalence and phenotypic features of polycystic ovary syndrome: a systematic review and meta-analysis. Hum Reprod 2016;31(12):2841–55.

[12] Joham AE, Teede HJ, Ranasinha S, et al. Prevalence of infertility and use of fertility treatment in women with polycystic ovary syndrome: data from a large community-based cohort study. J Womens Health (Larchmt) 2015;24(4):299–307.

[13] Hollinrake E, Abreu A, Maifeld M, et al. Increased risk of depressive disorders in women with polycystic ovary syndrome. Fertil Steril 2007;87:1369–76.

[14] Dokras A, Stener-Victorin E, Yildiz BO, et al. Androgen Excess- Polycystic Ovary Syndrome Society: position statement on depression, anxiety, quality of life, and eating disorders in polycystic ovary syndrome. Fertil Steril 2018;109(5):888–99.

[15] Estes SJ, Huisingh CE, Chiuve SE, et al. Depression, anxiety, and self-directed violence in women with endometriosis: a retrospective matched-cohort study. Am J Epidemiol 2021;190(5):843–52.

[16] Chen LC, Hsu JW, Huang KL, et al. Risk of developing major depression and anxiety disorders among women with endometriosis: a longitudinal follow-up study. J Affect Disord 2016;190:282–5.

[17] Gambadauro P, Carli V, Hadlaczky G. Depressive symptoms among women with endometriosis: a systematic review and meta-analysis. Am J Obstet Gynecol 2019; 220(3):230–41.

[18] Demartini B, Ranieri R, Masu A, et al. Depressive symptoms and major depressive disorder in patients affected by subclinical hypothyroidism: a cross-sectional study. J Nerv Ment Dis 2014;202(8):603–7.

[19] Fukao A, Takamatsu J, Arishima T, et al. Graves' disease and mental disorders. J Clin Transl Endocrinol 2019;19: 100207.

[20] Khizroeva J, Nalli C, Bitsadze V, et al. Infertility in women with systemic autoimmune diseases. Best Pract Res Clin Endocrinol Metab 2019;33(6):101369.

[21] Samuels MH. Psychiatric and cognitive manifestations of hypothyroidism. Curr Opin Endocrinol Diabetes Obes 2014;21(5):377–83.

[22] Maroufizadeh S, Omani-Samani R, Almasi-Hashiani A, et al. The reliability and validity of the patient health questionnaire-9 (PHQ-9) and PHQ-2 in patients with infertility. Reprod Health 2019;16(1):137.

[23] Ghaheri A, Omani-Samani R, Sepidarkish M, et al. The four-item patient health questionnaire for anxiety and depression: a validation study in infertile patients. Int J Fertil Steril 2020;14(3):234–9.

[24] Omani-Samani R, Ghaheri A, Navid B, et al. Prevalence of generalized anxiety disorder and its related factors among infertile patients in Iran: a cross-sectional study. Health Qual Life Outcomes 2018; 16(1):129.

[25] Verhaak CM, Lintsen AM, Evers AW, et al. Who is at risk of emotional problems and how do you know? Screening women going for IVF treatment. Hum Reprod 2010;25:1234–40.

[26] Pedro J, Vassard D, Hviid-Malling GM, et al. Infertility-related stress and the risk of antidepressants prescription in women: a 10-year register study. Hum Reprod 2019;34(8):1505–13.

[27] Verhaak CM, Smeenk JM, Evers AW, et al. Predicting emotional response to unsuccessful fertility treatment: a prospective study. J Behav Med 2005;28:181–90.
[28] Cousineau TM, Domar AD. Psychological impact of infertility. Best Pract Res Clin Obstet Gynaecol 2007; 21(2):293–308.
[29] Yoldemir T, Yassa M, Atasayan K. Comparison of depression between primary and secondary infertile couples. Gynecol Endocrinol 2020;36(12):1131–5.
[30] Galhardo A, Moura-Ramos M, Cunha M, et al. The infertility trap: how defeat and entrapment affect depressive symptoms. Hum Reprod 2016;31(2): 419–26.
[31] Milazzo A, Mnatzaganian G, Elshaug AG, et al. Depression and anxiety outcomes associated with failed assisted reproductive technologies: a systematic review and meta-analysis. PLoS One 2018;11:e0165805.
[32] Martins MV, Basto-Pereira M, Pedro J, et al. Male psychological adaptation to unsuccessful medical assisted reproduction treatments: a systematic review. Hum Reprod Update 2016;22:466–76.
[33] Massarotti C, Gentile G, Ferreccio C, et al. Impact of infertility and infertility treatments on quality of life and levels of anxiety and depression in women undergoing in vitro fertilization. Gynecol Endocrinol 2019; 35(6):485–9.
[34] Kiesswetter M, Marsoner H, Luehwink A, et al. Impairment in life satisfaction in infertility: associations with perceived stress, affectivity, partnership quality, social support and the desire to have a child. Behav Med 2020;46(2):130–41.
[35] Gana K, Jakubowska S. Relationship between infertility-related stress and emotional distress and marital satisfaction. J Health Psychol 2016;21(6):1043–54.
[36] Wilkins WM, Warnock JK, Serrano E. Depressive symptoms related to infertility and infertility treatments. Psychiatr Clin North Am 2010;33(2):309–21.
[37] Wischmann T, Scherg H, Strowitski T, et al. Psychosocial characteristics of women and men attending infertility counseling. Hum Reprod 2009;24:378–85.
[38] Huppelschoten AG, van Dongen AJCM, Verhaak CM, et al. Differences in quality of life and emotional status between infertile women and their partners. Hum Reprod 2013;28(8):2168–76.
[39] Chachamovich J, Chachamovich E, Ezer H, et al. Investigating quality of life and health-related quality of life among infertile men and women: findings from a couples-based study. Hum Reprod 2010;31: 101–10.
[40] Peterson BD, Newton CR, Rosen KH, et al. Gender differences in how men and women who are referred for IVF cope with infertility stress. Hum Reprod 2006; 21(9):2443–9.
[41] Pasch LA, Holley SR, Bleil ME, et al. Addressing the needs of fertility treatment patients and their partners: are they informed of and do they receive mental health services? Fertil Steril 2016;106(1):209–15.e.2.
[42] Holley SR, Pasch LA, Bleil ME, et al. Prevalence and predictors of major depressive disorder for fertility treatment patients and their partners. Fertil Steril 2015; 103(5):1332–9.
[43] Volgsten H, Ekselius L, Poromaa IS, et al. Personality traits associated with depressive and anxiety disorders in infertile women and men undergoing in vitro fertilization treatment. Acta Obstetricia et Gynecologica 2010;89:27–34.
[44] Gameiro S, Finnigan A. Long-term adjustment to unmet parenthood goals following ART: a systematic review and meta-analysis. Hum Reprod Update 2017;23:322–37.
[45] Vikstrom J, Josefsson A, Bladh M, et al. Mental health in women 20-23 years after IVF treatment: a Swedish cross-sectional study. BMJ Open 2015;5:1–8.
[46] Reis S, Xavier MR, Coelho R, et al. Psychological impact of single and multiple courses of assisted reproductive treatments in couples: a comparative study. Eur J Obstet Gynecol Reprod Biol 2013;171(1):61–6.
[47] Agostini F, Monti F, Paterlini M, et al. Effect of the previous reproductive outcomes in subfertile women after in vitro fertilization (IVF) and/or intracytoplasmic sperm injection (ICSI) treatments on perinatal anxious and depressive symptomatology. J Psychosom Obstet Gynaecol 2018;39(1):29–37.
[48] Hviid-Malling GM, Gronemann FH, Vassard D, et al. The association between antidepressant use and assisted reproductive technology (ART) treatment in Danish women: A national registry-based cohort study. Eur J Obstet Gynecol Reprod Biol 2021;258:401–8.
[49] Boivin J, Griffiths E, Venetis CA. Emotional distress in infertile women and failure of assisted reproductive technologies: metaanalysis of prospective psychosocial studies. BMJ 2011;342:d223.
[50] Maroufizadeh S, Karimi E, Vesali S, et al. Anxiety and depression after failure of assisted reproductive technology among patients experiencing infertility. Int J Obstet Gynecol 2015;130:253–6.
[51] Kjaer TK, Jensen A, Dalton SO, et al. Suicide in Danish women evaluated for fertility problems. Hum Reprod 2011;26(9):2401–7.
[52] Lundberg FE, Johansson AL, Ludvigsson JF. Mortality in 43,598 men with infertility - a Swedish nationwide population-based cohort study. Clin Epidemiol 2019; 11:645–57.
[53] Rooney KL, Domar AD. The relationship between stress and infertility. Dialogues Clin Neurosci 2018;20(1): 41–7.
[54] Grambsch P, Young EA, Meller WH, et al. Pulsatile luteinizing hormone disruption in depression. Psychoneuroendocrinology 2004;29(7):825–9.
[55] An Y, Wang Z, Ji H, et al. Pituitary-adrenal and sympathetic nervous system responses to psychiatric disorders in women undergoing in vitro fertilization treatment. Fertil Steril 2011;96:404–8.
[56] Haimovici F, Anderson JL, Bates GW, et al. Stress, anxiety, and depression of both partners in infertile couples

are associated with cytokine levels and adverse IVF outcome. Am J Reprod Immunol 2018;79(4):e12832.
[57] Rappaport MH, Nierenberg AA, Schettler PJ, et al. Inflammation as a predictive biomarker for response to omega-3-fatty acids in major depressive disorder: a proof-of-concept study. Mol Psychiatry 2016;21:71–9.
[58] Crawford NM, Hoff HS, Mersereau JE. Infertile women who screen positive for depression are less likely to initiate fertility treatments. Hum Reprod 2017;32(3): 582–7.
[59] Herbert DL, Lucke JC, Dobson AJ. Depression: an emotional obstacle to seeking medical advice for infertility. Fertil Steril 2010;94(5):1817–21.
[60] Domar AD, Rooney K, Hacker MR, et al. Burden of care is the primary reason why insured women terminate in vitro fertilization treatment. Fertil Steril 2018; 109(6):1121–6.
[61] Sejbaek CS, Hageman I, Pinborg A, et al. Incidence of depression and influence of depression on the number of treatment cycles and births in a national cohort of 42,880 women treated with ART. Hum Reprod 2013; 28:1100–9.
[62] Nicoloro-SantaBarbara J, Busso C, Moyer A, et al. Just relax and you'll get pregnant? Meta-analysis examining women's emotional distress and the outcomes of assisted reproductive technology. Soc Sci Med 2018;213: 54–62.
[63] Purewal S, Chapman SC, Akker OB. A systematic review and meta-analysis of psychological predictors of successful assisted reproductive technologies. BMC Res Notes 2017;10:711.
[64] Purewal S, Chapman SC, van den Akker OB. Depression and state anxiety scores during assisted reproductive treatment are associated with outcomes: a meta-analysis. Reprod Biomed Online 2018;36:646–57.
[65] Biringer E, Kessler U, Howard LM, et al. Anxiety, depression, and probability of live birth in a cohort of women with self-reported infertility in the HUNT 2 study and medical birth registry of Norway. J Psychosom Res 2018;113:1–7.
[66] Bostwick JR, Guthrie SK, Ellingrod VL. Antipsychotic-induced hyperprolactinemia. Pharmacotherapy 2009; 29(1):64–73.
[67] Park YM. Serum prolactin levels in patients with major depressive disorder receiving selective serotonin-reuptake inhibitor monotherapy for 3 months: a prospective study. Psychiatry Investig 2017;14(3):368–71.
[68] Montejo AL, Montejo L, Navarro-Cremades F. Sexual side-effects of antidepressant and antipsychotic drugs. Curr Opin Psychiatry 2015;28(6):418–23.
[69] Sjaarda LA, Radoc JG, Flannagan KS, et al. Urinary selective serotonin reuptake inhibitors across critical windows of pregnancy establishment: a prospective cohort study of fecundability and pregnancy loss. Fertil Steril 2020;114(6):1278–87.
[70] Dosiou C. Thyroid and fertility: recent advances. Thyroid 2020;30(4):479–86.
[71] Sylvester C, Menke M, Gopalan P. Selective serotonin reuptake inhibitors and fertility: considerations for couples trying to conceive. Harv Rev Psychiatry 2019;27(2): 108–18.
[72] Akioyamen LE, Minhas H, Holloway AC, et al. Effects of depression pharmacotherapy in fertility treatment on conception, birth, and neonatal health: a systematic review. J Psychosom Res 2016;84:69–80.
[73] Evans-Hoeker EA, Eisenberg E, Diamond MP, et al. Major depression, antidepressant use, and male and female fertility. Fertil Steril 2018;109(5):879–87.
[74] Cesta CE, Viktorin A, Olsson H, et al. Depression, anxiety, and antidepressant treatment in women: association with in vitro fertilization outcome. Fertil Steril 2016;105(6):1594–602.e3.
[75] Aussedat M, Jean-Louis J, Djahangirian O, et al. Clomiphene for the treatment of male infertility: a case report of mood change and a literature review. Curr Drug Saf 2017;12(3):209–15.
[76] Choi SH, Shapiro H, Robinson GE, et al. Psychological side-effects of clomiphene citrate and human menopausal gonadotrophin. J Psychosom Obstet Gynaecol 2005;26(2):93–100.
[77] Bloch M, Azem F, Aharonov I, et al. GnRH-agonist induced depressive and anxiety symptoms during in vitro fertilization-embryo transfer cycles. Fertil Steril 2011;95:307–9.
[78] Seeman MV. Transient psychosis in women on clomiphene, bromocriptine, domperidone and related endocrine drugs. Gynecol Endocrinol 2015;31(10):751–4.
[79] Snellen M, Power J, Blankley G, et al. Pharmacological lactation suppression with D2 receptor agonists and risk of postpartum psychosis: a systematic review. Aust NZ J Obstet Gynaecol 2016;56(4):336–40.
[80] Kenna H, Poon A, Lewis-de los Angeles CP, et al. Psychiatric complications of treatment with corticosteroids: review with case report. Psychiatry Clin Neurosci 2011; 65:549–60.
[81] Gaitzsch H, Benard J, Hugon-Rodin J, et al. The effect of mind-body interventions on psychological and pregnancy outcomes in infertile women: a systematic review. Arch Womens Ment Health 2020;23(4): 479–91.
[82] Ying L, Wu LH, Loke AY. The effects of psychosocial interventions on the mental health, pregnancy rates, and marital function of infertile couples undergoing in vitro fertilization: a systematic review. J Assist Reprod Genet 2016;33(6):689–701.
[83] Koszycki D, Bisserbe JC, Blier P, et al. Interpersonal psychotherapy versus brief supportive therapy for depressed infertile women: first pilot randomized controlled trial. Arch Womens Ment Health 2012; 15(3):193–201.
[84] Kalhori F, Masoumi SZ, Shamsaei F, et al. Effect of mindfulness-based group counseling on depression in infertile women: randomized clinical trial study. Int J Fertil Steril 2020;14(1):10–6.

[85] Patel A, Sharma PSVN, Kumar P. Application of mindfulness-based psychological interventions in infertility. J Hum Reprod Sci 2020;13(1):3–21.

[86] Kraaij V, Gamefski N, Schroevera M, et al. Cognitive coping, goal adjustment, and depressive and anxiety symptoms in people undergoing infertility treatment.; a prospective study. J Health Psychol 2010;15(6):876–86.

[87] Faramarzi M, Pasha H, Esmailzadeh S, et al. The effect of cognitive behavioral therapy and pharmacotherapy on infertility stress: a randomized controlled trial. Int J Fertil Steril 2013;7(3):199.

[88] Darwin Z, Greenfield M. The invisibility of LGBTQ people in reproductive and infant psychology. J Reprod Infant Psychol 2019;37(4):341–3.

[89] Johal JK, Gardner RM, Vaughn SJ, et al. Pregnancy success rates for lesbian women undergoing intrauterine insemination. F S Rep 2021;2(3):275–81.

[90] Charter R, Ussher J, Perz J, et al. The transgender parent: experiences and constructions of pregnancy and parenthood for transgender men in Australia. Int J Transgenderism 2018;19(1):64–77.

[91] Ross LE, Steele LS, Epstein R. Lesbian and bisexual women's recommendations for improving the provision of assisted reproductive technology services. Fertil Steril 2006;86(3):735–8.

[92] Boivin J, Schmidt L. Infertility-related stress in men and women predicts treatment outcome 1 year later. Fertil Steril 2005;83(6):1745–52.

[93] Hegyi BE, Kozinszky Z, Badó A, et al. Anxiety and depression symptoms in infertile men during their first infertility evaluation visit. J Psychosom Obstet Gynaecol 2019;40(4):311–7.

[94] Wdowiak A, Bień A, Iwanowicz-Palus G, et al. Impact of emotional disorders on semen quality in men treated for infertility. Neuro Endocrinol Lett 2017;38(1):50–8.

[95] Nørr L, Bennedsen B, Fedder J, et al. Use of selective serotonin reuptake inhibitors reduces fertility in men. Andrology 2016;4(3):389–94.

[96] Yau A, Friedlander RL, Petrini A, et al. Medical and mental health implications of gestational surrogacy. Am J Obstet Gynecol 2021;225(3):264–9.

[97] Centers for Disease Control and Prevention, American Society for Reproductive Medicine, Society for Assisted Reproductive Technology. 2016 assisted reproductive technology national summary report. Atlanta (GA): US Dept of Health and Human Services; 2018.

[98] Söderström-Anttila V, Wennerholm UB, Loft A, et al. Surrogacy: outcomes for surrogate mothers, children, and the resulting families-a systematic review. Hum Reprod Update 2016;22(2):260–76.

[99] Usadi RS, Merriam K. On-label and off-label drug use in the treatment of female infertility. Fertil Steril 2015;103:584–94.

[100] Diamond MP, Legro RS, Coutifaris C, et al. Letrozole, gonadotropin, or clomiphene for unexplained infertility. N Engl J Med 2015;373(13):1230–40.

[101] Rosenfeld CS, Shay DA, Vieira-Potter VJ. Cognitive effects of aromatase and possible role in memory disorders. Front Endocrinol (Lausanne) 2018;9:610.

[102] Cooperman AB, Benadiva C. Optimal usage of the GnRH antagonists: a review of the literature. Reprod Biol Endocrinol 2013;1:20.

[103] Stenbæk DS, Toftager M, Hjordt LV, et al. Mental distress and personality in women undergoing GnRH agonist versus GnRH antagonist protocols for assisted reproductive technology. Hum Reprod 2015;30(1):103–10.

[104] Stenbæk DS, Budtz-Jørgensen E, Pinborg A, et al. Neuroticism modulates mood responses to pharmacological sex hormone manipulation in healthy women. Psychoneuroendocrinology 2019;99:251–6.

[105] Skovlund CW, Morch LS, Kessing LV. Association of hormonal contraception with depression. JAMA Psych 2016;73(11):1154–62.

[106] Wang Y, Chen Q, Wang N, et al. Controlled ovarian stimulation using medroxyprogesterone acetate and hMG in patients with polycystic ovary syndrome treated for IVF: a double-blind randomized crossover clinical trial. Medicine (Baltimore) 2016;95(9):e2939.

[107] Erensoy H, Niafar M, Ghafarzadeh S. A pilot trial of metformin for insulin resistance and mood disturbances in adolescent and adult women with polycystic ovary syndrome. Gynecol Endocrinol 2019;35(1):72–5.

[108] Grall-Bronnec M, Sauvaget A, Perrouin F, et al. Pathological gambling associated with aripiprazole or dopamine replacement therapy: do patients share the same features? a review. J Clin Psychopharmacol 2016;36(1):63–70.

[109] Donarelli S, Lo Coco G, Gullo L, et al. The Fertility Quality of Life Questionnaire (FertiQoL) Relational subscale: psychometric properties and discriminant validity across gender. Hum Reprod 2016;31(9):2061–71.

[110] Ockhuijsen HDL, van Smeden M, van den Hoogen A, et al. Validation study of the SCREENIVF: an instrument to screen women or men on risk for emotional maladjustment before the start of a fertility treatment. Fertil Steril 2017;107(6):1370–9.

Child and Adolescent

Advances in Psychiatry and Behavioral Health 2 (2022) 133–140

ADVANCES IN PSYCHIATRY AND BEHAVIORAL HEALTH

Intensive Treatments for Youth with Obsessive-Compulsive Disorder and Anxiety Disorders

Caitlyn E. Maye, BS[a], Caitlin M. Pinciotti, PhD[b], Eric A. Storch, PhD[a,*]

[a]Department of Psychiatry and Behavioral Sciences, Baylor College of Medicine, 1977 Butler Boulevard, Suite 4-400 Houston, TX 77030, USA; [b]Rogers Behavioral Health System, 34700 Valley Road, Oconomowoc, WI 53066, USA

KEYWORDS

• Intensive treatment • Cognitive-behavioral therapy • Exposure and response prevention • Youth • OCD • Anxiety

KEY POINTS

- Intensive treatments for youth with OCD and anxiety are effective interventions.
- Intensive treatments vary from one extended session to numerous sessions.
- Telehealth treatment offers one modality for improving treatment access.

INTRODUCTION

Obsessive-compulsive disorder (OCD) is a debilitating psychiatric disorder, affecting about 2% to 3% youth [1,2]. Symptoms of OCD can generally be categorized into the following dimensions: symmetry and order, contamination/mental contamination, checking, taboo obsessions, and hoarding [3,4]. Symptoms of OCD can cause impairment and reduced quality of life [5] and tend to persist and even worsen without treatment [6]. Youth who have an earlier onset of this disorder often show more severe symptoms, higher rates of comorbidities of other psychiatric diagnoses, and greater chronicity [7]. In addition, OCD is associated with impairment within the home [8–10], among peers [11–13], and at school [14,15].

According to the Diagnostic and Statistical Manual of Mental Disorders, 5th Edition, anxiety disorders—a cluster of disorders that is separate from the obsessive-compulsive and related disorders and includes conditions such as generalized anxiety disorder, social anxiety disorder, and specific phobias, among others—are among the most common disorders affecting youth, with up to 10% of children and 20% of adolescents meeting criteria for an anxiety disorder at any one point in time [16]. Anxiety symptoms can include edginess or restlessness, increased fatigue, impaired concentration, irritability, consistent and pervasive worrying, increase in muscle tension, or sleep difficulties [17]. Having significant anxiety is associated with potential short-term and long-term negative outcomes. Youth with anxiety are more likely to have increased irritability, lower self-esteem, and significant academic impairment [18–20], and longitudinal research shows that these youth are at risk for nicotine dependence, illicit drug dependence, and higher depressive symptoms [21]. The societal impact of these disorders is noteworthy in both the short term and long term [22]. Although these disorders place significant burden on public health and accrue significant financial costs, many youth with anxiety disorders are untreated due to a lack of access to

*Corresponding author, *E-mail address:* eric.storch@bcm.edu

https://doi.org/10.1016/j.ypsc.2022.06.003
2667-3827/22/

evidence-based treatment or not receiving effective evidence-based treatment, thus perpetuating their symptoms [23]. Furthermore, anxiety disorders have been associated with disruption in multiple domains of youth's development and have been linked with the development of additional anxiety disorders, mood impairment, and substance use [23].

TREATMENT OF OBSESSIVE-COMPULSIVE DISORDER AND ANXIETY DISORDERS

Currently, effective treatments of anxiety disorders often use a cognitive behavioral therapy (CBT) approach. Specifically, for youth with OCD, the gold-standard, evidence-based cognitive behavioral treatment is exposure and response prevention (ERP) [24]. Within this framework, the therapist teaches the child to challenge anxious thoughts and exposes them in a hierarchical manner to their fears while encouraging the child to refrain from engaging in compulsions and avoidance. These exposures help challenge maladaptive beliefs about the likelihood and severity of feared outcomes and the child's ability to tolerate the anxiety that these situations elicit without relying on compulsions and avoidance to cope. Depending on the severity and needs of the child, treatment can be provided in multiple settings including outpatient (typically over 12–24 sessions) and higher levels of care (ie, intensive outpatient, partial hospitalization, and residential programs). Regardless of setting, treatment progresses in roughly the same fashion. Initially, patients are provided with psychoeducation about OCD and the course of treatment, whereas the clinician gathers information about the individual's presenting symptoms [25]. The patient and clinician then develop a hierarchy of internal and external stimuli that trigger the patient's obsessions. Patients typically move from less to most distressing situations and repeatedly confront situations in vivo and imaginably while refraining from engaging in compulsions/avoidance [25]. Through ERP, the patient learns that they can tolerate distress which the feared outcomes do not occur, how to manage anxious responses, and how to cope with uncertainty. The goal of treatment is to show the youth that they can handle distressing thoughts without needing to over-engage in those thoughts or perform an action to get rid of the distress. Like children with OCD, youth with anxiety disorders benefit from CBT with exposure therapy as well [26,27]. Exposure therapy provides an opportunity for extinction learning through exposure to anxiety provoking situations in a gradual manner, which reduces avoidance or safety behaviors that serve to maintain anxiety [28]. Overall, research indicates that CBT with exposure or ERP provides substantial reduction in symptoms for youth with OCD and anxiety disorders [26,29–31].

Although CBT with ERP is the gold-standard treatment for youth with OCD, CBT interventions seem to not be effective for some youth [23,31–33]. Furthermore, despite the documented adverse outcomes of youth with OCD, only a small number of youths receive effective evidence-based treatment of this disorder. Traditional CBT requires youth to attend 10 to 16 weekly 1-hour sessions, which may be challenging for working parents or when treatment scheduling conflicts with school hours. This barrier may exacerbate systemic disparities for families that are marginalized or from lower socioeconomic statuses because of a lack of access of care, ability to take time away from work, or the financial burden. In addition to the potential financial and time burden CBT places on families of youth with OCD or anxiety disorders, there is a lack of trained therapists who specialize in working with youth with OCD and/or anxiety disorders. Given the burden that OCD and anxiety have on the individual and the serious potential impact on public health [34–36], effective evidence-based treatments are critical to help youth and families.

INTENSIVE TREATMENT FOR YOUTH WITH OCD AND ANXIETY DISORDERS

One approach to increase the availability and feasibility of evidence-based treatments for youth with OCD and anxiety disorders is to modify existing treatments to be administered in a shorter amount of time. This could help alleviate the burden on families who must travel sometimes quite far to the nearest clinic for the duration of treatment. Intensive treatments can range in duration from one single session of treatment to daily sessions over a small number of days or weeks. Although these treatments reduce the number of sessions or the period of time when sessions are delivered, they maintain fidelity to the core elements of traditional CBT of implementing cognitive restructuring/challenging of catastrophic thinking and graduated exposure [37]. Intensive treatment for youth with OCD was initially proposed as being more effective than the traditional standard CBT treatment because of the barriers that traditional CBT presents [38]. Intensive treatment approaches may increase patients' motivation because it is less of a time commitment than traditional treatment, and its short duration allows it to be the patient's primary focus [39]. Because of the brevity of the intensive format (ie, several times per week over a short period of time), this treatment can serve as a remedy to some barriers that accompany standard CBT. For example, intensive treatment alleviates barriers for families living outside the geographical location where a specialized therapist is available. In addition, families who have engaged in suboptimal treatment may benefit from intensive treatment. Intensive treatment approaches may lead to increased or sustained treatment gains because of having the family focus on treatment solely during the short duration of treatment and an increase in opportunities to practice exposure sessions [40,41]. Several intensive treatment protocols have been developed for multiple youth anxiety disorders, such as specific phobias [42], separation anxiety disorder [43], and OCD [41,44].

Since the earliest work on intensive treatment protocols for anxiety and OCD, the data continue to show that intensive treatment is an effective alternative to traditional CBT. Storch and colleagues [41] initially conducted a randomized controlled clinical trial of intensive CBT for youth with OCD. Participants were randomized to either standard CBT condition of 14 weekly sessions or to an intensive CBT condition involving 90-minute CBT sessions every weekday for 3 weeks with at least one caregiver present for all sessions. Results found that intensive CBT was as effective as standard weekly treatment, and the results were maintained over a 3-month follow-up period [41]. However, some patients required additional care of 1-month posttreatment to maintain treatment goals, which suggest the potential need for additional booster sessions in the form of telehealth, when geographically needed, or in-person sessions following the intensive treatment [41]. Since this initial randomized clinical study, subsequent studies have examined the efficacy of a variety of intensive approaches to treat youth with OCD or anxiety disorders [43,45–48].

Ost and Ollendick [37] found support for the hypothesis that intensive treatment is as effective as standard CBT for youth with OCD and anxiety disorders in a meta-analysis of brief, intensive CBT interventions for youth with anxiety disorders, including OCD. Twenty-three randomized controlled trials that were either "brief" (reduced number of sessions compared with standard CBT), concentrated (more than one session per week during a fairly short-time period), or intensive (brief and concentrated)" were included [37]. Results found that brief, intensive, and concentrated treatments were effective in comparison to wait-list control conditions, placebo control conditions (eg, education, support, nondirective therapy), and to standard, full CBT interventions. These effects were maintained up to 1-year following treatment. This meta-analysis found that brief, intensive, and concentrated interventions led not only to successful treatment response but also 54% remission rates and 64% recovery rates [37]. In addition, low attrition rates among brief, intensive, and concentrated treatments provided evidence of their acceptability among the majority of youth and their families [37]. Although this meta-analysis found promising results for brief, intensive, and concentrated treatments for youth, no studies were examined that used intensive treatments for youth with generalized anxiety disorder or selective mutism [37]. In addition, 13 of the 23 randomized clinical controlled trials that were examined were for specific phobias. The meta-analysis found moderate effects for post-traumatic stress disorder and OCD studies (three each) and minimal effects for panic disorder, social anxiety disorder, separation anxiety disorder, and mixed anxiety disorders (one study each), thus suggesting the need for additional trials to be conducted for youth with the latter anxiety diagnoses to fully determine the efficacy of intensive treatment approaches in future meta-analyses.

To date, several brief and intensive treatments have been conducted and tested with youth who have OCD. Whiteside and colleagues [44] developed a 5-day intensive CBT treatment. Parents were required to be present at all sessions, which consisted of 10 individual 50 to 75-minute sessions across 5 days (two sessions per day). This protocol focused on training parents how to help guide their child through exposure exercises without the therapist so that they can become "exposure coaches" who will continue to facilitate exposures after returning home [44]. The 5-day intensive CBT treatment was found to be comparable to standard CBT or 3-week intensive CBT treatment programs [44]. To increase the availability for evidence-based exposure therapy, Whiteside and colleagues expanded on this protocol to a group-based format for youth with OCD and childhood anxiety disorders. This group-based intensive treatment was implemented over 5 days and consisted of parent-coached exposure over nine 90 to 120-minute group sessions and one 30-minute individual appointment. The goals of this treatment protocol were (1) providing psychoeducation from a cognitive behavioral perspective to parents on how avoidance and rituals maintain childhood anxiety disorders and OCD, (2) assisting parents via exposures in a reduction of symptoms among their children, and (3) training parents to coach their youth through exposures. The feasibility of this program was retrospectively examined; across all anxiety disorders and OCD, patients had decreased symptoms, impairment, and avoidance [49]. In addition, the Bergen 4-day concentrated exposure treatment has been used for youth with OCD and found to be effective [50,51]. This treatment is conducted over 4 days in groups of three to six participants with a 1:1 patient to therapist ratio, with the main approach of this treatment being "LEan into The anxiety" technique. This technique's goal is to help teach patients to approach the trigger for anxiety and discomfort and lean into those feelings rather than avoiding them [50,51]. Studies using this intensive treatment approach find that youth with OCD show a decrease in symptoms after participating in this 4 day treatment, with gains maintained at 12 months and 4 years after treatment [50,51]. Overall, the work by the investigators suggest the feasibility of using a brief and intensive treatment approach for youth with OCD [44] as well as a transdiagnostic group-based approach for youth with a variety of anxiety disorders and OCD [49]. These protocols indicate that these treatments may increase access for families with youth who have childhood anxiety disorders or OCD, which may not be otherwise feasible if not for being delivered in this condensed amount of time.

These studies suggest that intensive treatment approaches may provide an evidence-based option for youth with anxiety disorders or OCD with greater symptom severity. Although past research has emphasized symptom reduction and remission rates as outcome for these treatment approaches, it was not until recent work by Sperling and colleagues [52] that researchers examined daily functioning as an outcome for families and youth with OCD or childhood anxiety disorders in intensive treatments. Youth ages 8 to 19 years and their caregivers [52] were enrolled in an intensive outpatient group-based treatment program. Treatment consisted of youth attending 4 days per week for a minimum of 4 weeks, with the option to extend for any number of full weeks. Caregivers attended a separate weekly 50-minute group-based session that taught parents skills to support their child's treatment and attended a weekly 45-minute meeting that offered parents support and provided a time to discuss logistical concerns (eg, discharge plans). Results from this study found that youth and parents observed less functional impairment over the course of the treatment, and youth were able to spend more time with family and friends and attend school [52]. In addition, youth who reported comorbid depressive symptoms at the beginning of treatment reported a decrease in their depression at discharge [52]. This study highlights the importance of evaluating treatment success above and beyond symptom reduction. Specifically, although this study found that youth who participated in this group-based intensive treatment reported symptom relief, it is one of the first studies to highlight the importance of examining adaptive behavior as a treatment outcome.

VARIABILITY WITHIN INTENSIVE TREATMENT

Intensive treatment for youth with childhood anxiety disorders and OCD often varies in the approach, modality, and length of treatment. One-session treatment (OST) was initially developed to treat specific phobias [53]. This treatment approach involves cognitive restructuring, in vivo exposure, participant modeling, reinforced practice, and psychoeducation in one 3-hour session. Intensive treatments that are based on OST provide more opportunity for extinction of fear due to there being a greater number of ERP exercises through a more continuous and rapid exposure to feared stimuli [54]. In a case study involving an individual with OCD, Farrell and Miller [54] modeled their intensive treatment for youth with OCD based-on OST, where the patient and family completed two 3.5 hour long sessions spaced 1 week apart and followed up with the family with four 1-hour telehealth sessions for the following month. This case study found that the patient showed reduced symptoms and assessment scores for OCD decreased [54]. The follow-up controlled baseline design studies of Farrell and Miller's intensive treatment approach found that there continued to be reductions on all measures and patients reported improvement in symptoms [55]. In addition, a recent study examined the potential efficacy D-cycloserine (DCS) relative to placebo for youth with OCD, with both groups receiving intensive exposure therapy [56]. Following a brief psychoeducation session, participants from both groups received 3 weekly 3-hour ERP sessions, with at least one being conducted at home, and a final 2-hour booster session focusing on ERP and relapse prevention after 1 month [56]. Results from this study did not find a statistically significant difference between groups at any time point (post-session, 1 month after session, 3 months after session, and 6 months after session), suggesting no augmenting effects of DCS at posttreatment or any time point after [56]. These results suggest that intensive and time-limited approaches for youth with OCD or anxiety disorders show promising results and may provide greater access and relief to youth and families with OCD and anxiety disorders.

Studies vary on the duration of sessions, parental involvement, setting where the intensive treatment takes place and number of sessions for youth with OCD anxiety disorders enrolled in intensive treatment. Specifically, in a study by Whiteside and colleagues [49], the investigators expanded their intensive treatment protocol to a group-based format for mixed childhood anxiety disorders and OCD. The treatment was completed over 5 days, including nine 90 to 120-minute group sessions and one 30-minute individual session with at least two clinicians (sometimes a third trainee was also present). In a similar duration, an intensive treatment was delivered to youth with CBT during 5 consecutive days for 5 hours per day in the Netherlands and Switzerland [57]. The ratio of patients to therapists was 2:1 with each group having six to eight patients in each group. Parents attended one session of psychoeducation on OCD and CBT and were highly encouraged (but not required) to attend one block of ERP during the week [57]. Alternatively, Storch and colleagues [41] conducted a randomized control trial for youth with OCD and the intensive protocol included attending individual CBT sessions every weekday for 3 weeks consecutively, for a total of 14 sessions. Angelosante and colleagues [58] delivered an outpatient intensive CBT program for adolescents with panic disorder, which was delivered daily over 8 days. Parents were included and taught parenting skills for aiding their adolescent with panic disorder. Although the previously described studies varied in session length, number of sessions, and caregiver involvement, collectively the results continue to indicate that intensive treatment for youth with OCD and anxiety disorders is as effective as standard CBT. Similarly, although most intensive treatment approaches have been conducted in an outpatient setting, some studies have examined intensive CBT treatment for youth with OCD in a residential setting [59,60]. Results from these studies find that intensive CBT treatments held in residential treatment settings are as effective compared with standard CBT while providing advantages for youth who are treatment-resistant or may need a very rapid response [46,61]. As noted above, intensive treatment approaches vary in the duration, family involvement, and setting; yet, therapist contact time remains relatively stable, averaging about 9 hours [62]. However, research indicates that these treatment approaches remain as effective as standard CBT treatment for youth with OCD and anxiety disorders.

TELEHEALTH WITHIN INTENSIVE TREATMENT

Currently, it is becoming increasingly common to offer standard CBT via telehealth and is found to be as effective as in-person treatment [63,64]. However, little research has been conducted to determine the efficacy of a telehealth-based intensive treatment for youth with OCD and anxiety. Farrell and colleagues [65] delivered an intensive CBT treatment, which consisted of one 60-minute education session and two intensive ERP sessions in person followed by a 3-week "e-therapy maintenance" program. Each telehealth maintenance phone call, via Skype, lasted about 45 minutes and the therapist, child, and parents reviewed exposure practice that week, addressed any challenges, and discussed homework compliance with exposure practice. During these e-therapy calls, therapists encouraged the patient to engage in one ERP session during the call to maintain progress [65]. Results from this novel study found that 60% of patients were in remission of symptoms, 80% of the sample reliably improved on almost all measures except measures of self-reported anxiety, and at 6-month follow-up 70% of patients were in remission of symptoms [65]. A case study of a fully web-based intensive family-based treatment showed a reduction in OCD symptoms for the patient [66]. This case study described a child patient with OCD who participated in an intensive treatment with a parent twice a day for 5 days via web camera. The intensive treatment was similar to the previously described intensive treatment approaches, such that it was family-based, and sessions were delivered twice a day for 60 to 75 minutes and lasted for 5 days [49,57]. Results from this case study found that the patient showed reductions in symptoms; however, these were not statistically significant [66]. These studies show promising results that aspects of intensive treatment can be delivered effectively via telehealth. However, further research is warranted to compare a fully web-based telehealth intensive treatment to an in-person intensive treatment for youth with OCD and anxiety disorders to confirm these findings on a larger scale.

FUTURE DIRECTIONS

Brief and intensive CBT approaches for youth with OCD and anxiety disorders have shown to be effective in reducing symptoms, remission rates, and improving daily functioning for families and patients compared with standard CBT treatment [37,41,44,57,67]. To date, these studies have mostly focused on non-

Hispanic white samples. Future studies should focus on recruiting more representative and diverse samples to understand if these effects generalize to different races and ethnicities. In addition, studies to date have primarily consisted of samples from family incomes that are above the US median, indicating a gap in research in treatment for families across all incomes [41,67]. Future research is warranted to explore the efficacy of these treatments for families from lower socioeconomic statuses. Finally, although research is beginning to examine intensive treatment approaches via telehealth, to the authors' knowledge, only a few studies have evaluated the efficacy of telehealth-based intensive treatment for youth with OCD and anxiety disorders. As telehealth interventions mitigate logistical barriers for many families, additional research with larger sample sizes is warranted to determine the full efficacy of telehealth-based intensive treatment.

SUMMARY

We highlight that using intensive treatment produces similar posttreatment effects as the standard gold-standard treatment for youth with OCD and anxiety disorders. Specifically, intensive treatment still uses the same content as standard CBT (ie, cognitive restructuring, psychoeducation, exposure therapy with response prevention) but does so in a shorter amount of sessions. Using telehealth will likely continue to develop into a typical method to treat youth with OCD and anxiety disorders, which warrants research to continue to evaluate the efficacy of web-based intensive treatment approaches for youth with OCD and anxiety disorder [68–70]. Therefore, clinicians should continue to stay current with telehealth modalities to deliver mental health services.

CLINICS CARE POINTS

- Intensive treatment for youth with anxiety disorders and OCD is an effective treatment for this population.
- Delivery of intensive treatment, via telehealth or in-person, both are effective.

FUNDING DETAILS

This research did not receive any specific grant from funding agencies in the public, commercial, or not-for-profit sectors.

DISCLOSURE

Ms C.E. Maye, Dr C.M. Pinciotti report no disclosures. Dr E.A. Storch receives grant support from NIH, the Ream Foundation, Greater Houston Community Foundation, International OCD Foundation, and Texas Higher Education Coordinating Board. He receives book royalties from Elsevier, Springer, American Psychological Association, Jessica Kingsley, Oxford, and Lawrence Erlbaum. He holds stock in NView, where he serves on the clinical advisory board. He was a consultant for Levo Therapeutics and is currently a consultant for Biohaven Pharmaceuticals and Brainsway. He cofounded and receives payment from Rethinking Behavioral Health, which is a consulting firm that provides support for implementing evidence-based psychological treatment strategies.

REFERENCES

[1] Kessler RC, Chiu WT, Demler O, et al. Prevalence, severity, and comorbidity of 12-month DSM-IV disorders in the National Comorbidity Survey Replication. Arch Gen Psychiatry 2005;62(6):617–27.

[2] Ruscio AM, Stein DJ, Chiu WT, et al. The epidemiology of obsessive-compulsive disorder in the National Comorbidity Survey Replication. Mol Psychiatry 2010; 15(1):53–63.

[3] Cervin M, Miguel EC, Güler AS, et al. Towards a definitive symptom structure of obsessive–compulsive disorder: a factor and network analysis of 87 distinct symptoms in 1366 individuals. Psychol Med 2021;1–13.

[4] Hasler G, Pinto A, Greenberg BD, et al. Familiality of factor analysis-derived YBOCS dimensions in OCD-affected sibling pairs from the OCD Collaborative Genetics Study. Biol Psychiatry 2007;61(5):617–25.

[5] Kugler BB, Lewin AB, Phares V, et al. Quality of life in obsessive-compulsive disorder: the role of mediating variables. Psychiatry Res 2013;206(1):43–9.

[6] Stewart SE, Stack DE, Farrell C, et al. Effectiveness of intensive residential treatment (IRT) for severe, refractory obsessive-compulsive disorder. J Psychiatr Res 2005; 39(6):603–9.

[7] Taylor S. Early versus late onset obsessive-compulsive disorder: evidence for distinct subtypes. Clin Psychol Rev 2011;31(7):1083–100.

[8] Cooper M. Obsessive-compulsive disorder: Effects on family members. Am J Orthop 1996;66(2):296–304.

[9] Piacentini J, Bergman RL, Keller M, et al. Functional impairment in children and adolescents with obsessive-compulsive disorder. J Child Adolesc Psychopharmacol 2003;13(Suppl 1):S61–9.

[10] Valderhaug R, Ivarsson T. Functional impairment in clinical samples of Norwegian and Swedish children and adolescents with obsessive-compulsive disorder. Eur Child Adolesc Psychiatry 2005;14(3):164–73.

[11] Allsopp M, Verduyn C. Adolescents with obsessive-compulsive disorder: a case note review of consecutive patients referred to a provincial regional adolescent psychiatry unit. J Adolesc 1990;13(2):157–69.

[12] Storch EA, Ledley DR, Lewin AB, et al. Peer victimization in children with obsessive-compulsive disorder: relations with symptoms of psychopathology. J Clin Child Adolesc Psychol 2006;35(3):446–55.

[13] Weidle B, Jozefiak T, Ivarsson T, et al. Quality of life in children with OCD with and without comorbidity. Health Qual Life Outcomes 2014;12:152.

[14] Honjo S, Hirano C, Murase S, et al. Obsessive-compulsive symptoms in childhood and adolescence. Acta Psychiatr Scand 1989;80(1):83–91.

[15] Toro J, Cervera M, Osejo E, et al. Obsessive-compulsive disorder in childhood and adolescence: a clinical study. J Child Psychol Psychiatry 1992;33(6):1025–37.

[16] Essau CA, Ollendick TH. The Wiley-Blackwell handbook of the treatment of childhood and adolescent anxiety. Chichester (England): John Wiley & Sons; 2013.

[17] Association AP. Diagnostic and statistical manual of mental disorders : DSM-5. Arlington, VA: American Psychiatric Association; 2013.

[18] Fowler S, Szabó M. The emotional experience associated with worrying in adolescents. J Psychopathology Behav Assess 2013;35(1):65–75.

[19] Maldonado L, Huang Y, Chen R, et al. Impact of early adolescent anxiety disorders on self-esteem development from adolescence to young adulthood. J Adolesc Health 2013;53(2):287–92.

[20] Nail JE, Christofferson J, Ginsburg GS, et al. Academic impairment and impact of treatments among youth with anxiety disorders. Child Youth Care Forum 2015; 44(3):327–42.

[21] Woodward LJ, Fergusson DM. Life course outcomes of young people with anxiety disorders in adolescence. J Am Acad Child Adolesc Psychiatry 2001;40(9):1086–93.

[22] Lynch FL, Dickerson JF, Clarke G, et al. Incremental cost-effectiveness of combined therapy vs medication only for youth with selective serotonin reuptake inhibitor-resistant depression: treatment of SSRI-resistant depression in adolescents trial findings. Arch Gen Psychiatry 2011;68(3):253–62.

[23] Higa-McMillan CK, Francis SE, Rith-Najarian L, et al. Evidence Base Update: 50 Years of Research on Treatment for Child and Adolescent Anxiety. J Clin Child Adolesc Psychol 2016;45(2):91–113.

[24] Storch EA, Merlo LJ. Obsessive-compulsive disorder: strategies for using CBT and pharmacotherapy. J Fam Pract 2006;55(4):329–33.

[25] Stines LR, Feeny NC, Foa EB. Emotional disorders: treatment. In: Squire LR, editor. Encyclopedia of neuroscience. Oxford: Academic Press; 2009. p. 929–32.

[26] McGuire JF, Piacentini J, Lewin AB, et al. A meta-analysis of cognitive behavior therapy and medication for child obsessive-compulsive disorder: moderators of treatment efficacy, response, and remission. Depress anxiety 2015;32(8):580–93.

[27] Reid AM, Guzick AG, Fernandez AG, et al. Exposure therapy for youth with anxiety: Utilization rates and predictors of implementation in a sample of practicing clinicians from across the United States. J Anxiety Disord 2018;58:8–17.

[28] Craske MG, Treanor M, Conway CC, et al. Maximizing exposure therapy: an inhibitory learning approach. Behav Res Ther 2014;58:10–23.

[29] Ale CM, McCarthy DM, Rothschild LM, et al. Components of cognitive behavioral therapy related to outcome in childhood anxiety disorders. Clin Child Fam Psychol Rev 2015;18(3):240–51.

[30] Whiteside SP, Ale CM, Young B, et al. The feasibility of improving CBT for childhood anxiety disorders through a dismantling study. Behav Res Ther 2015;73:83–9.

[31] James AC, James G, Cowdrey FA, et al. Cognitive behavioural therapy for anxiety disorders in children and adolescents. Cochrane Database Syst Rev 2013;6:Cd004690.

[32] Ollendick TH, King NJ. Evidence-based treatments for children and adolescents: issues and commentary. In: Child and adolescent therapy: cognitive-behavioral procedures. 4th ed. New York, NY, US: Guilford Press; 2012. p. 499–519.

[33] Reynolds S, Wilson C, Austin J, et al. Effects of psychotherapy for anxiety in children and adolescents: a meta-analytic review. Clin Psychol Rev 2012;32(4):251–62.

[34] DuPont RL, Rice DP, Shiraki S, et al. Economic costs of obsessive-compulsive disorder. Med Interf 1995;8(4): 102–9.

[35] Freeman J, Garcia A, Frank H, et al. Evidence base update for psychosocial treatments for pediatric obsessive-compulsive disorder. J Clin Child Adolesc Psychol 2014;43(1):7–26.

[36] Markarian Y, Larson MJ, Aldea MA, et al. Multiple pathways to functional impairment in obsessive-compulsive disorder. Clin Psychol Rev 2010;30(1):78–88.

[37] Öst L-G, Ollendick TH. Brief, intensive and concentrated cognitive behavioral treatments for anxiety disorders in children: A systematic review and meta-analysis. Behav Res Ther 2017;97:134–45.

[38] Foa EB, Steketee G. Behavioral treatment of phobics and obsessive-compulsives. In: Psychotherapists in clinical practice: cognitive and behavioral perspectives. New York, NY, US: Guilford Press; 1987. p. 78–120.

[39] Grabill K, Storch EA, Geffken GR. Innovations in CBT interventions for anxious youth-intensive cognitive-behavioral therapy for pediatric OCD. Behav Therapist 2007; 30(1):19.

[40] Schmidt RA, Bjork RA. New conceptualizations of practice: common principles in three paradigms suggest new concepts for training. Psychol Sci 1992;3(4): 207–18.

[41] Storch EA, Geffken GR, Merlo LJ, et al. Family-based cognitive-behavioral therapy for pediatric obsessive-compulsive disorder: comparison of intensive and

weekly approaches. J Am Acad Child Adolesc Psychiatry 2007;46(4):469–78.

[42] Ollendick TH, Ost LG, Reuterskiöld L, et al. One-session treatment of specific phobias in youth: a randomized clinical trial in the United States and Sweden. J Consult Clin Psychol 2009;77(3):504–16.

[43] Santucci LC, Ehrenreich JT, Trosper SE, et al. Development and Preliminary Evaluation of a 1-Week Summer Treatment Program for Separation Anxiety Disorder. Cogn Behav Pract 2009;16(3):317–31.

[44] Whiteside SP, McKay D, De Nadai AS, et al. A baseline controlled examination of a 5-day intensive treatment for pediatric obsessive-compulsive disorder. Psychiatry Res 2014;220(1–2):441–6.

[45] Ehrenreich JT, Santucci LC. Special series: Intensive cognitive-behavioral treatments for child and adolescent anxiety disorders. Cogn Behav Pract 2009;16(3):290–3.

[46] Hojgaard DRMA, Schneider SC, La Buissonniere-Ariza V, et al. Predictors of treatment outcome for youth receiving intensive residential treatment for obsessive-compulsive disorder (OCD). Chichester (England): Cognitive Behaviour Therapy; 2019.

[47] Jónsson H, Kristensen M, Arendt M. Intensive cognitive behavioural therapy for obsessive-compulsive disorder: a systematic review and meta-analysis. J Obsessive-Compulsive Relat Disord 2015;6:83–96.

[48] Tolin DF, Whiting S, Maltby N, et al. Intensive (Daily) behavior therapy for school refusal: a multiple baseline case series. Cogn Behav Pract 2009;16(3):332–44.

[49] Whiteside SPH, Dammann JE, Tiede MS, et al. Increasing availability of exposure therapy through intensive group treatment for childhood anxiety and OCD. Behav modification 2018;42(5):707–28.

[50] Hansen B, Kvale G, Hagen K, et al. The Bergen 4-day treatment for OCD: four years follow-up of concentrated ERP in a clinical mental health setting. Cogn Behav Ther 2019;48(2):89–105.

[51] Hansen B, Hagen K, Öst L-G, et al. The bergen 4-Day OCD treatment delivered in a group setting: 12-month follow-up. Front Psychol 2018;9:639.

[52] Sperling J, Boger K, Potter M. The impact of intensive treatment for pediatric anxiety and obsessive-compulsive disorder on daily functioning. Clin Child Psychol Psychiatry 2020;25(1):133–40.

[53] Ost LG. One-session treatment for specific phobias. Behav Res Ther 1989;27(1):1–7.

[54] Farrell LJ, Milliner EL. Intensive cognitive behavioural treatment for obsessive compulsive disorder in children and adolescents. Psychopathology Rev 2014;a1(1):182–8.

[55] Farrell LJ, Sluis R, Waters AM. Intensive treatment of pediatric OCD: the case of Sarah. J Clin Psychol 2016;72(11):1174–90.

[56] Farrell LJ, Waters AM, Tiralongo E, et al. Efficacy of D-cycloserine augmented brief intensive cognitive-behavioural therapy for paediatric obsessive-compulsive disorder: A randomised clinical trial. Depression and Anxiety 2022;39(6):461–73.

[57] Wolters LH, Ball J, Brezinka V, et al. Brief intensive cognitive behavioral therapy for children and adolescents with OCD: two international pilot studies. J Obsessive-Compulsive Relat Disord 2021;29:100645.

[58] Angelosante AG, Pincus DB, Whitton SW, et al. Implementation of an intensive treatment protocol for adolescents with panic disorder and agorophobia. Cogn Behav Pract 2009;16(3):345–57.

[59] Björgvinsson T, Wetterneck CT, Powell DM, et al. Treatment outcome for adolescent obsessive-compulsive disorder in a specialized hospital setting. J Psychiatr Pract 2008;14(3):137–45.

[60] Leonard RC, Franklin ME, Wetterneck CT, et al. Residential treatment outcomes for adolescents with obsessive-compulsive disorder. Psychother Res 2016;26(6):727–36.

[61] Geller DA, March J. Practice parameter for the assessment and treatment of children and adolescents with obsessive-compulsive disorder. J Am Acad Child Adolesc Psychiatry 2012;51(1):98–113.

[62] Team POTSP. Cognitive-behavior therapy, sertraline, and their combination for children and adolescents with obsessive-compulsive disorder: the Pediatric OCD Treatment Study (POTS) randomized controlled trial. JAMA 2004;292(16):1969–76.

[63] Orsolini L, Pompili S, Salvi V, et al. A systematic review on telemental health in youth mental health: focus on anxiety, depression and obsessive-compulsive disorder. Medicina 2021;57(8):793.

[64] Pinciotti CM, Bulkes NZ, Horvath G, et al. Efficacy of intensive CBT telehealth for obsessive-compulsive disorder during the COVID-19 pandemic. J Obsessive-Compulsive Relat Disord 2022;32:100705.

[65] Farrell LJ, Oar EL, Waters AM, et al. Brief intensive CBT for pediatric OCD with E-therapy maintenance. J Anxiety Disord 2016;42:85–94.

[66] Ojserkis R, Morris B, McKay D. Pediatric obsessive-compulsive disorder: an illustration of intensive family-based treatment delivered via web camera. Clin Case Stud 2014;13(1):68–79.

[67] Storch EA, Merlo LJ, Larson MJ, et al. Impact of comorbidity on cognitive-behavioral therapy response in pediatric obsessive-compulsive disorder. J Am Acad Child Adolesc Psychiatry 2008;47(5):583–92.

[68] Palo A, D'Souza JM. The impact of COVID-19 on the treatment of obsessive-compulsive disorder. Bull Menninger Clin 2022;86(1):35–47.

[69] Ros-DeMarize R, Chung P, Stewart R. Pediatric behavioral telehealth in the age of COVID-19: Brief evidence review and practice considerations. Curr Probl Pediatr Adolesc Health Care 2021;51(1):100949.

[70] Peros OM, Webb L, Fox S, et al. Conducting exposure-based groups via telehealth for adolescents and young adults with social anxiety disorder. Cogn Behav Pract 2021;28(4):679–89.

Advances in Psychiatry and Behavioral Health 2 (2022) 141–153
ADVANCES IN PSYCHIATRY AND BEHAVIORAL HEALTH

Moving Beyond the Clinic

Leveraging Telehealth Strategies to Address Youth Mental Health Challenges

Gabrielle F. Freitag, MS, Anya E. Urcuyo, BA, Jonathan S. Comer, PhD*
Center for Children and Families, Department of Psychology, Florida International University, Center for Children and Families, 11200 South West 8th Street, Miami, FL 33199, USA

KEYWORDS
• Telehealth • Technology • Child • Mental health care • Treatment delivery • Videoconference

KEY POINTS

- Telehealth approaches hold great promise and potential for expanding the reach and scope of youth mental health care.
- Clinical trials have found telehealth can be useful, effective, and well-tolerated in the treatment of a wide range of youth mental health concerns.
- Pandemic-era emergency orders and relaxed regulations facilitated a large-scale telehealth rollout by removing several telehealth barriers; telehealth practices surged during the COVID-19 pandemic.
- Barriers to telehealth persist; many of the populations underserved by telehealth are the same populations underserved by brick-and-mortar care.
- Ensuring equitable access to telehealth is critical for telehealth to actualize its potential for reaching new populations that have been underserved by office-based care.

INTRODUCTION

Child and adolescent mental health problems constitute an enormous public health concern. Up to 40% of youth will suffer from a diagnosable mental disorder by the time they reach adulthood [1], and countless others will experience various traumatic events, life stress, experiences of marginalization, or difficulties with mood or behavior that are also linked with serious clinical impairments [2,3]. Youth mental health challenges are associated with academic, peer, and family dysfunction [4], and earlier onset is typically associated with worse prognosis. Accordingly, broad equitable access to effective youth mental health care is critical.

Although the past 20 years have witnessed remarkable progress in the development and evaluation of youth mental health interventions designed for office-based delivery [5], considerable barriers persist in the accessibility and acceptability of these supported interventions. At the broadest level, there are an insufficient number of mental health providers. Kazdin and Blase [6] speculated that even if we were to double the mental health workforce, there would still not be enough providers to address the mental health needs at a population level with traditional 1:1 care. Geographic disparities in the mental health workforce further constrain the availability of care for many, as mental health providers tend to concentrate in metropolitan regions and academic hubs [7], rendering over 5000 regions in the United States as mental health professional shortage areas [8]. Forty US states have

*Corresponding author, *E-mail address:* jocomer@fiu.edu

https://doi.org/10.1016/j.ypsc.2022.06.004
2667-3827/22/

less than 7 psychiatric nurses for every 100,000 residents [9]. Over two-thirds of US counties have less than 5 licensed psychologists, and roughly three-quarters of US counties have less than 10 licensed psychologists [10]. Transportation obstacles, stigma-related concerns about visiting a mental health clinic, and treatment costs driven up by brick-and-mortar expenses further limit the reach of traditional outpatient mental health care for many [7]. Of course, in recent years, the COVID-19 pandemic and associated stay-at-home guidelines further exacerbated the care availability crisis, abruptly putting traditional office-based care out of reach for most of the population.

To address barriers to traditional office-based care, clinical innovators have increasingly leveraged technology to extend the reach and scope of child and adolescent mental health care. Considerable empirical literature has now come to support *telehealth* treatment formats, in which synchronous interactive communication technologies, such as videoconferencing, are used to afford real-time interactions between patients and providers for the remote delivery of care that is typically delivered in office settings [11–18]. Providers can now remotely deliver therapist-led care, in real time, regardless of the patient's geographic proximity to the provider's office. Relative to traditional office-based care, telehealth approaches to mental health care also have potential to overcome stigma-related concerns many have about visiting a mental health clinic by treating families in the privacy of their home.

Telehealth strategies are gaining acceptance and empirical support in the treatment of youth mental health challenges, and they are assuming an increasingly prominent role in the delivery of youth mental health services and supports. During the COVID-19 pandemic, the field saw a sharp uptick in the use of telehealth strategies to remotely deliver children's mental health care and parenting interventions [12,19–22], and looking to the years ahead, there is a strong indication that telehealth is set to remain a major vehicle for the delivery of children's mental health care.

Against this backdrop, we provide an overview of telehealth approaches that extend the reach and scope of children's mental health care. Throughout, we cover the rationale, history, practice trends, and supporting evidence for telehealth strategies. We also discuss key administrative, logistical, ethical, and policy-related considerations for telehealth providers working with children and families, and we conclude with an eye toward future directions in this promising and growing area of practice and research.

TELEHEALTH AND YOUTH MENTAL HEALTH CARE: HISTORY, EMPIRICAL SUPPORT, AND TRENDS

Telehealth treatment, or telemedicine, refers to the use of interactive, synchronous communication technologies, such as videoconferencing platforms, to deliver a real-time, provider-led health care that is typically delivered in-person. Of note, this increasingly embraced conceptualization of telehealth does not include asynchronous or self-administered technology-based options, such as self-guided mobile apps, self-paced digital intervention technologies with minimal therapist involvement, or digital applications that use passive sensing and machine learning to continuously monitor, process, and intervene on moment-to-moment states.

The use of telehealth for the specific delivery of mental health care has been alternatively referred to as telepsychiatry [23], behavioral telehealth [7], and telemental health [24] throughout the literature. For the present purposes, we use the broader term "telehealth" to generically refer to all such services and to acknowledge the interdisciplinary nature of the work that mental health workers provide.

Telehealth: A Brief History

The concept of using technology to remotely deliver real-time, interactive health care was first written about in the 1920s by Hugo Gernsback, an early radio technology pioneer and the father of science fiction. Gernsback predicted the practice of telehealth in his fictionalized, but prophetic, extrapolation of where radio technologies could take medical care across the next 50 years. In a piece published in his scientific pulp magazines *Science and Invention* and *Radio News*, Gernsback envisioned doctors of the future who would be able to see into a patient's home on a screen while using radio technology to remotely communicate in real-time with the patient. While interacting on the screen, it was described that these "radio doctors" would manipulate controls on a fictitious instrument in their office that Gernsback referred to as a *teledactyl* (from the Greek, meaning "far arms") that would allow the doctor to physically "interact" with the patient. Specifically, the doctor would operate the teledactyl in their office which would manipulate a robotic device in the patient's room in exactly the same manner. This would enable the doctor to "feel" the patient at a distance and would facilitate remote assessment, diagnosis, and treatment [25].

In the 1950s, the field saw the first application of remote technologies for the actual practice of health care. Specifically, innovators at the University of Nebraska used the two-way interactive television technology to transmit psychiatric evaluations across Nebraska medical school campuses for therapy consultations and to extend the reach of education and training. In the 1960s, Massachusetts General Hospital (MGH) in Boston, MA, established the first telehealth practice when they set up a remote medical station at the airport and used the closed-circuit, interactive telecommunications technology to enable MGH clinicians to provide psychiatric care for patients without their having to visit the hospital [26]. Descriptions of this MGH telehealth service marked the first appearance in the literature of the term "telepsychiatry."

Despite advances in telehealth innovations across the mid-to-late twentieth century, it was not until the turn of the century, with rapidly broadening availability and sophistication of telecommunication technologies, which telehealth approaches to mental health care began to gain broader feasibility and credibility. Clinical innovators were beginning to use scientific methods to empirically evaluate telehealth applications for the delivery of mental health care.

Modern Telehealth Trends in Mental Health Care

Relative to other health care subdisciplines, mental health care has been thought to be particularly amenable to a teleconferencing format, given the discipline's primary emphasis on audio and visual information. The first two decades of the twenty-first century were marked by an accumulating body of empirical literature supporting the use of telehealth strategies for delivering mental health care [12,13,27–31], but only a very small proportion of mental health providers were adopting telehealth in their own practices. At the time, regulatory policies presented obstacles to the broad adoption of telehealth, discouraging providers from using telehealth with their patients. Before 2020, for example, most insurance providers would not reimburse for telehealth services, especially when such services were delivered to patients in their homes. Consequently, at the time, telehealth services were mostly available only to patients paying for mental health services out-of-pocket, to patients receiving services as part of research participation, or to patients treated as part of group-level care delivered outside of individual fee-for-service reimbursement. As a result, communities of color and patients experiencing resource insecurity were particularly underserved by telehealth innovations [12]. In addition, at this time, most providers were concerned that offering telehealth services could leave them vulnerable to serious professional and personal penalties, should a hacking incident or other unforeseen technology-related confidentiality breach occur.

Despite policy and reimbursement obstacles to telehealth, throughout the 2010s, an increasing number of clinical evaluations and controlled trials began to populate the literature and provide rigorous support for the use of telehealth to deliver provider-led mental health care [11–13,27,28,32,33]. The vast majority of these studies found that telehealth approaches were useful, effective, and well tolerated in the treatment of a wide range of youth mental health concerns. Meta-analyses that have quantitatively synthesized the empirical literature on telehealth have found telehealth to be associated with a highly significant, positive, and relatively large-sized effect on pretreatment versus posttreatment outcomes [11,14–18]. Telehealth approaches have exhibited the largest effects when the treatment is based in cognitive-behavioral therapy, and when it is targeting affective disorders or delivering parenting interventions [13,14,28]. Research has also typically found that telehealth services are associated with maintenance of gains across time [13,34]. Moreover, the adult literature has found larger effects of telehealth for female patients than for male patients [11], but this gender effect has not been supported in the child literature.

On average, families participating in telehealth report experiencing significantly fewer barriers to care (eg, scheduling and keeping appointments) than do families participating in traditional office-based care [13,28]. Meta-analyses that have pooled the results of clinical trials that directly compared telehealth to traditional office-based care have typically found no significant overall differences between the two modalities with regard to overall improvements [11,14–17]. In fact, some clinical trials have found telehealth approaches to *outperform* traditional office-based care. For example, Comer and colleagues [13] randomly assigned families of young children with behavior problems to receive a well-established parenting intervention—Parent–Child Interaction Therapy (PCIT) [35]—either in the office or over the Internet using videoconferencing (Internet-delivered PCIT [iPCIT]). In the iPCIT telehealth condition, families used webcams to stream their child's behavior and family interactions from their home, whereas providers remotely delivered parent coaching in real time via parent-worn Bluetooth earpieces. In contrast, in office-based PCIT, families came to the clinic and their therapist provided walkie-talkie bug-in-the-ear coaching from behind a one-way mirror. Most outcomes were comparable across the families receiving PCIT in the office versus via telehealth, but independent evaluators who were masked to each family's treatment condition rated a higher proportion of posttreatment "excellent responders" among families who received the telehealth condition [13]. Results such as these have been interpreted to suggest that under some circumstances, for some clinical problems and some youth and families, telehealth approaches may not only increase the reach of care but may also improve the ecological validity of care by treating children and families in their natural settings—in the situations that are most problematic [12,13,36].

In the early months of 2020, when the COVID-19 pandemic took hold of North America, the field saw perhaps the largest and most abrupt transformation of clinical practice in the history of mental health care. When the pandemic hit, mental health needs surged in the general population, particularly among youth, as a result of virus fears and COVID-related financial instability, life disruption, and isolation. Pandemic-related surges in mental health needs were accompanied by stay-at-home orders that abruptly curtailed the feasibility and safety of traditional office-based mental health care. Virtual schooling put the availability of mental health care particularly out of reach for youth, given that before the pandemic over one-third of youth in mental health care were receiving these services in school settings [37]. At a moment of unprecedented mental health need in the population, providers found themselves without their traditional tools for treating patients.

To maintain continuity of care for those receiving mental health care and to address the newly emerging pandemic-related mental health challenges in the population, several emergency orders were enacted in the United States at the federal, state, and private levels, and several reimbursement policies were expanded to facilitate a large-scale transition to telehealth. For example, emergency orders were enacted that effectively waived penalties against health care workers if good faith efforts to provide telehealth during the pandemic resulted in an unintentional breach in confidentiality. Consumer-grade teleconferencing equipment and platforms could now be used to deliver care without the same level of concern about provider liability. In addition, federal, state, and most private insurance plans quickly adjusted their policies to allow reimbursement for telehealth appointments.

These expanded policies and relaxed regulations removed several pre-pandemic obstacles and set the stage for broad telehealth implementation [38,39]. Among health care subdisciplines, mental health care saw particularly surging telehealth usage [40]. Although before the pandemic only about one in every 10 surveyed mental health providers were using telehealth strategies in their practices [41], just a few weeks after the pandemic-era emergency policies were enacted, roughly 80% of surveyed mental health providers had already transitioned almost entirely to telehealth practice [42]. By about a half a year into the pandemic, telehealth practice was ubiquitous, with only about 5% of surveyed mental health workers exclusively seeing their patients in the office [41]. Moreover, half a year into the pandemic, most surveyed mental health workers (ie, 90%) predicted they would still use telehealth to treat their patients long after the crisis of the pandemic was over [41]. At the time of this writing, most of mental health workers are still continuing to use telehealth strategies to see at least some of their patients.

KEY CONSIDERATIONS AND CAUTIONS FOR TELEHEALTH PRACTICE WITH CHILDREN AND FAMILIES

The COVID-19 pandemic forced the field to abruptly transform the delivery and formatting of outpatient mental health care. Although it is remarkable how quickly outpatient mental health care transitioned to a largely telehealth model in the early months of the pandemic, in the context of an urgent public health crisis it was not possible for most providers to complete formal telehealth training before launching into practice. In fact, most outpatient mental health providers reported that despite transitioning to telehealth services, they did not think sufficiently trained to provide proper telehealth care [43]. Although telehealth had been steadily growing for 20 years as a defined practice with expert standards [24,44], when the pandemic forced most outpatient providers to newly go online, actual practices were not always aligned with existing telehealth practice guidelines. With telehealth here to stay, we turn our attention now to several key cautions and considerations for post-pandemic telehealth practice.

Telehealth's Long-Term Regulatory Landscape Remains Unclear

Regulatory practices and policies in health care shifted under emergency orders during the COVID-19 pandemic to enable large-scale uptake of telehealth practices. However, the post-pandemic regulatory landscape for telehealth remains unclear. For example, to facilitate an immediate transition to telehealth across the United States, the Department of Health and

Human Services Office for Civil Rights temporarily relieved certain patient privacy restrictions to allow for broader accessibility of services [45–47]. This relaxed legislation enabled providers to temporarily use consumer-grade equipment and platforms to conduct telehealth treatment in ways that were not always compatible with standards of the Health Insurance Portability Accountability Act (HIPAA). Under this relaxed regulation, many pandemic-era providers became accustomed to using telehealth equipment and platforms that only offered minimal encryption (eg, FaceTime on a personal device) to maintain needed continuity of care.

Given ongoing uncertainty around which pandemic-era emergency orders will become permanent policies, providers are advised to have alternative plans ready for their telehealth work that will conform with pre-pandemic privacy guidelines [12]. This is critical from a patient privacy perspective. Although relaxed regulations during the pandemic may have eliminated liability concerns for many providers who were previously hesitant about telehealth, unsecure practices still pose serious confidentiality risks and ethical questions. In addition, providers must be prepared should emergency pandemic-era policies related to telehealth abruptly reverse [12]. A priority will need to be placed on restoring secure telehealth practices that are consistent with consensus guidelines for telehealth confidentiality [24,44], including the use of equipment and platforms that facilitate compliance with HIPAA standards. For example, privacy regulations require that a telehealth provider hold a special individualized contract, called a business associates agreement (BAA), with the videoconferencing platform company they use that outlines how each party is responsible for safeguarding patient information. It is an HIPAA violation to practice telehealth without holding an individualized BAA with the videoconferencing platform being used. Hames and colleagues [48] further recommend providers always connect to a virtual private network, which offers an additional layer of security. Moreover, when possible, Ethernet cable connections are preferred over Wi-Fi connections to the Internet.

Although telehealth frees the provider and the patient from many geographic constraints, it also introduces important new issues about practice jurisdiction. Because each state (or province or territory) has a responsibility and authority to protect the citizens in its jurisdiction, each state (or province or territory) develops their own occupational legislation to identify and credential "qualified" providers and to discipline incompetent, unethical, or phony providers. Accordingly, providers must procure a professional license for every state, province, or territory where they wish to practice—and this is no different for the practice of telehealth. Practice jurisdiction for telehealth is typically determined by the location of the patient at the time of service, regardless of where the provider is located. Just because one can technically "reach" a patient in another state, province, or territory by teleconference does not mean that one has the professional and legal authority to do so.

With many patients and providers quarantining out-of-state during the pandemic, some providers became accustomed to practicing telehealth across state lines, despite the reality of state-based professional licensing. That said, the 2005 Public Readiness and Emergency Preparedness Act (PREP Act) allows US federal laws to preempt state and local laws when a federal public health emergency has been declared. When the COVID-19 pandemic was declared a federal emergency, many interpreted this to mean that for the duration of the declared emergency, it was acceptable to practice telehealth across state lines for the greater national good—that state laws were moot if they prevented "qualified persons" (such as mental health providers licensed in other states) from conducting essential practices and needed services during the emergency. Of course, pandemic-era emergency orders created some confusion with regard to practice jurisdictions.

Fortunately, most states are now modernizing their laws surrounding occupational licenses and practice jurisdiction to allow for greater flexibility. Interstate compacts that allow for reciprocal professional licensing between specific states are increasingly facilitating multistate practice [49,50]. Leading national interstate compacts relevant to mental health care include the Interstate Medical Licensure Compact for physicians, the Psychology Interjurisdictional Compact (PSYPACT) for psychologists, and the Nurse Licensure Compact for nurses. Each of these compacts allows for mutual recognition of licenses across member states. At present, PSYPACT has 33 participating states that have enacted legislation to join PSYPACT, and several additional states are in the process of introducing PSYPACT legislation. The National Association of Social Workers is also developing an interstate licensure compact that will enhance the exchange of social worker licensure verification, as well as professional investigatory and disciplinary information, between member states.

Before the pandemic, most payers did not reimburse for telehealth services unless the patient lived in a federally designated health care shortage region. For the minority of patients who were authorized for reimbursement of telehealth services, most insurance companies and public payers further required that the patient had to be in a "clinically supervised" setting—that is, a setting with health care professionals on-site. Accordingly, a mental health provider could bill insurance when remotely conducting telehealth with a rural-dwelling family if the family was situated in their child's pediatrician's office or school nurse's office during the call, but the insurance claim would be denied if the rural-dwelling family was situated in their own home during the call. However, at the beginning of the pandemic, the Centers for Medicare and Medicaid Services expanded their list of covered telehealth services to newly include telehealth services for everyone (not just those in rural or indigenous communities) and to newly include telehealth services delivered directly to patients in their own homes. Continuing to provide telehealth coverage for all, regardless of geography or location, will be critical for maximizing the impact and value of post-pandemic telehealth practices.

ALLIANCE AND PROCESSES IN TELEHEALTH

As mental health providers increasingly use telehealth strategies to reach children and families, it is important to consider how psychotherapeutic processes may (or may not) be impacted by the technological aspects of telehealth. Technology-based disruptions in telehealth can be frustrating for patients and for providers, can disrupt the flow of treatment, and can compromise the quality and effectiveness of a session. With modern technology, these disruptions can be minimal, but they can also be quite substantial when outdated technology is used, when participants have minimal experience with the technology or have a low threshold for tolerating technological disruptions and hassles. In addition, some patients and providers may feel less connected when not interacting together in the same space, whereas others experience little-to-no differences between the quality of in-person versus virtual interactions. Accordingly, issues of treatment process, therapeutic alliance, and treatment acceptability are critical in the conduct of telehealth, as these factors often predict individual differences in telehealth engagement and premature drop-out.

In the initial years of telehealth applications to mental health care, ratings of therapeutic alliance were reported to be somewhat lower than ratings of therapeutic alliance in office-based care [51]. However, as teleconferencing has become relatively standard for an increasing proportion of the population, disparities in reported alliance across telehealth and office-based care seem to have disappeared. An increasing body of research finds that on average, telehealth formats for the delivery of youth mental health care are associated with very high levels of patient/family satisfaction and therapeutic alliance, comparable to what is reported for office-based care [12,13,27,28,52–57]. Of note, pre-pandemic providers often reported somewhat lower expectations for telehealth and lower ratings of the therapeutic alliance than did their patients [58]. However, provider ratings of telehealth acceptability and therapeutic alliance have improved as the COVID-19 pandemic led to relaxed regulations as well as broader telehealth uptake [42]. It is important to note that almost the entire literature base examining therapeutic alliance in telehealth has relied on patient- and provider-report questionnaires. To complement the existing work in this area, studies are needed that have trained coders watch recorded sessions of telehealth and office-based care and independently rate observable indicators of therapeutic alliance (eg, coder ratings of the warmth of therapist–child interactions; coder ratings of collaboration, child participation, or engagement).

It is important to consider how some unique aspects of telehealth can specifically interfere with the therapeutic process [58,59]. Just as careful thought must be put into designing a therapy office for office-based care, telehealth providers must be thoughtful about the user experience and how the tele-environment will present itself. One of the first things a telehealth provider must do in treatment is set appropriate expectations and prepares the patient or family for the likelihood of dropped or disrupted calls. When patients are dissatisfied with or drop out of telehealth-delivered mental health services, the most common reason they give is frustration with technology-related issues [43].

It is also important to have clear backup plans for continuing provider–patient communication in the event that a call is dropped (eg, "if one of us loses our Internet connection or if our videoconference call is dropped, I will call your telephone number from my telephone. If that does not work, we should each text each other."). Telehealth providers must also develop contingency plans for *emergencies* with their patients and families, such as if the child or family disconnects the meeting and the therapist is concerned the child might imminently hurt themself or that the caregivers might imminently hurt the child physically (eg, "As a condition of treatment, if I have reason to be worried about the welfare or safety of anyone in your home and I cannot get in touch with you, I will contact the numbers you have provided me for your child's pediatrician and for your neighbor. Can you confirm that you agree to this plan?").

Videoconferencing etiquette highlights the importance of appropriate lighting. Allowing for some natural lighting optimizes the videoconferencing experience, and too much overhead lighting can cast shadows on faces that interfere with communication. Ideally, the telehealth provider is facing a light source in their office (eg, facing toward a window so natural light shines in their face; using a ring light or facing a goose neck lamp to create a vanity lighting effect with limited shadows). When possible, patients and families should do the same. Camera placement also requires consideration. If a session entails mostly conversation, to approximate eye contact the camera should be placed directly in front of each participant at eye level. If it is important for the provider to see the child's full body or if the child is moving around a lot (eg, when working with a hyperactive child), then the child's camera may be better placed to capture the full room rather than as a close-up shot of their face. Similarly, if the telehealth provider needs to observe family interactions or if the provider is coaching a caregiver through a Bluetooth earpiece, although they interact with their child (eg, iPCIT) [13], the family's camera should be set up to capture the full room or interaction space.

Telehealth providers and patients often have to be somewhat more deliberate in conversation turn-taking, as even slight transmission delays may result in accidental cross talk that can come across as insensitive or rude. In addition, just as in traditional office-based care, the telehealth provider must make sure they have silenced all push notifications on their various devices. Providers and patients who are accustomed to multitasking while sitting at their computer may find it hard to stay "present" and may have to intentionally refrain from checking other things, such as emails, while at their computer. Moreover, sorting through papers during an office-based session may not create much noise, but over videoconferencing or on a telephone call, paper rustling near a microphone and can be extremely loud and frustrating for the other party. When one needs to sort through papers during a telehealth session, it is recommended that they temporarily mute themselves.

When mental health services are conducted in a traditional office setting, the patient and provider are located in the same room and each party is aware of who is present. In contrast, the provider of telehealth care has a relatively limited control over the patient's environment. Because telehealth participants can only see the parts of each other's rooms that are in view of the camera, it is important for each party to announce who, if anyone else, is in the room or within earshot. This is critical for maintaining trust, in addition to protecting patient privacy and confidentiality. Patients and families may feel less comfortable speaking freely if they are not fully clear and confident about who can see or hear them. Parties should also notify each other as soon as anyone new enters their room (eg, child: "My abuela just walked in.").

Some have argued that the computer-mediated nature of telehealth clinical encounters compromises the extent to which telehealth providers can form and access empathy for their patients. Grondin and colleagues [60], for example, provide a useful review of technology-related factors that can negatively impact "connection" and empathy in computer-mediated clinical interactions, such as low richness of communication, delayed interaction, or poor transmission quality. Whereas Grondin and colleagues [60] address ways in which computer-mediated interactions can "filter out" important pieces of information that are readily afforded in traditional office-based care (eg, nonverbal signals), in our work we consider the other side of the coin—emphasizing ways in which telehealth strategies can also "filter in" important information *not* readily afforded in traditional office-based care. Specifically, we have argued that telehealth can offer opportunities for *enhanced* interpersonal understanding—that is, "augmented empathy" [36]—by offering an improved vicarious "entry" into a patient's world in ways that can facilitate improved awareness, understanding, and/or sensitivity to the patient's or family's perspective, feelings, and motivations [36].

Specifically, traditional office-based care has the patient step out of the usual contexts of their world and into the provider's professional context, which filters *out* much of the contextual details that can directly inform a broadened understanding of the patient, their experiences, and their environments. The patient in office-based care is inundated with multisensory details about the *provider's* work context and work experience (eg, how messy the provider keeps their desk, the temperature of the room in which the provider works, how distressed other patients in the provider's waiting room seem, how friendly other staff at the office seem). At the same time, the office-based provider's experience of the *patient* and their life is mostly decontextualized, aside from what limited details the patient offers verbally. In contrast, telehealth can treat patients and families in situ (eg, in their own home), which offers a direct window for providers into patients' and families' lives. With a telehealth format, the provider can observe natural family dynamics and everyday occurrences that may offer key contextual insights into a patient's difficulties or clearer appreciations of how challenging or stressful life may be for a caregiver, for example, experiencing the ongoing sound of car horns and emergency sirens in the background, a loudly barking pet, extensive clutter in the house, a crying sibling in the home needing simultaneous attention, other adults in the house who do not jump in to help the primary caregiver with any childcare or household needs, and so forth. To some providers, such information can be distracting or upsetting and can interfere with getting through all intended session material. However, a trained telehealth provider can leverage this vicarious "entry" into the family's everyday experience to gain a better understanding of and appreciation for how overwhelming home and family life may be for the caregiver or child. When used correctly, jointly "experiencing" distractions and hassles in the patient's world can facilitate richer collaborative problem-solving and improve engagement and understanding.

Using telehealth to work with children and families in their natural settings can also help the provider develop a more complete portrait of the clinical problem(s) they are treating [36]. For example, it is not rare for the caregiver of a child with behavior problems in office-based treatment to complain that their child "acts like an angel" at the provider's office but is "a terror" at home. The telehealth provider, in contrast, is able to observe more naturalistic samplings of child behavior, family interactions, and functional contingencies.

Cultural Considerations, Digital Divides, and Ongoing Disparities in Telehealth

It is hoped that broadening telehealth practices will help the field better engage youth from marginalized backgrounds—such as racial, ethnic, and language-minoritized youth, rural youth, and youth from indigenous communities—who have been underserved by traditional office-based mental health care [61]. Indeed, telehealth offers opportunities to overcome many key barriers and deliver mental health services to diverse new populations. It is important to recognize that just because a provider can use technology to overcome logistical obstacles and interact with a new population does not mean that the provider is prepared with the appropriate cultural knowledge and humility to work with this new population [12]. At present, there is a dearth of literature on culturally responsive telehealth care [61,62].

Overcoming geographic divides is not the same as overcoming cultural divides. This has been an important finding from extensive telehealth work conducted with rural indigenous populations [63,64]. As in all mental health care [65], telehealth providers must learn and respect the local customs, traditions, and values of each patient's community, consider the cultural context of the patient's problems and help-seeking, engage in continual self-reflection regarding one's own positions of privilege and bias, and leverage any of the patient's cultural strengths into treatment. There is a critical need for training standards and guidelines that help providers effectively integrate a culturally conscious lens, cultural humility, and cultural strengths throughout telehealth care, similar to what we have seen advocated for in traditional office-based mental health care [65–68]. Furthermore, community partnerships invested in overcoming accessibility gaps for marginalized populations are needed to address how telehealth can address complex interactions among oppressive systems, racism, and daily stress [67].

Digital divides currently constrain the reach of telehealth and perpetuate inequities. Disparities in access to technology persist across different racial, ethnic, geographic, and economic groups. At present, communities of color, rural populations, and families living with resource insecurity are significantly less likely than their non-marginalized counterparts to own a computing device or to have reliable access to high-speed Internet [23,61,69,70]. Ethnic and racial minoritized individuals with serious mental illness are at particularly elevated risk for technological exclusion [71]. Internet accessibility challenges are a primary factor in people not seeking out telehealth services [72,73], and such challenges have been cited as a key barrier to broad telehealth adoption among rural and indigenous communities. Currently, only about 60% of individuals in rural communities in the United States have access to broadband Internet [74]. During the COVID-19 pandemic, when telehealth was the only format available among many for outpatient mental health care, digital divides played a role in amplifying preexisting health inequities [75–78].

Encouragingly, there is evidence that many racial and ethnic digital divides are starting to disappear, especially for younger generations [77]. However, disparities in technological literacy and usage still persist [61]. For many patients, conducting video telehealth may not be an option and telehealth may need to be conducted over the telephone. On a smartphone, video calls use up a lot of data, and thus patients who do not have cellular data plans, or patients with fixed or limited cellular data plans, may also not be able to stream video during telehealth care [79].

Telehealth requires a private, safe, and quiet room or space in which the child and/or caregiver(s) can speak freely and openly. This can be particularly challenging when treating resource-insecure families living in smaller dwellings and when treating immigrant and refugee families living in more crowded dwellings with several generations of extended family [23,80]. Given that children of color disproportionately live in resource-insecure households [81,82], assisting families to identify private spaces for child telehealth is critical for helping overcome racial and ethnic disparities in mental health. Moreover, even when private spaces in the home are available, households with undocumented family members may have deportation concerns that make them hesitant about letting an outsider "into" their home. Despite the particular benefits that child and family telehealth can have when delivered to the home setting (eg, refs 13,27,28), if a private space cannot be located in the home, if the family is hesitant about their home being on camera, or if the family does not have the necessary equipment for telehealth, the family or provider may do well to pursue whether a private room with a computer and/or phone can be reserved at the child's school, local library, or neighborhood center.

ARE WE EXPANDING THE REACH OF CARE YET? TELEHEALTH RHETORIC VERSUS REALITY

Currently, there is a relative mismatch between the *rhetoric* that characterizes the promise of telehealth and the *reality* of who telehealth is actually serving [12,83]. A primary argument for telehealth that has been lauded by telehealth proponents and emphasized in policy decisions has focused on the format's ability to overcome obstacles to care and reach *new* populations underserved by traditional office-based mental health care. Despite a majority of outpatient mental health providers transitioning to telehealth during the COVID-19 pandemic, it is not yet clear whether telehealth options actually did much during the pandemic to *expand* the reach of mental health services to *new* populations beyond those who were already accessing mental health services before the pandemic [12].

At present, many of the populations underserved by telehealth are the same populations underserved by brick-and-mortar mental health care [77,84]. Telehealth must make significant advances in offsetting service disparities before it can be deemed a realistic public health strategy for expanding the reach of children's mental health care. For telehealth to succeed, the practice has to do more than simply offer more convenient options and alternative treatment formats for those children and families already able to access traditional mental health care. Extensive community-engaged partnerships and research efforts are needed to examine barriers to telehealth in racial, ethnic, and language-minoritized families, rural families, resource-insecure families, and families from indigenous communities. The key factors to explore in the pursuit of telehealth equity include pragmatic obstacles such as Internet connectivity and equipment costs, cultural divides, institutional mistrust, and systemic inequities [12]. The large-scale federal, state, and private investments are needed to expand access to high-speed Internet to rural and underserved regions.

SUMMARY AND CONCLUDING THOUGHTS

Advancing technologies, increasingly sophisticated methods for remote telecommunications, broadening Internet accessibility, and the COVID-19 pandemic have collectively led to a rapid transformation in youth mental health care practices. At this point, telehealth approaches to the treatment of child mental health problems are shown to be well supported and well tolerated, typically exhibit comparable outcomes to office-based care and are associated with fewer perceived barriers to care by patients and families. In addition to expanding the reach and acceptability of care, there is some evidence that telehealth can expand the ecological validity of care by treating children and families in their natural settings.

It has been said that "necessity is the mother of innovation." When the COVID-19 pandemic began, a majority of children's mental health providers, out of sheer necessity, began adopting telehealth practices with their patients in a matter of weeks [85], despite the reality that most of them had no telehealth training [12]. When stay-at-home guidelines, emergency orders, and relaxed regulations finally launched telehealth into the mainstream of clinical practice, most providers were not practicing telehealth in accordance with existing telehealth standards. Throughout this article, we have outlined the key considerations and cautions for responsible telehealth practices in youth mental health care. As the field prepares for post-pandemic practices, it is important to recognize that telehealth holds great potential for overcoming key barriers to youth mental health services, but concerted efforts are needed to ensure we are not overcoming traditional barriers only to encounter new ones [84]. Disparities in technological access and usage persist along racial, ethnic, and geographic lines, constraining the reach of telehealth and threatening to perpetuate and amplify existing disparities, rather than overcome them. Ensuring equitable access to telehealth options and ensuring culturally responsive telehealth practices are critical if telehealth is to actualize its potential for reaching new populations that have been underserved by traditional office-based mental health care.

CLINICS CARE POINTS

- Telehealth offers opportunities to extend the reach of services and can improve the ecological validity of care by treating children and families in their natural settings.
- Telehealth providers must procure a license for every state, province, or territory they deliver services to. Telehealth practice jurisdiction is typically determined by location of patient at time of service.
- Licensure laws are modernizing to allow for greater flexibility. Interstate compacts that allow for reciprocal professional licensing between specific states are increasingly facilitating multistate telehealth practice.
- Regulatory policies shifted under emergency orders during the COVID-19 pandemic to enable large-scale telehealth uptake. However, the post-pandemic regulatory landscape for telehealth remains unclear.
- Overcoming geographic divides is not the same as overcoming cultural divides. Telehealth providers must integrate a culturally conscious lens and operate from a position of cultural humility and continuous self-reflection throughout their work.

DISCLOSURE

Dr. J.S. Comer receives research funding from NIH, SAMHSA, and PCORI. He also earns textbook royalties from Macmillan Learning, and an editorial stipend from the Association for Behavioral and Cognitive Therapies. Ms G.F. Freitag and Ms A.E. Urcuyo have nothing to disclose.

REFERENCES

[1] Merikangas KR, He JP, Burstein M, et al. Lifetime prevalence of mental disorders in U.S. adolescents: results from the National Comorbidity Survey Replication–Adolescent Supplement (NCS-A). J Am Acad Child Adolesc Psychiatry 2010;49(10):980–9.

[2] Lewis SJ, Arseneault L, Caspi A, et al. The epidemiology of trauma and post-traumatic stress disorder in a representative cohort of young people in England and Wales. Lancet Psychiatry 2019;6(3):247–56.

[3] McLaughlin KA, Koenen KC, Hill ED, et al. Trauma exposure and posttraumatic stress disorder in a national sample of adolescents. J Am Acad Child Adolesc Psychiatry 2013;52(8):815–30.e14.

[4] Ezpeleta L, Keeler G, Erkanli A, et al. Epidemiology of psychiatric disability in childhood and adolescence. J Child Psychol Psychiatry 2001;42(7):901–14.

[5] Southam-Gerow MA, Prinstein MJ. Evidence base updates: the evolution of the evaluation of psychological treatments for children and adolescents. J Clin Child Adolesc Psychol 2014;43(1):1–6.

[6] Kazdin AE, Blase SL. Rebooting psychotherapy research and practice to reduce the burden of mental illness. Perspect Psychol Sci 2011;6(1):21–37.

[7] Comer JS, Barlow DH. The occasional case against broad dissemination and implementation: retaining a role for specialty care in the delivery of psychological treatments. Am Psychol 2014;69(1):1–18.

[8] Health Resources & Services Administration. Shortage areas. HRSA Data Warehouse. 2018. Available at: https://data.hrsa.gov/tools/shortage-area. Accessed May 21, 2022.

[9] University of Michigan Behavioral Health Workforce Research Center. Mapping supply of the U.S. Psychiatric workforce. Ann Arbor (MI): UMSPH; 2018.

[10] Lin L, Stamm K, Christidis P. County-level analysis of U.S. Licensed psychologists and health indicators. Washington, DC: American Psychological Association Center for Workforce Studies; 2015–2016. Available at: https://www.apa.org/workforce/publications/15-county-analysis. Accessed May 21, 2022.

[11] Batastini AB, Paprzycki P, Jones ACT, et al. Are videoconferenced mental and behavioral health services just as good as in-person? A meta-analysis of a fast-growing practice. Clin Psychol Rev 2021;83:101944.

[12] Comer JS. Rebooting Mental Health Care Delivery for the COVID-19 Pandemic (and Beyond): Guiding Cautions as Telehealth Enters the Clinical Mainstream. Cogn Behav Pract 2021;28(4):743–8.

[13] Comer JS, Furr JM, Miguel EM, et al. Remotely delivering real-time parent training to the home: An initial randomized trial of Internet-delivered parent-child interaction therapy (I-PCIT). J Consult Clin Psychol 2017;85(9):909–17.

[14] Fernandez E, Woldgabreal Y, Day A, et al. Live psychotherapy by video versus in-person: A meta-analysis of efficacy and its relationship to types and targets of treatment. Clin Psychol Psychother 2021;28(6):1535–49.

[15] Greenwood H, Krzyzaniak N, Peiris R, et al. Telehealth versus face-to-face psychotherapy for less common mental health conditions: systematic review and meta-

analysis of randomized controlled trials. JMIR Ment Health 2022;9(3):e31780.
[16] McLean SA, Booth AT, Schnabel A, et al. Exploring the efficacy of telehealth for family therapy through systematic, meta-analytic, and qualitative evidence. Clin Child Fam Psychol Rev 2021;24(2):244–66.
[17] Osenbach JE, O'Brien KM, Mishkind M, et al. Synchronous telehealth technologies in psychotherapy for depression: a meta-analysis. Depress Anxiety 2013;30(11):1058–67.
[18] Shigekawa E, Fix M, Corbett G, et al. The current state of telehealth evidence: a rapid review. Health Aff (Millwood) 2018;37(12):1975–82.
[19] Barnett ML, Sigal M, Green Rosas Y, et al. Therapist experiences and attitudes about implementing internet-delivered parent-child interaction therapy during COVID-19. Cogn Behav Pract 2021;28(4):630–41.
[20] Garcia D, Blizzard AM, Peskin A, et al. Rapid, full-scale change to virtual PCIT during the COVID-19 pandemic: implementation and clinical implications [published correction appears in prev sci. 2021 apr 1. Prev Sci 2021;22(3):269–83.
[21] Gurwitch RH, Salem H, Nelson MM, et al. Leveraging parent-child interaction therapy and telehealth capacities to address the unique needs of young children during the COVID-19 public health crisis. Psychol Trauma 2020; 12(S1):S82–4.
[22] Sullivan ADW, Forehand R, Acosta J, et al. COVID-19 and the acceleration of behavioral parent training telehealth: current status and future directions. Cogn Behav Pract 2021;28(4):618–29.
[23] Folk JB, Schiel MA, Oblath R, et al. The transition of academic mental health clinics to telehealth during the COVID-19 pandemic. J Am Acad Child Adolesc Psychiatry 2022;61(2):277–90.
[24] Myers K, Nelson EL, Rabinowitz T, et al. American Telemedicine Association Practice Guidelines for Telemental Health with Children and Adolescents. Telemed J E Health 2017;23(10):779–804 [Erratum appears in Telemed J E Health 2020;26(8):1071].
[25] Novak M. Telemedicine predicted in 1925. Smithsonian Magazine. 2012. Available at: https://www.smithsonianmag.com/history/telemedicine-predicted-in-1925-124140942/. Accessed May 21, 2022.
[26] Institute of Medicine (US). Committee on evaluating clinical applications of telemedicine. In: Field MJ, editor. Telemedicine: a guide to assessing telecommunications in health care. Washington (DC): National Academies Press (US); 1996.
[27] Carpenter AL, Pincus DB, Furr JM, et al. Working from home: an initial pilot examination of videoconferencing-based cognitive behavioral therapy for anxious youth delivered to the home setting. Behav Ther 2018;49(6): 917–30.
[28] Comer JS, Furr JM, Kerns CE, et al. Internet-delivered, family-based treatment for early-onset OCD: A pilot randomized trial. J Consult Clin Psychol 2017;85(2):178–86.
[29] Hilty DM, Ferrer DC, Parish MB, et al. The effectiveness of telemental health: a 2013 review. Telemed J E Health 2013;19(6):444–54.
[30] Myers K, Vander Stoep A, Lobdell C. Feasibility of conducting a randomized controlled trial of telemental health with children diagnosed with attention-deficit/hyperactivity disorder in underserved communities. J Child Adolesc Psychopharmacol 2013;23(6): 372–8.
[31] Myers K, Vander Stoep A, Zhou C, et al. Effectiveness of a telehealth service delivery model for treating attention-deficit/hyperactivity disorder: a community-based randomized controlled trial. J Am Acad Child Adolesc Psychiatry 2015;54(4):263–74.
[32] Himle MB, Freitag M, Walther M, et al. A randomized pilot trial comparing videoconference versus face-to-face delivery of behavior therapy for childhood tic disorders. Behav Res Ther 2012;50(9):565–70.
[33] McGrath PJ, Lingley-Pottie P, Thurston C, et al. Telephone-based mental health interventions for child disruptive behavior or anxiety disorders: randomized trials and overall analysis. J Am Acad Child Adolesc Psychiatry 2011;50(11):1162–72.
[34] Coughtrey AE, Pistrang N. The effectiveness of telephone-delivered psychological therapies for depression and anxiety: A systematic review. J Telemed Telecare 2018;24(2): 65–74.
[35] Eyberg SM, Funderburk BW. Parent-child interaction therapy protocol. Gainesville (FL): PCIT International; 2011.
[36] Comer JS, Timmons AC. The other side of the coin: Computer-mediated interactions may afford opportunities for enhanced empathy in clinical practice. Clin Psychol Sci Pract 2019;26:e12308.
[37] Merikangas KR, He JP, Burstein M, et al. Service utilization for lifetime mental disorders in U.S. adolescents: results of the National Comorbidity Survey-Adolescent Supplement (NCS-A). J Am Acad Child Adolesc Psychiatry 2011;50(1):32–45.
[38] Cantor J, McBain RK, Kofner A, et al. Telehealth adoption by mental health and substance use disorder treatment facilities in the COVID-19 Pandemic. Psychiatr Serv 2022;73(4):411–7.
[39] Zhu JM, Myers R, McConnell KJ, et al. Trends In Outpatient Mental Health Services Use Before And During The COVID-19 Pandemic. Health Aff (Millwood) 2022; 41(4):573–80.
[40] Uscher-Pines L, McCullough C, Dworsky MS, et al. Use of Telehealth Across Pediatric Subspecialties Before and During the COVID-19 Pandemic. JAMA Netw Open 2022;5(3):e224759.
[41] Sammons MT, VandenBos GR, Martin JN, et al. Psychological Practice at Six Months of COVID-19: A Follow-Up to the First National Survey of Psychologists During the Pandemic. J Health Serv Psychol 2020;46:145–54.

[42] Sammons MT, VandenBos GR, Martin JN. Psychological practice and the COVID-19 crisis: A rapid response survey. J Health Serv Psychol 2020;46:51–7.
[43] Mazziotti R, Rutigliano G. Tele-mental health for reaching out to patients in a time of pandemic: provider survey and meta-analysis of patient satisfaction. JMIR Ment Health 2021;8(7):e26187.
[44] Joint Task Force for the Development of Telepsychology Guidelines for Psychologists. Guidelines for the practice of telepsychology. Am Psychol 2013;68(9):791–800.
[45] U.S. Department of Health and Human Services' Office for Civil Rights. BULLETIN: HIPAA privacy and novel coronavirus. 2020. Available at: https://www.hhs.gov/sites/default/files/february-2020-hipaa-and-novel-coronavirus.pdf. Accessed May 21, 2022.
[46] U.S. Department of Health and Human Services' Office for Civil Rights. OCR eases HIPAA telehealth enforcement for COVID-19 emergency. 2020. Available at: https://www.aha.org/news/headline/2020-03-18-ocr-eases-hipaa-telehealth-enforcement-covid-19-emergency. Accessed May 21, 2022.
[47] U.S. Department of Health and Human Services' Office for Civil Rights. Notification of Enforcement Discretion for Telehealth. 2021. Available at: https://www.hhs.gov/hipaa/for-professionals/special-topics/emergency-preparedness/notification-enforcement-discretion-telehealth/index.html. Accessed May 21, 2022.
[48] Hames JL, Bell DJ, Perez-Lima LM, et al. Navigating uncharted waters: Considerations for training clinics in the rapid transition to telepsychology and telesupervision during COVID-19. J Psychotherapy Integration 2020;30(2):348–65.
[49] Bell DJ, Self MM, Davis C, et al. Health service psychology education and training in the time of COVID-19: Challenges and opportunities. Am Psychol 2020;75(7):919–32.
[50] Shachar C, Engel J, Elwyn G. Implications for telehealth in a postpandemic future: regulatory and privacy issues. JAMA 2020;323(23):2375–6.
[51] Norwood C, Moghaddam NG, Malins S, et al. Working alliance and outcome effectiveness in videoconferencing psychotherapy: a systematic review and noninferiority meta-analysis. Clin Psychol Psychother 2018;25(6):797–808.
[52] Jenkins-Guarnieri MA, Pruitt LD, Luxton DD, et al. Patient perceptions of telemental health: systematic review of direct comparisons to in-person psychotherapeutic treatments. Telemed J E Health 2015;21(8):652–60.
[53] Myers KM, Valentine JM, Melzer SM. Feasibility, acceptability, and sustainability of telepsychiatry for children and adolescents. Psychiatr Serv 2007;58(11):1493–6.
[54] Myers KM, Valentine JM, Melzer SM. Child and adolescent telepsychiatry: utilization and satisfaction. Telemed J E Health 2008;14(2):131–7.
[55] Simpson SG, Reid CL. Therapeutic alliance in videoconferencing psychotherapy: a review. Aust J Rural Health 2014;22(6):280–99.
[56] Lopez A, Schwenk S, Schneck CD, et al. Technology-Based Mental Health Treatment and the Impact on the Therapeutic Alliance. Curr Psychiatry Rep 2019;21(8):76.
[57] Sloan DM, Gallagher MW, Feinstein BA, et al. Efficacy of telehealth treatments for posttraumatic stress-related symptoms: A meta-analysis. Cogn Behav Ther 2011;40(2):111–25.
[58] Goldstein F, Glueck D. Developing rapport and therapeutic alliance during telemental health sessions with children and adolescents. J Child Adolesc Psychopharmacol 2016;26(3):204–11.
[59] Shore JH. Telepsychiatry: videoconferencing in the delivery of psychiatric care. Am J Psychiatry 2013;170(3):256–62.
[60] Grondin F, Lomanowska AM, Jackson PL. Empathy in computer-mediated interactions: A conceptual framework for research and clinical practice. Clin Psychol Sci Pract 2019;26(4):17.
[61] Ramos G, Chavira DA. Use of technology to provide mental health care for racial and ethnic minorities: evidence, promise, and challenges. Cogn Behav Pract 2022;29(1):15–40.
[62] Hilty DM, Gentry MT, McKean AJ, et al. Telehealth for rural diverse populations: telebehavioral and cultural competencies, clinical outcomes and administrative approaches. Mhealth 2020;6:20.
[63] Dawson AZ, Walker RJ, Campbell JA, et al. Telehealth and indigenous populations around the world: a systematic review on current modalities for physical and mental health. Mhealth 2020;6:30.
[64] Goss CW, Richardson WJB, Dailey N, et al. Rural American Indian and Alaska Native veterans' telemental health: A model of culturally centered care. Psychol Serv 2017;14(3):270–8.
[65] Sanchez AL, Comer JS, La Roche M. Enhancing the responsiveness of family-based therapy through culturally informed case conceptualization and treatment planning. Cogn Behav Pract 2021. https://doi.org/10.1016/j.cbpra.2021.04.003.
[66] Lau AS. Making the Case for Selective and Directed Cultural Adaptations of Evidence-Based Treatments: Examples From Parent Training. Clin Psychol Sci Pract 2006;13(4):295–310.
[67] Pina AA, Polo AJ, Huey SJ. Evidence-based psychosocial interventions for ethnic minority youth: the 10-year update. J Clin Child Adolesc Psychol 2019;48(2):179–202.
[68] Martyr MA, Kivlighan DM III, Ali SR. The role of telepsychology training clinics in addressing health disparities with rural Latinx immigrant communities. Translational Issues Psychol Sci 2019;5(4):346–54.
[69] Cortelyou-Ward K, Atkins DN, Noblin A, et al. Navigating the digital divide: barriers to telehealth in rural areas. J Health Care Poor Underserved 2020;31(4):1546–56.
[70] Pruitt Z, Chapin KP, Eakin H, et al. Telehealth During COVID-19: Suicide Prevention and American Indian

Communities in Montana. Telemed J E Health 2022;28(3):325–33.
[71] Spanakis P, Peckham E, Mathers A, et al. The digital divide: amplifying health inequalities for people with severe mental illness in the time of COVID-19. Br J Psychiatry 2021;219(4):529–31.
[72] Benda NC, Veinot TC, Sieck CJ, et al. Broadband internet access is a social determinant of health! Am J Public Health 2020;110(8):1123–5.
[73] Zhang D, Shi L, Han X, et al. Disparities in telehealth utilization during the COVID-19 pandemic: Findings from a nationally representative survey in the United States. J Telemed Telecare 2021. https://doi.org/10.1177/1357633X211051677 1357633X211051677.
[74] Schueller SM, Hunter JF, Figueroa C, et al. Use of digital mental health for marginalized and underserved populations. Curr Treat Options Psych 2019;6:243–55.
[75] Aisbitt GM, Nolte T, Fonagy P. Editorial Perspective: The digital divide – inequalities in remote therapy for children and adolescents. Child Adolesc Ment Health 2022. https://doi.org/10.1111/camh.12545.
[76] Saeed SA, Masters RM. Disparities in Health Care and the Digital Divide. Curr Psychiatry Rep 2021;23(9):61.
[77] Fortuna LR, Tolou-Shams M, Robles-Ramamurthy B, et al. Inequity and the disproportionate impact of COVID-19 on communities of color in the United States: The need for a trauma-informed social justice response. Psychol Trauma 2020;12(5):443–5.
[78] Atske S, Perrin A. Home broadband adoption, computer ownership vary by race, ethnicity in the U.S. Pew Research Center. 2021. Available at: https://www.pewresearch.org/fact-tank/2021/07/16/home-broadband-adoption-computer-ownership-vary-by-race-ethnicity-in-the-u-s/. Accessed May 19, 2022.
[79] Perrin PB, Rybarczyk BD, Pierce BS, et al. Rapid telepsychology deployment during the COVID-19 pandemic: A special issue commentary and lessons from primary care psychology training. J Clin Psychol 2020;76(6):1173–85.
[80] Grieco-Page H, Black CJ, Berent JM, et al. Beyond the Pandemic: Leveraging Rapid Expansions in U.S. Telemental Health and Digital Platforms to Address Disparities and Resolve the Digital Divide. Front Psychiatry 2021;12:671502.
[81] Coleman-Jensen A, Rabbitt MP, Gregory CA, et al. Household food security in the United States in 2016, ERR-237. Washington, DC: U.S. Department of Agriculture, Economic Research Service; 2017.
[82] Odoms-Young A, Bruce MA. Examining the Impact of Structural Racism on Food Insecurity: Implications for Addressing Racial/Ethnic Disparities. Fam Community Health 2018;41(Suppl 2 food insecurity and obesity): S3–6.
[83] Chou T, Comer JS, Turvey CL, et al. Technological considerations for the delivery of real-time child telemental healthcare. J Child Adolesc Psychopharmacol 2016;26(3):192–7.
[84] Pierce BS, Perrin PB, Tyler CM, et al. The COVID-19 telepsychology revolution: A national study of pandemic-based changes in US mental health care delivery. Am Psychol 2021;76(1):14–25.
[85] Yang J, Landrum MB, Zhou L, et al. Disparities in outpatient visits for mental health and/or substance use disorders during the COVID surge and partial reopening in Massachusetts. Gen Hosp Psychiatry 2020;67:100–6.

Advances in Psychiatry and Behavioral Health 2 (2022) 155–172

ADVANCES IN PSYCHIATRY AND BEHAVIORAL HEALTH

Common Treatment Elements of Manualized Evidence-Based Treatments for Youth Anxiety Disorders

Sandra L. Cepeda, MS[1], Hannah L. Grassie, BA[1], Jill Ehrenreich-May, PhD*

Department of Psychology, University of Miami, 5665 Ponce De Leon Drive, Coral Gables, FL 33146, USA

KEYWORDS

• Adolescence • Anxiety disorders • Cognitive behavioral therapy • Acceptance and commitment therapy • Common treatment elements

KEY POINTS

- A review of evidence-based treatment manuals for youth anxiety disorders suggests that existent programs share more similarities than differences in techniques commonly used.
- The common treatment strategies found across all reviewed programs for youth anxiety can be largely categorized into educational, cognitive, behavioral, and caregiver-focused techniques.
- Clinicians are encouraged to use at minimum the core techniques of psychoeducation, cognitive flexibility, and exposure-based strategies in treating youth with anxiety disorders.

INTRODUCTION

Overview of anxiety disorders in youth

Anxiety is one of the world's leading causes of disability in young people, with symptoms of anxiety disorders often emerging by ages 11 to 17 years [1]. Anxiety disorders commonly co-occur both with other anxiety disorders (eg, comorbid generalized anxiety disorder [GAD] and specific phobias [SP]) and with other internalizing disorders (eg, comorbid GAD and major depressive disorder) [2]. There is recent evidence to suggest that the prevalence of youth internalizing disorders has been increasing over the past 2 decades and in particular over the course of the coronavirus disease 2019 pandemic [3–5]. Youth anxiety, whether presenting as a singular or comorbid disorder, is associated with heightened impairment across several functional domains (eg, family, school, peers) [6,7] and increased risk for negative psychosocial outcomes lasting into adulthood [8,9]. As such, the effective treatment of youth anxiety disorders and associated concerns is a considerable public health concern.

Psychotherapy for youth anxiety disorders generally involves targeting increased education about the function of anxiety, along with its associated maladaptive thought patterns and avoidance behaviors. The most common psychological intervention for youth anxiety disorders is cognitive behavioral therapy (CBT). CBT aims to modify not only maladaptive thought and behavioral patterns but also the interconnection between these cognitive behavioral domains through skill practice, such as cognitive restructuring and exposure. CBT is an evidence-based treatment (EBT) for anxiety disorders in children and adolescents, as demonstrated across more than 40 randomized controlled trials,

[1] Denotes shared first authorship.

*Corresponding author, *E-mail address:* j.ehrenreich@miami.edu

https://doi.org/10.1016/j.ypsc.2022.06.005

where the majority of youth receiving CBT for anxiety have shown significant reductions in both symptoms and overall clinical severity at posttreatment [10–12]. The efficacy of CBT has been demonstrated not only for youth with a single anxiety disorder but also for those with numerous anxiety disorders [13], as well as those with co-occurring anxiety, neurodevelopmental, and/or externalizing disorders [14]. Although less common and extensively evaluated, acceptance and commitment therapy (ACT) is also used to treat youth anxiety disorders. ACT is considered a "third wave" behavioral therapy that integrates a range of unique behavioral and cognitive strategies to increase distress tolerance and minimize unnecessary avoidance. Similar to CBT, ACT targets distressing thoughts and problematic behaviors; however, such goals are achieved through principles of psychological flexibility, acceptance, and mindfulness [15]. ACT has demonstrated efficacy in treating anxiety disorders in adults [16–18] and obsessive-compulsive disorder (OCD) in youth [19,20]; however, the empirical base for such efficacy in youth is still growing. A host of studies have demonstrated comparable outcomes among ACT and CBT in treating youth anxiety disorders [15,19,21].

Most CBT approaches for youth target either a single anxiety disorder (eg, social anxiety disorder [SOC], panic disorder [PD]) [22,23] or are designed with a limited range of anxiety disorders in mind (eg, SOC, GAD, separation anxiety disorder [SAD]) [24]. There are also other CBT-informed protocols that target both anxiety and other forms of youth psychopathology simultaneously—often referred to as transdiagnostic treatment approaches. Transdiagnostic treatment approaches contain multiple common elements or shared treatment principles—similar to those found in single-problem CBT approaches and in ACT and provide guidance or planning assistance to clinicians for how to also target commonly comorbid youth disorders, such as depression, OCD, trauma, or conduct problems, along with anxiety [25]. Some transdiagnostic treatments are theorized to operate through higher-order factors that may be modifiable targets across disorders, whereas others take a more empirical approach to selection of treatment strategies to be deployed across youth problem sets.

Overall, a plethora of EBT manuals exist with CBT and ACT elements for youth anxiety. Similar to a transdiagnostic approach to treatment, the aim of this review is to highlight the shared or common elements of these manualized interventions for youth anxiety disorders, with a focus on helping practitioners navigate between existent treatments and crafting a personalized course of intervention most appropriate for a given child and family. The goal is to provide a descriptive review and tabular presentation of the key evidence-based techniques commonly used across both single-domain and transdiagnostic interventions for youth anxiety.

APPROACH

To construct a review of existent treatments, the authors reviewed the Oxford Clinical Psychology library [26], the California Evidence-Based Clearinghouse for Child Welfare (CEBC) [27], and the *Journal of Clinical Child and Adolescent Psychology* EBT archives [28,29] for published or publicly available manuals that focused on the treatment of anxiety disorder in youth, either as a singular or as a co-occurring disorder. Specifically, the authors focused on manualized treatment protocols that targeted any anxiety disorders in children and adolescents based on *Diagnostic and Statistical Manual of Mental Disorders, Fifth Edition*, classification: SAD, selective mutism, SOC, GAD, SP, PD, and agoraphobia [30]. The search resulted in 14 EBT manuals that met the following criteria: (1) the intervention involved child-and/or a combination of parent- and child-directed strategies, (2) the intervention targeted youth aged 18 years or younger with anxiety, and (3) the intervention was written in English. Although other manuals certainly exist in a range of languages, sufficient author fluency in a range of languages would have been required to include these and provide appropriate treatment strategy comparisons. Manuals that focused on the treatment of youth emotional-behavioral concerns broadly, without direct mention of anxiety, were excluded. One exception was made to include an ACT protocol in the authors' review, given the growing empirical support and interest among clinicians in using this psychotherapeutic approach to treat anxiety disorders in children [15,21].

As seen in Table 1, the common elements of 15 selected treatment programs are reviewed: ACT, Brief Behavioral Therapy for Anxiety and Depression (BBT) [51], Building Confidence [52], Coping Cat [24], Cool Kids Anxiety Program [53], FIRST [54], FRIENDS [55], Integrated Behavior Therapy for Selective Mutism (IBTSM) [56], Mastery of Anxiety and Panic for Adolescents (MAP-A) [22], Modular Approach to Therapy for Children (MATCH) [57], Mindfulness-Based Cognitive Therapy for Children (MBCT-C) [36], Modular Cognitive-behavior Therapy for Childhood Anxiety Disorders (MCBT-C) [58], Social Effectiveness Therapy for Children (SET-C) [23], Stand Up, Speak Out [59], and Unified Protocols for Transdiagnostic Treatment of

TABLE 1
Overview of selected treatment manuals for youth anxiety

Program	Manuals	Core Modules	Relevant Citations	Target Age range	Target Diagnoses
ACT for Youth Anxiety	-	• Psychoeducation on anxiety; values and feelings; introduction to acceptance and mindfulness • Mindfulness Practice • Introduction to Cognitive Defusion; Mindful thinking • Body Scanning • Introduction to stepladders; Graded exposures • Judging versus describing; letting go of negative self-judgements • Problem-solving skills building; Social skills training • Reviewing goals; Planning for the future	Hancock et al,[15] 2018	7–17	Any anxiety disorder
BBT	Brief Behavioral Therapy for Anxiety and Depression in Youth: Therapist guide	• Understanding Stress and Mood • Relax Your Self and Your World • Problem-Solving Plans • Developing and Implementing the Master Plan (graded engagement activities, problem-solving) • Relapse Prevention • Reinforcement and Rewards	Weersing et al, [51] 2021	8–16	Any anxiety disorder; depression
Building Confidence	Child Anxiety Disorders: A Family-Based Treatment Manual for Practitioners	• Psychoeducation; Functional analysis; Rapport building • KICK Plan: K step, *Know* When You're Nervous	Wood et al [52], 2008	6–11	Any anxiety disorder; OCD

(*continued on next page*)

TABLE 1
(*continued*)

Program	Manuals	Core Modules	Relevant Citations	Target Age range	Target Diagnoses
		• KICK Plan: I step, *Identify* Icky Thoughts and Encourage Independence • KICK Plan: C step, *Calm* Your Thoughts • Exposure Hierarchy; Exposure Therapy • KICK Plan: Second K step, *Keep* Practicing/Rewards • Family Therapy Modules: Problem Solving; Finding New Roles, Talk Time			
Coping Cat	Cognitive-Behavioral Therapy for Anxious Children: Therapist Manual	• Building rapport; treatment orientation • Identifying anxious feelings; somatic responses to anxiety • Relaxation training • Identifying anxious self-talk; Learning to challenge thoughts • Reviewing anxious and coping self-talk; developing problem-solving skills • Introducing self-evaluation; self-reward • Exposure tasks	Kendall & Hedtke [24] 2006	7–13	Any anxiety disorder; OCD
Cool Kids	The Cool Kids Child and Adolescent Anxiety Program: Therapist Manual	• Psychoeducation • Realistic Thinking • Parenting Anxiety • Exposure • Problem Solving • Social Skills; Assertiveness	Rapee et al., [53] 2006	7–17	Any anxiety disorder; OCD

(*continued on next page*)

TABLE 1
(*continued*)

Program	Manuals	Core Modules	Relevant Citations	Target Age range	Target Diagnoses
		• Sustaining Progress; Reviewing goals • Maintaining gains and coping with setbacks			
FIRST	FIRST: A Principle-Guided Approach to Evidence-Based Youth Psychotherapy	• Feeling Calm (self-calming, relaxation) • Increasing Motivation (differential attention, praise, rewards) • Repairing Thoughts (cognitive restructuring) • Solving Problems • Trying the Opposite (graded exposure, behavioral activation)	Weisz & Bearman, [54] 2016	6–15	Any anxiety disorder; depression; conduct problems
FRIENDS	FRIENDS Program for Children: Group Leaders Manual	• Psychoeducation • F - Feeling Worried • R - Relax and feel good • I - Inner thoughts • E – Explore plans • N - Nice work so reward yourself • D - Don't forget to practice • S - Stay Calm	Barrett et al., [55] 2000	6–16	Any anxiety disorder
IBTSM	Treatment for Children with Selective Mutism: An Integrative Behavioral Approach	• Introduction to Treatment; Rapport building • Reward System; Feelings Chart • Talking Ladder • Exposure Practice • Introduction of Transfer of Control • Relapse Prevention and Graduation	Bergman, [56] 2013	4–8	Selective mutism
MAP-A	Mastery of Anxiety and Panic for Adolescents, Therapist Guide: Riding the Wave	• Introduction to Treatment and Three-Component Model	Pincus et al, [22] 2008	12–17	Panic disorder; agoraphobia

(*continued on next page*)

TABLE 1
(*continued*)

Program	Manuals	Core Modules	Relevant Citations	Target Age range	Target Diagnoses
		• Physiology of Panic; Breathing Awareness • Probability Overestimation; Catastrophic Thinking • Thinking Like a Detective • Interoceptive/Situational Exposures; Safety Behaviors • Relapse Prevention			
MATCH	Modular Approach to Therapy for Children with Anxiety, Depression, Trauma, or Conduct problems (MATCH-ADTC)	• *Anxiety Modules:* Psychoeducation; Fear Ladder; Practice (exposures); Maintenance; Cognitive STOP • *Depression Modules:* Problem Solving; Activity Selection; Relaxation; Quick Calming; Cognitive BLUE; Plans for Coping • *Conduct Modules:* One-on-one time; Praise; Active ignoring; Effective Instruct; Rewards; Time out	Chorpita & Weisz, [57] 2009	6–15	Any anxiety disorder; depression; trauma; conduct problems
MBCT-C	Mindfulness-based Cognitive Therapy for Anxious Children: A Manual for Treating Childhood Anxiety	• Being on Automatic Pilot • Being Mindful is Simple, but it is Not Easy! • Who Am I? • A Taste of Mindfulness • Music to Our Ears • Sound Expressions • Practice Looking • Strengthening the Muscle of Attention • Touching the World with Mindfulness • What the Nose Knows	Semple & Lee, [35] 2008	8–12	Any anxiety disorder

(*continued on next page*)

TABLE 1
(continued)

Program	Manuals	Core Modules	Relevant Citations	Target Age range	Target Diagnoses
		• Life is Not a Rehearsal • Living with Presence, Compassion, Awareness			
MCBT-C	Modular Cognitive-Behavioral therapy for Childhood Anxiety Disorders: Guides to Individualized Evidence-based Treatment	• Learning about Anxiety • Making a Fear Ladder • Imaginal/In Vivo Exposures • Maintenance and Relapse Prevention • Cognitive Restructuring: Probability overestimation; Catastrophic thinking; STOP • Social Skills Training • Working with Parents: Active ignoring; Rewards; Time-Out	Chorpita, [58] 2006	7–17	Any anxiety disorder
SET-C	Social Effectiveness Therapy for Children and Adolescents (SET-C): Therapist Guide	• Psychoeducation • Social Skill Training • Peer Generalization • In Vivo Exposure	Beidel et al, [23] 2003	7–12	Social phobia
Stand Up, Speak Out	Cognitive-Behavioral Therapy for Social Phobia in Adolescents: Stand up, Speak out, Therapist Guide	• Skill Building Psychoeducation • Cognitive-behavioral Model of Social Anxiety • Automatic thoughts; Rational responses • Social Problem Solving; Cognitive Restructuring • Social Skills; Assertiveness Training • Support System • Exposures • Relapse Prevention	Albano et al., [59] 2008	13–18	Social phobia

(continued on next page)

TABLE 1
(*continued*)

Program	Manuals	Core Modules	Relevant Citations	Target Age range	Target Diagnoses
UP-C/A	Unified Protocols for Transdiagnostic Treatment of Emotional Disorders in Children and Adolescents: Therapist Guide	• Building and Keeping Motivation • Getting to Know Your Emotions and Behaviors • Introduction to Emotion-focused Behavioral Experiments • Awareness of Physical Sensations • Being Flexible in Your Thinking • Awareness of Emotional Experiences • Situational Emotion Exposure • Reviewing Accomplishments and Looking Ahead • Parenting the Emotional Adolescent	Ehrenreich-May et al [39] 2017	7–17	Any anxiety disorder; OCD; depression; trauma; stress-related disorders; tic disorders

Abbreviations: BBT, Brief Behavioral Therapy for Anxiety and Depression; MAP-A, Mastery of Anxiety and Panic for Adolescents; MATCH, Modular Approach to Therapy for Children; MCBT-C, Modular Cognitive-behavior Therapy for Childhood Anxiety Disorders; SET-C, Social Effectiveness Therapy for Children; UP-C/A, Unified Protocols for Transdiagnostic Treatment of Emotional Disorders in Children and Adolescents.

Emotional Disorders in Children and Adolescents (UP-C/A) [39]. Table 2 presents the core techniques from each of the 15 domain-specific and transdiagnostic treatment programs for youth anxiety.

COMMON TREATMENT STRATEGIES

Educational techniques

Psychoeducation is a common, foundational strategy found across all 15 domain-specific and transdiagnostic interventions for youth anxiety. Broadly, psychoeducation can be categorized into 2 stages—one that introduces the structure and goals of treatment and the other that introduces the theoretical underpinnings of emotions. For the first stage, the exact educational content and overview of treatment depends on the specific manual; however, most clinicians begin by explaining the general nature of the intervention (eg, underlying theory, number of sessions, in-session and at-home activities, and the role of parents in treatment). Following, clinicians work with the youth (herein also referred to as "the client") to identify specific treatment goals that consist of attainable, measurable outcomes (eg, less avoidance of an anxiety-provoking trigger) and are relevant to individual's needs. These specific goals are then commonly used to inform and monitor the youth's progress over the course of treatment.

In educating clients on the theoretical underpinnings of emotions, many manuals start by emphasizing how emotions are natural, normal, and harmless. In terms of anxiety specifically, clinicians may highlight to clients that anxiety or worry are normative emotional responses to potential future threats and are important from an evolutionary standpoint (ie, prepares the body to respond swiftly to real or imagined dangers). Another key feature in this stage of psychoeducation is the accurate identification and labeling of emotional experiences and affective states. To enhance emotion identification skills, clinicians teach clients about the

TABLE 2
Core techniques from domain-specific and transdiagnostic treatment programs for youth anxiety

	ACT for youth anxiety	**BBT**	**Building Confidence**	**Coping Cat**	**Cool Kids**	**FIRST**	**FRIENDS**	**IBTSM**
Target age range	7–17	8–16	6–11	7–13	7–17	6–15	6–16	4–8
Domain-specific treatment	-	-	X	X	X	-	X	X
Transdiagnostic treatment	X	X	-	-	-	X	-	-
Foundational/educational strategies								
Psychoeducation	X	X	X	X	X	X	X	-
Progress monitoring	-	X	-	X	-	X	-	-
Cognitive strategies								
Identification of negative self-talk	-	-	X	X	X	-	X	-
Cognitive reappraisal	-	-	X	X	X	X	X	-
Mindfulness/ acceptance/ cognitive diffusion/ self-as-context	X	-	-	-	-	-	-	-
Awareness of somatic sensations	X	-	-	X	-	-	X	-
Problem solving	X	X	-	X	X	X	X	-
Behavioral strategies								
Exposures/committed action	X	X	X	X	X	X	X	X
Relapse prevention	-	X	-	-	X	X	-	X
Social/assertiveness skills training, peer generalization experiences	X	-	-	-	X	-	X	-
Additional strategies								
Relaxation skills	-	X	X	X	X	X	X	-
Self-reward	-	-	X	X	-	-	X	-
Values identification	X	-	-	-	-	-	-	-

(continued on next page)

TABLE 2
(continued)

	ACT for youth anxiety	BBT	Building Confidence	Coping Cat	Cool Kids	FIRST	FRIENDS	IBTSM
Caregiver strategies								
Psychoeducation	-	-	X	X	-	-	X	X
Parenting emotional behaviors (eg, accommodation, criticism, inconsistency, overprotection, anxiety management)	-	-	-	-	X	-	X	-
Motivational techniques/differential reinforcement (eg, labeled praise, active/planned ignoring, reward system)	-	X	X	-	-	X	X	X

	MAP-A	MATCH	MBCT-C	MCBT-C	SET-C	Stand up, speak out	UP-C/A
Target age range	12–17	6–15	8–12	7–17	7–12	13–18	7–17
Domain-specific treatment	X	-	-	X	X	X	-
Transdiagnostic treatment	-	X	X	-	-	-	X
Foundational/educational strategies							
Psychoeducation	X	X	X	X	X	X	X
Progress monitoring	X	X	-	X	-	X	X
Cognitive strategies							
Identification of negative self-talk	-	-	-	-	-	X	X
Cognitive reappraisal	X	X	-	X	-	X	X
Mindfulness/acceptance/cognitive diffusion/self-as-context	-	-	X	-	-	-	X
Awareness of somatic sensations	X	-	X	-	-	-	X
Problem solving	-	X	-	-	-	X	X
Behavioral strategies							
Exposures/committed action	X	X	-	X	X	X	X
Relapse prevention	X	X	-	X	-	X	X

(continued on next page)

TABLE 2
(continued)

	MAP-A	MATCH	MBCT-C	MCBT-C	SET-C	Stand up, speak out	UP-C/A
Social/assertiveness skills training, peer generalization experiences	-	-	-	X	X	X	-
Additional strategies							
Relaxation skills	X	X	X	-	-	-	-
Self-reward	-	-	-	-	-	-	-
Values identification	-	-	-	-	-	-	-
Caregiver strategies							
Psychoeducation	-	X	-	-	X	-	X
Parenting emotional behaviors (eg, accommodation, criticism, inconsistency, overprotection, anxiety management)	-	-	-	-	-	-	X
Motivational techniques/ differential reinforcement (eg, labeled praise, active/planned ignoring, reward system)	-	X	-	X	-	-	X

Abbreviation: FIRST, the FIRST program.

3 parts of an emotional experience: cognitions (eg, thoughts), physiological sensations (eg, bodily experiences), and behaviors (eg, goal-directed behavior to minimize subjective distress). Last, most manuals that adopt a CBT framework also emphasize the antecedents and consequences of such emotional experiences. Given that experiential avoidance of unpleasant situations is a core behavioral feature of anxiety disorders [30], clinicians typically educate clients on how avoidance behaviors are negatively reinforced by short-term reductions in distress (often termed the *cycle of avoidance*).

ACT-informed programs for youth anxiety [15] provide psychoeducation in a similar manner to traditional CBT in that clients are still introduced to the structure of treatment and educated on the theoretical underpinnings of anxiety. However, as expected, discussions with clients are predominantly centered on ACT components (eg, psychological inflexibility, use of acceptance and mindfulness as alternatives to managing distressing thoughts/feelings) rather than those of traditional CBT. To demonstrate ACT elements, clinicians regularly use metaphors, such as the *Chinese Finger Trap* metaphor [31], which draws a parallel between attempting to pull one's fingers free from a Chinese finger trap (which in turn makes it get tighter) and resisting/pulling away from uncomfortable emotions (which in turn increase emotional discomfort). Through this metaphor and experiential learning, clients learn the importance of accepting and leaning into discomfort. During the early stages of ACT, clinicians also begin to work with the client on identifying and discussing the importance of their values to the treatment course. Identification of values makes up a core component of the ACT model, and this initial discussion with the client is analogous to the goal-setting portion of psychoeducation that is typical of many CBT-based manuals.

Notably, MBCT-C also provides psychoeducation to clients in a manner similar to ACT. Like ACT, MBCT-C underscores the importance of acceptance around the thoughts, feelings, and behaviors that make up an emotional experience. Clinicians typically begin by orienting clients to program expectations, introducing mindfulness, and how practicing mindful awareness can be helpful in learning to respond effectively to intense emotions. Specifically, in educating clients to the nature of mindfulness-based treatment, clinicians typically illustrate to clients that as their awareness and acceptance of experiences grows over time, significant changes in their thoughts and behaviors may also occur [35].

There are numerous important considerations to be made when providing psychoeducation of anxiety disorders and treatment of such disorders. To begin, it is important that clinicians are culturally humble, such that they foster an environment in which the clients (and/or their caregivers) are comfortable sharing their conceptualization of anxiety disorders and psychotherapy through the lens of their culture. The Culture Formulation Interview (CFI) [30] may be a valuable tool in achieving this goal. The CFI "aim[s] to clarify key aspects of the presenting clinical problem from the point of view of the individual and other members of the individual's social network (ie, family, friends, or others involved in current problem). This includes the problem's meaning, potential sources of help, and expectations for services" [30]. In addition to conceptualizing an individual's anxiety through their own culture and lived experiences, clinicians should set treatment goals that are consistent with the client's individual and cultural values and beliefs.

Cognitive techniques

Cognitive strategies are largely present across youth anxiety interventions and target negative or unpleasant thoughts that may arise in the context of anxiety or distress. As can be seen in Table 2, explicit cognitive strategies are used in all but 3 manuals (IBTSM, BBT, SET-C), although cognitive changes (eg, changes in threat appraisal) may be more distal consequents of the behavioral strategies used in these manuals. Cognitive strategies in youth CBT approaches are generally based on Beck's cognitive model [36], which poses that biased self-relevant thoughts, evaluations, and beliefs play an important role in the development and persistence of psychopathological states. Across cognitive strategies, the goal is to manage self-talk-related distress such that the youth can select more helpful or approach-oriented behavioral strategies relative to the trigger stimulus or situation. Largely, cognitive strategies are designed to enhance cognitive flexibility or willingness to consider a variety of possible threat interpretations related to evocative stimuli. Such flexibility can be achieved through strategies such as reappraisal, mindfulness, tolerance of uncomfortable cognitions/physiological sensations, and problem solving.

Cognitive reappraisal (also termed cognitive restructuring) is one of the hallmark techniques of CBT, whereby youths are taught to identify, evaluate, and modify negative cognitions [36]. The goal of cognitive reappraisal is to replace maladaptive thoughts, evaluations, and beliefs with neutral or more adaptive ones [38]. As demonstrated in Table 2, cognitive reappraisal is a common strategy used across a variety of therapeutic interventions for anxiety disorders. In fact, many of the reviewed programs use similar methods to teach cognitive reappraisal to clients, including the Building Confidence program, Coping Cat, Cool Kids, UP-C/A, MCBT-C, MAP-A, MATCH, and the Stand Up, Speak Out program. In almost all 8 of these manuals, clinicians will begin by orienting clients to the concept of automatic thought or self-talk, particularly in the context of an emotional experience. Manuals like Coping Cat, Cool Kids, and the Building Confidence program highlight the use of an illustrative activity to further orient clients on the topic, whereby clients are presented with cartoons and asked to fill in any possible thoughts for a given character. These cartoons may also be used to educate clients on the differences between anxious self-talk and coping self-talk. Similarly, UP-C/A uses optical illusions or images that contain more than one interpretation to demonstrate automatic thoughts to clients and introduce the concept of flexible thinking.

The next shared cognitive reappraisal practice found across all 8 of these manuals is the idea of teaching clients to "think like a detective" as a means of evaluating automatic thoughts or anxious self-talk. Specifically, the first step in detective thinking typically involves working with clients to identify examples of interpretations that could be categorized as cognitive errors or "thinking traps" (eg, catastrophizing, probability overestimation, and so on). Then, clinicians have clients gather and evaluate evidence for that interpretation. Manuals such as Coping Cat and UP-C/A illustrate the use of specific self-questioning techniques to guide clients through this process (eg, having clients ask themselves, *do I know for sure this is going to happen? what has happened before? what is the worst thing that could happen?*) [24,39]. As a final step, clients are encouraged to identify an alternative interpretation or more realistic outcome, as well as consider their ability to cope should the feared outcome occur.

Problem solving is a common consequent-based strategy that often follows cognitive reappraisal as the next skill introduced to clients and blends both cognitive and behavioral components. As shown in Table 2, 9 of the reviewed manuals include problem solving as a core technique in treatment. Problem solving involves the client identifying an evocative incident/situation and thinking flexibly to generate numerous potential solutions. Furthermore, problem-solving strategies typically follow a set structure that encourages clients to consider the pros and cons, along with anticipated behavioral outcomes associated with each solution.

Mindful awareness techniques are also common cognitive strategies [33,35]. Mindfulness strategies aim to increase present-moment awareness (being in the here-and-now), increase acceptance of anxious distress instead of placing judgment on the subjective experience (eg, negative self-talk), and promote goal-directed action. Such aims are pillars of ACT's overall goal of fostering acceptance or diffusion of unpleasant self-talk and committing to making necessary, value-driven behavioral changes to reduce distress [40]. One component of mindfulness, awareness of somatic sensations, involves helping clients to recognize, and in turn tolerate, the physiological reactions that often co-occur with anxious cognitions. Such tolerance of anxiety-related physiological discomfort is often achieved through interoceptive exposure. Here, clients are given the opportunity to evoke and experience anxiety-related physical sensations in a safe situation, such as the clinician's office, through a series of planned symptom-induction tasks that are devoid of the typical situational triggers of such sensations (eg, moving one's head from side to side to evoke a sense of dizziness). Experiencing uncomfortable somatic experiences in a safe setting during interoceptive exposure allows clients to recognize whether these exercises prompt any catastrophic cognitions about their bodily sensations and, if so, to help sever the link between such sensations and subsequent cognitions over repeated practices.

Although the aforementioned cognitive strategies may appear to be quite different, particularly cognitive reappraisal and mindfulness-based strategies, they have the shared outcome of minimizing distress through noticing, and then challenging or accepting negative self-talk. Select manuals, such as the UP-C/A and MAP-A, present both reappraisal and mindful awareness. In such an instance, the timing of each strategy may be particularly important. For example, cognitive reappraisal may be more effective in the antecedent time frame, during which youth can identify and challenge negative anticipatory self-talk [32]. Moreover, in the antecedent time frame, the child's cognitive load may be lower because they have yet to enter the anxiety-evoking situation and thus engaging in the steps of threat reappraisal may be easier and more likely to promote approach-oriented behaviors. On the other hand, youth may be more readily able to apply mindfulness strategies, such as reorienting to the present and accepting unpleasant self-talk and physiological sensations across various timepoints of an evocative situation (antecedent, response, consequence). Mindfulness strategies may be particularly applicable in the consequence time frame to minimize negative postevent processing and negative self-referential rumination.

Importantly, the application of cognitive strategies should be considered within cultural contexts. Although youth with elevated anxiety tend to aberrantly perceive nonthreatening situations as potentially threatening [41], real threat is a relative concept that is greatly impacted by one's lived experiences and societal (mis) treatment of communities. Experiences with discrimination, bullying, and media depictions of danger for a particular cultural or other marginalized group may need to be considered in working with youth from such communities. In such instances, it is important for mental health professionals to practice cultural humility and foster a safe, collaborative environment in which youth can express their threat perceptions.

Behavioral techniques

While cognitive strategies target thoughts associated with an emotional experience, behavioral techniques address maladaptive behavioral responses. A common goal of behavioral strategies is for anxious youth to reduce the frequency of maladaptive behavior, such as avoidance or withdrawal, engage in approach-oriented behavior toward distressing stimuli, and learn to tolerate or cope with any discomfort associated with the anxiety. Among the 15 reviewed programs, all but MBCT-C incorporate at least 1 behavioral technique—with exposure presenting as the most used strategy across treatments. This observation is not surprising given that exposure is a hallmark of anxiety treatment and potentially the most potent technique in terms of positive anxiety treatment outcomes [34,37]. In fact, the use of increased exposure tasks in treatment has been specifically linked with greater improvement in childhood anxiety [42,43].

There are a range of exposure strategies included across the reviewed programs (eg, in vivo, interoceptive, and imaginal exposures), and all generally involve the client approaching evocative stimuli, tolerating resulting discomfort, and being rewarded for such tolerance. Exposure is often completed in a gradual manner, whereby clinicians work with clients to develop a fear hierarchy of situations/stimuli, ranging from those that cause the least to those that cause most anxious distress. Here, clients first approach lesser distressing stimuli on their fear hierarchy and practice tolerating the associated unpleasant thoughts and physiological sensations. Such tolerance is often achieved through implementing mindfulness strategies, including nonjudgmentally accepting cognitions related to the evocative stimulus and remaining flexible in one's appraisal of a potential threat situation. Once clients can successfully approach the evocative stimulus without an excessive anxiety response and/or avoidance behavior, they then move up the fear hierarchy to approach a slightly more distressing stimulus.

Importantly, there are various schools of thought regarding the underlying mechanisms of exposure therapy for anxiety. Exposure therapy is based on models of classical fear conditioning [44] whereby an initial stimulus (eg, dog bite; unconditioned stimulus [US]) produces a fear response (unconditioned response [UR]) and the emotional response becomes a learned reaction (conditioned response [CR]) that is elicited by related stimuli (eg, all dogs; conditioned stimuli [CS]) through stimulus generalization. Owing to the aversiveness of the CR, fearful individuals may avoid the CS (all dogs) and develop the belief that the CR can only be prevented through avoidance, thus reinforcing both the fear and avoidant response. Extinction theory purports that the association between the CR and CS (eg, anxious reaction to all dogs) can be weakened through repeated exposure to the CS in the absence of the US (eg, exposure to dogs without getting bitten). One school of thought suggests that exposure works through inhibitory learning [45], such that the client comes to develop a new association between the US and CS (the dog that bit them and all other dogs) whereby the CS no longer predicts the US and in turn reduces the frequency of the CR. Essentially, through repeated exposure to the evocative stimuli without negative outcomes, the client learns not to associate the feared stimuli with related or neutral stimuli [46]. A second camp of thought purports that the association between the CR and CS is weakened in exposure through habituation [47], such that there is a natural reduction in the emotional response after repeated exposures to the CS.

These differences in thinking regarding the mechanism of change in exposure may play out in functional differences in how an exposure is conducted with youth clients. For example, if inhibitory learning is the goal of exposure, then exposure stimuli may be presented as naturalistically as possible, with purposeful variations in intensity and no need to wait for habituation to occur before moving to subsequent exposures. If habituation is the goal, then a clinician would typically wait for the youth's distress to return to more tolerable level before moving on to other exposures and may be more likely to proceed through a hierarchy in a graduated manner. Youth manuals currently present education about exposure that primarily references extinction learning and habituation, because research on inhibitory learning is newer and not as extensive in youth samples. For younger children, there may be some initial treatment-engagement value in conducting some exposures in which distress will demonstrably decrease and promote positive affect about success in exposure. Nonetheless, some stimuli (eg, social interactions) are brief or fleeting and naturally lend themselves better to youth exposures that focus on inhibitory learning principles. It is anticipated that inhibitory learning will increasingly be represented in new and revised youth CBT manuals in the future.

Committed action, which is one of the 6 core processes of ACT, also stems from a similar framework to exposure, whereby clients engage in persistent value consistent behaviors, regardless of any presenting psychological barriers (eg, distressing thoughts, feelings) that may hinder achieving said behaviors [40]. Specifically, in ACT for youth anxiety, clients engage in exposures as a means of cultivating committed action that falls in line with their chosen values [15]. Rather than focusing on fear ratings, exposure work in ACT uses willingness (or acceptance of discomfort) as an indicator for moving up the fear hierarchy.

Notably, there is also a suite of behavioral strategies used in manuals that target social anxiety-related behaviors, in particular (eg, Coping Cat, Cool Kids, FRIENDS, MCBT-C, SET-C, and Stand Up, Speak Out). Youth with social anxiety typically avoid social interactions due to fear of negative evaluation, and thus the clinician's objective is to increase approach behavior toward said interactions. Such approach behavior can be achieved through techniques, such as social assertiveness training, whereby the child learns skills for social interactions and communicating with others with the end goal of making friends and building their social networks. Many social anxiety interventions adopt a group modality and leverage group members in exposures such that youth can practice social skills with other group members.

Caregiver-focused techniques

Across most psychological interventions for youth, regardless of domain, caregivers play an important role in facilitating attendance and engagement, understanding therapeutic content, and completing outside session activities. Moreover, certain interventions specifically engage parents by providing caregiver-directed strategies to minimize youth distress or disrupt unproductive parent-child interactions. Although the amount of caregiver-focused content varies across different manuals, almost all the reviewed treatments involve some component of caregiver-directed strategies (ie, with exception to ACT, MAP-A, MBCT-C, and the Stand Up, Speak Out program). Broadly, the observed caregiver-directed strategies can be classified as psychoeducation, modification of less productive parenting behaviors, and strategies to increase the frequency of approach-oriented behaviors and to decrease the frequency of avoidance behaviors. Regardless of the specific technique, caregiver-directed strategies share the common goal of recruiting the caregiver in a therapeutic process to minimize youth's anxious distress and avoidance.

As one of the most rudimentary caregiver-directed strategies, psychoeducation is a common technique provided to caregivers across 7 of the reviewed manuals. Parent-directed psychoeducation is largely similar to the previously described youth-directed psychoeducation. This technique is particularly important because it ensures that the caregiver and youth share a common conceptualization of anxiety and its treatment. Although not as common, a second class of caregiver-directed strategies observed in 3 of the reviewed manuals (ie, UP-C/A, Cool Kids, and FRIENDS) involves identifying and modifying caregiver behavior that may be maintaining youth anxiety and associated behaviors. For instance, in the parent module of the UP-C/A, caregivers are introduced to 4 common emotional parenting behaviors: overprotection/accommodation, criticism, inconsistency, and excessive modeling of intense emotions/avoidance. The clinician presents caregivers with examples of each, followed by a discussion on the potential consequences of these behaviors and different actions that can be used instead as effective, supportive responses to child distress.

The third class of caregiver-directed strategies, inclusive of motivational techniques and differential reinforcement, involves teaching the caregiver specific strategies and systems that aim to increase the frequency of desirable behaviors and decrease the frequency of undesirable behaviors via reward learning principles. Among the reviewed manuals, 8 focus on teaching caregivers at least some form of motivational technique or differential reinforcement strategy over the course of treatment (ie, BBT, Building Confidence, FIRST, FRIENDS, IBTSM, MATCH, MCBT-C, UP-C/A). Generally, across these manuals, the most common type of strategies taught to caregivers is to attend to desired or approach-oriented behaviors (eg, through labeled praise and/or reward systems) and not attend to undesirable or avoidant behaviors (eg, through active/planned ignoring).

As with all other treatment strategies, caregiver-directed techniques should be considered in the context of the caregiver's culture and lived experiences. The previously mentioned considerations for youth-directed psychoeducation, such as the CFI, and youth-directed reappraisal should also be applied when working with caregivers. Moreover, different communities may have differing expectations for the caregiver-child relationship. In particular, caregiver accommodation may be appropriate and normative in certain instances and cultural contexts. For example, caregiver accommodation in the form of speaking for a socially anxious child may be more normative and less maladaptive for children who have recently immigrated to a new country and are learning the language, compared with socially anxious nonimmigrant children who are fluent in the language. Furthermore, caregivers cosleeping with a child high in anxiety may be engaging in unhelpful accommodation that reinforces the child's anxiety in certain cultural contexts, whereas such behavior may be considered normative parenting behavior in other cultural contexts [48]. The authors recommend that clinicians foster a transparent and collaborative relationship with caregivers whereby discussions of cultural considerations are openly and comfortably discussed.

Although this review focuses primarily on child-directed treatments, there are several parent-directed manuals for youth anxiety worth highlighting as well. Supportive Parenting for Anxious Childhood Emotions (or SPACE) is one example of a parent-led treatment program, designed to provide caregivers with a step-by-step guide for helping their child confront anxiety and OCD-related concerns [49]. A main focus of the SPACE program is to help caregivers identify their own parenting responses to their child's anxiety (eg, accommodation) and replace unhelpful responses with supportive responses that foster a greater sense of self-efficacy in their child. Another example is the Helping Your Anxious Child (HYAC) bibliotherapy program for parents [50]. HYAC is based on the Cool Kids Anxiety Program and focuses on directly teaching parents the skills needed to coach their own child through managing their anxiety. In this program, the parent takes on the role as therapist and guides the child through structured activities, following similar core techniques as described in Cool Kids (eg, detective thinking, problem solving, social skills training, graded exposures).

SUMMARY AND DISCUSSION

The purpose of this review is to highlight commonalities and differences in widely available EBTs for youth anxiety disorders. Overall, given that all these treatment approaches share the theoretic frameworks underlying CBT, mindfulness, and ACT, it is no surprise that the similarities across programs reviewed well outpace their differences. In fact, the similarities in these approaches might suggest to practitioners that any one version of a CBT or ACT manual for youth anxiety or a transdiagnostic treatment that incorporates such strategies may be useful across anxiety disorders in this age group. Although nuanced differences in the presentation, stimuli, and proposed use of these different manuals exist, the authors' review suggests that most practitioners may select materials from any of these programs and potentially combine them with preferred materials from other EBT manuals for anxiety in youth with ease to chart a personalized, culturally relevant, and appealing version of such intervention materials for a given child or family. However, to avoid lessening the efficacy of such approaches through more anecdotal combinations of materials, practitioners are encouraged to ensure they are providing at minimum core techniques of psychoeducation, cognitive flexibility, and exposure-based strategies to youth with anxiety to promote clinically significant improvements in this symptom cluster both immediately and through generalization of such strategies in the longer term.

CLINICS CARE POINTS

- Evidence-based treatment manuals for youth anxiety share common psychoeducation, cognitive flexibility, and exposure-based strategies.
- Given the shared overlap in treatment strategies, any one of the reviewed manuals may be efficacious in treating youth with anxiety disorders.
- Practitioners might consider combining preferred treatment materials regarding core elements of these manuals.
- Providers should foster a treatment environment that is culturally humble and responsive in providing these core strategies.

DISCLOSURE

Ms Cepeda and Ms Grassie have no known conflicts of interest to disclose. Dr Ehrenreich-May is the first author of the therapist guide and workbooks for the Unified Protocols for Transdiagnostic Treatment of Emotional Disorders in Children and Adolescents (UP-C and UP-A) and receives a royalty from these publications. Dr Ehrenreich-May (also) receives payments for UP-C and UP-A clinical trainings, consultation, and implementation support services.

REFERENCES

[1] Fichter MM, Kohlboeck G, Quadflieg N, et al. From childhood to adult age: 18-year longitudinal results and prediction of the course of mental disorders in the community. Soc Psychiatry Psychiatr Epidemiol 2009; 44(9):792–803.

[2] Garber J, Brunwasser SM, Zerr AA, et al. Treatment and prevention of depression and anxiety in youth: test of cross-over effects. Depress Anxiety 2016;33(10): 939–59.

[3] Ghandour RM, Sherman LJ, Vladutiu CJ, et al. Prevalence and treatment of depression, anxiety, and conduct problems in US children. J Pediatr 2019;206:256–67. e253.

[4] Twenge JM, Joiner TE. US Census Bureau-assessed prevalence of anxiety and depressive symptoms in 2019 and during the 2020 COVID-19 pandemic. Depress Anxiety 2020;37(10):954–6.

[5] Racine N, McArthur BA, Cooke JE, et al. Global prevalence of depressive and anxiety symptoms in children and adolescents during COVID-19: a meta-analysis. JAMA Pediatr 2021;175(11):1142–50.

[6] Grover RL, Ginsburg GS, Ialongo N. Psychosocial outcomes of anxious first graders: a seven-year follow-up. Depress Anxiety 2007;24(6):410–20.

[7] Ialongo N, Edelsohn G, Werthamer-Larsson L, et al. The significance of self-reported anxious symptoms in first grade children: Prediction to anxious symptoms and adaptive functioning in fifth grade. J Child Psychol Psychiatry 1995;36(3):427–37.

[8] Essau CA, Lewinsohn PM, Olaya B, et al. Anxiety disorders in adolescents and psychosocial outcomes at age 30. J Affect Disord 2014;163:125–32.

[9] Last CG, Hansen C, Franco N. Anxious children in adulthood: a prospective study of adjustment. J Am Acad Child Adolesc Psychiatry 1997;36(5):645–52.

[10] Seligman LD, Ollendick TH. Cognitive-behavioral therapy for anxiety disorders in youth. Child Adolesc Psychiatr Clin N Am 2011;20(2):217–38.

[11] Sigurvinsdóttir AL, Jensínudóttir KB, Baldvinsdóttir KD, et al. Effectiveness of cognitive behavioral therapy (CBT) for child and adolescent anxiety disorders across different CBT modalities and comparisons: a systematic review and meta-analysis. Nord J Psychiatry 2020;74(3):168–80.

[12] Crowe K, McKay D. Efficacy of cognitive-behavioral therapy for childhood anxiety and depression. J Anxiety Disord 2017;49:76–87.

[13] Ollendick TH, Jarrett MA, Grills-Taquechel AE, et al. Comorbidity as a predictor and moderator of treatment outcome in youth with anxiety, affective, attention deficit/hyperactivity disorder, and oppositional/conduct disorders. Clin Psychol Rev 2008;28(8):1447–71.

[14] Ollendick TH, Ost LG, Reuterskiöld L, et al. Comorbidity in youth with specific phobias: impact of comorbidity on treatment outcome and the impact of treatment on comorbid disorders. Behav Res Ther 2010;48(9):827–31.

[15] Hancock KM, Swain J, Hainsworth CJ, et al. Acceptance and commitment therapy versus cognitive behavior therapy for children with anxiety: Outcomes of a randomized controlled trial. J Clin Child Adolesc Psychol 2018;47(2):296–311.

[16] Ossman WA, Wilson KG, Storaasli RD, et al. A preliminary investigation of the use of acceptance and commitment therapy in group treatment for social phobia. Int J Psychol Psychol Ther 2006;6(3):397–416.

[17] Hayes SA, Orsillo SM, Roemer L. Changes in proposed mechanisms of action during an acceptance-based behavior therapy for generalized anxiety disorder. Behav Res Ther 2010;48(3):238–45.

[18] Dalrymple KL, Herbert JD. Acceptance and commitment therapy for generalized social anxiety disorder: a pilot study. Behav Modif 2007;31(5):543–68.

[19] Barney JY, Field CE, Morrison KL, et al. Treatment of pediatric obsessive compulsive disorder utilizing parent-facilitated acceptance and commitment therapy. Psychol Sch 2017;54(1):88–100.

[20] Armstrong AB, Morrison KL, Twohig MP. A preliminary investigation of acceptance and commitment therapy for adolescent obsessive-compulsive disorder. J Cogn Psychother 2013;27(2):175–90.

[21] Swain J, Hancock K, Dixon A, et al. Acceptance and commitment therapy for children: a systematic review of intervention studies. J Context Behav Sci 2015;4(2): 73–85.

[22] Pincus DB, Ehrenreich JT, Mattis SG. Mastery of anxiety and panic for adolescents, therapist guide: riding the wave. New York, NY: Oxford University Press; 2008.

[23] Beidel DC, Turner SM, Morris TL. Social effectiveness therapy for children and adolescents (SET-C): therapist guide. Toronto, Ontario: MHS; 2003.

[24] Kendall PC, Hedtke K. Cognitive-behavioral therapy for anxious children: Therapist manual. 3rd edition. Ardmore, PA: Workbook Publishing; 2006.

[25] Marchette LK, Weisz JR. Practitioner review: empirical evolution of youth psychotherapy toward transdiagnostic approaches. J Child Psychol Psychiatry 2017;58(9): 970–84.

[26] Oxford University Press. Oxford clinical Psychology homepage. 2022. Available at: https://www.oxfordclinicalpsych.com/. Accessed February, 2022.

[27] California Evidence-Based Clearinghouse for Child Welfare. CEBC home page. 2022. Available at: https://www.cebc4cw.org/. Accessed February, 2022.

[28] Higa-McMillan CK, Francis SE, Rith-Najarian L, et al. Evidence base update: 50 years of research on treatment for child and adolescent anxiety. J Clin Child Adolesc Psychol 2016;45(2):91–113.

[29] Silverman WK, Pina AA, Viswesvaran C. Evidence-based psychosocial treatments for phobic and anxiety disorders in children and adolescents. J Clin Child Adolesc Psychol 2008;37(1):105–30.

[30] American Psychiatric Association. Diagnostic and statistical manual of mental disorders. 5th edition. Washington, DC: Author; 2013.

[31] Hayes SC, Strosahl KD, Wilson KG. Acceptance and commitment therapy: an experiential approach to behavior change. New York, NY: Guilford Press; 1999.

[32] Gross JJ. Antecedent-and response-focused emotion regulation: divergent consequences for experience, expression, and physiology. J Pers Soc Psychol 1998;74(1): 224–37.

[33] Herbert JD, Formanv EM. Mindfulness and acceptance techniques. In: Hofmann SG, Dozois DJ, Rief W, editors. The wiley handbook of cognitive behavioral therapy, 1. West Sussex, UK: Wiley-Blackwell; 2013. p. 131–56.

[34] Peris TS, Caporino NE, O'Rourke S, et al. Therapist reported features of exposure tasks that predict differential treatment outcomes for youth with anxiety. J Am Acad Child Adolesc Psychiatry 2017;56(12):1043–52.

[35] Semple RJ, Lee J. Treating anxiety with mindfulness: Mindfulness-based cognitive therapy for children. In: Greco LA, Hayes SC, editors. Acceptance and mindfulness interventions for children, adolescents and families. Oakland, CA: Context Press/New Harbinger Publications; 2008. p. 94–134.

[36] Beck AT. Cognitive therapy and the emotional disorders. New York, NY: International Universities Press; 1976.

[37] Stewart E, Frank H, Benito K, et al. Exposure therapy practices and mechanism endorsement: a survey of specialty clinicians. Prof Psychol Res Pr 2016;47(4):303.

[38] Clark DA. Cognitive restructuring. In: Hofmann SG, Dozois DJ, Rief W, editors. The wiley handbook of cognitive behavioral therapy, 1. West Sussex, UK: Wiley-Blackwell; 2013. p. 23–44.

[39] Ehrenreich-May J, Kennedy SM, Sherman JA, et al. Unified protocols for transdiagnostic treatment of emotional disorders in children and adolescents: therapist guide. New York, NY: Oxford University Press; 2017.

[40] Hayes SC, Strosahl KD, Wilson KG. Acceptance and commitment therapy: the process and practice of

mindful change. 2nd edition. New York, NY: Guilford press; 2012.

[41] Puliafico AC, Kendall PC. Threat-related attentional bias in anxious youth: a review. Clin Child Fam Psychol 2006;9(3):162–80.

[42] Peris TS, Compton SN, Kendall PC, et al. Trajectories of change in youth anxiety during cognitive-behavior therapy. J Consult Clin Psychol 2015;83(2):239–52.

[43] Whiteside SP, Sim LA, Morrow AS, et al. A meta-analysis to guide the enhancement of CBT for childhood anxiety: exposure over anxiety management. Clin Child Fam Psychol 2020;23(1):102–21.

[44] Pavlov PI. Conditioned reflexes: an investigation of the physiological activity of the cerebral cortex. Ann Neurosci 2010;17(3):136–41.

[45] Craske MG, Treanor M, Conway CC, et al. Maximizing exposure therapy: an inhibitory learning approach. Behav Res Ther 2014;58:10–23.

[46] Bouton ME. Context, time, and memory retrieval in the interference paradigms of Pavlovian learning. Psychol Bull 1993;114(1):80–99.

[47] Baker A, Mystkowski J, Culver N, et al. Does habituation matter? Emotional processing theory and exposure therapy for acrophobia. Behav Res Ther 2010;48(11):1139–43.

[48] Milan S, Snow S, Belay S. The context of preschool children's sleep: racial/ethnic differences in sleep locations, routines, and concerns. J Fam Psychol 2007;21(1):20.

[49] Lebowitz ER. Breaking Free of Child Anxiety and OCD: a scientifically proven program for parents. New York, NY: Oxford University Press; 2020.

[50] Rapee R, Wignall A, Spence S, et al. Helping your anxious child: a step-by-step guide for parents. Oakland, CA: New Harbinger Publications; 2008.

[51] Weersing VR, Gonzalez A, Rozenman M. Brief Behavioral Therapy for anxiety and depression in youth: Therapist guide. New York, NY: Oxford University Press; 2021.

[52] Wood JJ, McLeod BD. Child anxiety disorders: A family-based treatment manual for practitioners. New York, NY: WW Norton & Co; 2008.

[53] Rapee RM, Lyneham HJ, Schniering CA, et al. The Cool Kids Child and Adolescent Anxiety Program: Therapist manual. Sydney, Australia: Centre for Emotional Health, Macquarie University; 2006.

[54] Weisz JR, Bearman SK. FIRST: A principle-guided approach to evidence-based youth psychotherapy. Cambridge, MA: Harvard University; 2016.

[55] Barrett PM, Lowry-Webster H, Turner C. FRIENDS program for children: Group leaders manual. Brisbane, Australia: Australian Academic Press; 2000.

[56] Bergman RL. Treatment for children with selective mutism: An integrative behavioral approach. New York, NY: Oxford University Press; 2013.

[57] Chorpita BF, Weisz JR. Modular approach to therapy for children with anxiety, depression, trauma, or conduct problems (MATCH-ADTC). Satellite Beach, FL: PracticeWise; 2009.

[58] Chorpita BF. Modular cognitive-behavioral therapy for childhood anxiety disorders. New York, NY: Guildford Press; 2007.

[59] Albano AM, DiBartolo PM. Cognitive-behavioral therapy for social phobia in adolescents: Stand up, Speak out, therapist guide. New York, NY: Oxford University Press; 2007.

Geriatrics

Advances in Psychiatry and Behavioral Health 2 (2022) 173–181

ADVANCES IN PSYCHIATRY AND BEHAVIORAL HEALTH

Promotion of Psychological Well-Being in Later Life and Prevention of Late-Life Mental Disorders

Nancy A. Pachana, PhD, FAPS, FASSA

School of Psychology, The University of Queensland, Brisbane, Queensland 4072, Australia

KEYWORDS

• Aging • Mental health • Wellbeing • Assessment • Intervention • Culture

KEY POINTS

- Healthy aging encompasses the intrinsic capacity of the individual situated within their environmental context, optimally viewed within a lifespan developmental context.
- Understanding relevant cultural factors is vital for effective diagnosis, assessment, and interventions aimed at restoring and maintaining psychological well-being.
- Successful negotiation of transition points across the lifespan (eg, retirement) is vital for successful aging, particularly with regard to maintaining social connectivity.
- The placement of the therapist as well as the patient within the larger interpersonal and cultural contexts is important for treatment success, as is the examination of their own views of the maturational process as it affects the presenting problem and possible intervention strategies.
- Increasingly, community-based interventions for promoting positive aging are being implemented; the evidence base on these, while still not well-developed, is promising.

INTRODUCTION

The United Nations has declared 2021 to 2030 to be the Decade of Healthy Aging, with the goal of improving the lives of older people, their families, and their communities—a goal requiring international action as well as national and community initiatives [1]. The World Health Organization's (WHO's) *World Report on Aging and Health* [2] underpinned the call to action to meet the opportunities and challenges of shifting demographics. A larger proportion of older people globally requires new thinking—on the diversity of background, health, and functioning of these citizens, how public health initiatives need to guard against ageist stereotypes of later life, and how social changes globally impact what it means to be old, and to age well, in the 21st century [2]. Most importantly, the mental health professionals themselves need to focus on working with older people to support and maintain well-being in later life, rather than focus exclusively on disease and disability.

While a global pandemic was not on the agenda for this important decade, coronavirus disease 19 has had a profound impact on how we look at these issues of later life. The marginalization of older persons, particularly those in nursing homes, has resulted in isolation, loss of autonomy, and restriction of health care [3]. Ageist statements within the media rose in many nations [4]. Mental health concerns for those in later life rose, again particularly for persons in aged care facilities. However, here at least there has been some better news, with data

E-mail address: n.pachana@psy.uq.edu.au

https://doi.org/10.1016/j.ypsc.2022.05.007

supporting the resilience of older persons to the global pandemic and its aftermath [5]. These events throw into even more stark relief the need to address the rights of older persons and to invest in the aging population, across health care, lifelong learning, and age-friendly environmental contexts [2]. This in turn enhances both health and social connectivity, which are intimately tied to psychological well-being in later life, as well as aiding in the prevention of mental disorders in older persons.

The WHO concept of healthy aging has been built on the appreciation of the interplay between the intrinsic capacity of the individual (physical and mental capabilities) situated within their environmental context (factors in that individual's extrinsic world) that together make up that person's functional ability. It is this functional ability that enables "people to do and to be what they have reason to value" [2]. Within a mental health context, the question that arises is what factors might be at play at a more nuanced, lifespan level to lead to better outcomes with respect to psychological well-being. Expanding on the familiar biopsychosocial contextual framework, factors of increasing relevance as highlighted in the literature, but equally familiar within the zeitgeist of the modern world, are issues of culture, the influence of technology, both economic and social resources, and genetic and epigenetic factors, and are shown in Fig. 1 [6].

The holistic framework offered in Fig. 1 encompasses factors at the individual level, such as genetics, and includes proximate and distal events, resources, and risk and protective factors. This developmental regulation is reflected in a host of gerontological theories underpinning the psychological theories of aging (eg, Baltes' selective optimization with compensation) [7] which have as their goal understanding the ways in which individuals age more or less successfully. Within such a framework as presented in Fig. 1, psychological interventions at both an individual and a public health level should be viewed as planned developmental regulation, influencing the trajectory of healthy aging within a mental health context. The efficacy of such interventions to a certain extent is underpinned by their appreciation of the entirety of the holistic framework in which individuals experience biopsychosocial development and their own aging. Given the interconnectedness of the world and the increased appreciation for generational traumas to be carried forward, for example, we can see in Fig. 1 how a historical-cultural context as well as the influence of technology must not be ignored in terms of a developmental, lifespan context.

CULTURAL CONSIDERATIONS FOR MENTAL WELL-BEING IN LATER LIFE

As mentioned in the *World Report on Aging and Health* [2] and as shown in Fig. 1, cultural considerations play a key role in psychological well-being.

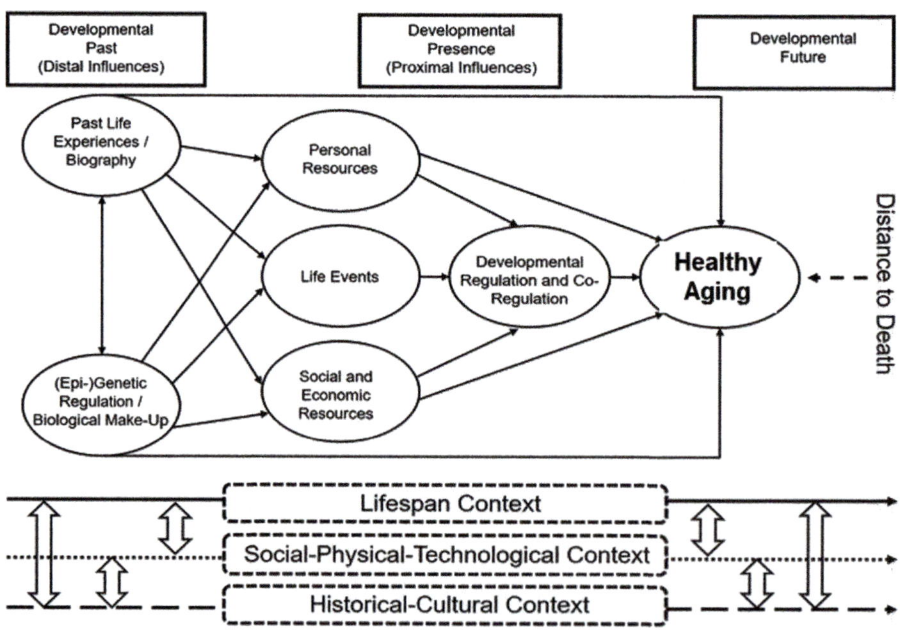

FIG. 1 A biopsychosocial and contextual model of healthy aging.

Investigating, diagnosing, assessing, and treating mental health disorders, as well as having an appreciation and understanding of what the experience of mental well-being constitutes, requires a cultural lens. Both mental well-being and ill-being may be thought of as the products of social-ecological contexts, including culture *in situ* as well as cultural considerations for migrants and displaced persons, for example. Such a multisystemic view accords well with the diversity of later life and how risk and protective factors may lead to a variety of mental health outcomes [8]. Cultural considerations also affect how mental health and illness are understood, how health-seeking behaviors are expressed, and how health care practitioners and systems include or exclude certain groups and their beliefs [9].

Recently there has been much criticism of the lack of diversity within clinical trials, including within mental health contexts; for example, despite an increase in countries globally participating in clinical drug trials, the overwhelming majority of participants in those trials remain white, despite data suggesting differences in drug efficacy depending on ancestry [10]. But there is also recent evidence of shifts with respect to the consideration of diversity and inclusion within mental health research. Groups in the mental health area have proposed criteria for cultural adaptation in psychological intervention trials [11]. Diversity beyond culture, such as suggestions for increased reporting of sexual orientation and gender diversity within clinical trials, has also been forthcoming [12].

Various instantiations of culture require consideration in effective clinical practice. In a mental health context, attunement to culture is important; lack of attention to culture may cause harm. For example, application of a test instrument developed in one distinct culture but applied in another can result in assessment bias and misdiagnosis [13]. For example, in a wide-ranging review, older adults representing racial and ethnic minorities reported higher pain intensity and prevalence than non-Hispanic white older adults [14]. Culture has been cited as an influential context for older adults' sexual health and well-being [15] and for mental help-seeking behaviors [16]. These disparate examples underscore how cultural considerations come into play in the context of usual clinical practice; unfortunately, the amount of research on the intersection of age and culture within clinical practice is less robust than for midlife, but this is literature that is growing. Considerations of culture are critical in ensuring clinical decision-making takes into account such contextual factors with respect to treatment plans and adequately addressing patient concerns. Early career practitioners may wish to seek specific mentoring around cultural issues, including intersectional cohort and cultural issues, to improve their understanding of how best to navigate unfamiliar circumstances within their patients.

One group that has been neglected with respect to the promotion of psychological well-being later in life is the First Nations People. Spread across 90 countries and representing over 5000 different cultures, First Nations People, at over 476 million individuals, make up 6.2% of the global population [17]. Older adults within this population are fast growing, understudied and underserved, and with lower longevity and higher morbidity than their nonindigenous counterparts [18]. Their inclusion in considerations of well-being and mental health in later life is overdue but growing. Although in almost all countries, indigenous peoples make up a small percentage of the population, their inclusion in understanding mental health issues and policies is heartening where it occurs. In New Zealand, Māori health models have influenced that country's health care system (including health research) since the mid-1980s (eg, the *Whare Tapa Whā* model of health [19]). Recent work has looked at Māori understandings of dementia and the assessment of cognitive function [20]. The family (*whanau*) is central to life in Māori culture and central to how health and mental health services are delivered. Keys to understanding both brain health and dementia from a Māori perspective included a sense of connection (eg, to place and extended family) and individual considerations (eg, spirituality, identity and role) [20]. These elements figure prominently in the *Whare Tapa Whā* model, confirming its relevance as a model of health; moreover, these considerations play an important role in how services (eg, mental health, hospice) can be informed by the cultural priorities of older Māori [20].

PROMOTION OF PSYCHOLOGICAL WELL-BEING THROUGH LIFE TRANSITIONS

Life events often play a large role in mental well-being or distress. Understanding how certain life events which are more common in later life affect well-being is critical in clinical practice. But this must be considered not simply from a stereotypical perspective. For example, older adults often cope with bereavement better than younger cohorts, given that loss of a partner is more expected at advanced ages, and peers have often been through a similar life event and can offer support [21]. As another example, not all older adults living alone are lonely; not all older persons with apparent social connections perceive and receive adequate social support [22]. An individual's context is key; their chronologic age less so.

However, some life transitions are more difficult for older persons. The need to cease driving is an event few plan for but one which can have a profound negative effect on general health, mental health, and social engagement, with additional risks for premature institutionalization [23] as well as social identity [24]. In fact, older drivers rate loss of driving as more significant than loss of a friend in one study [25]. People who cease driving in an unsupported manner risk reduced community participation, significant mental health declines, negative changes to self-identity, fractured relationships with spouses and family members, and increased social isolation [24,26]. Supported transitions involving key networks of health professionals as well as family and friends are vital for successful transition to nondriving status [27].

Retirement poses another transition point for older adults, and how it affects well-being depends on its context and timing. Up to a quarter of retirees find this transition highly stressful and experience reductions in well-being and quality of life [28]. Premature exit from the work force, lack of perceived or actual retirement planning, and managing social relationships (both the loss or work relationships and the potential lack of post-retirement relationships) play a role in how well an individual adjusts to retirement but also suggests intervention strategies [29]. The maintenance of existing social connections and group memberships, as well as having the skills to develop new relationships and connect with groups that can provide support, leisure outlets, and meaningful social bonds, is key for mental well-being post retirement [30]. The intervention GROUPS 4 HEALTH provides guidance to older adults in developing and embedding group ties so as to protect and enhance their mental well-being; this program has been used to address multiple mental health issues including depression, loneliness, and adjustment to retirement [29,31].

CONTEXTUAL APPROACHES TO THE PROMOTION OF MENTAL WELL-BEING IN LATER LIFE

Having discussed several contextual issues (ie, culture, life transitions) relevant to older adults' mental well-being, positioning these within a clinical framework within which to guide practice is useful. The Contextual Adult Lifespan Theory for Adapting Psychotherapy (CALTAP) model [32,33] is a transtheoretical way of understanding older patients from a lifespan perspective. The CALTAP model contains the following themes: developmental aging, social context, cohort differences, and cultural issue; these encompass an individual's physical, cognitive, emotional, and interpersonal functioning, along with their conceptualization of sources and causes of their own distress, as well as the relationship between the patient and the treating clinician (Fig. 2).

Within the model, *both the patient and the clinician's* model of developmental aging is included, as each party's views of the aging process and its contribution to well-being or distress is important. For example, if either the patient or the clinician views depression as a normal part of aging, this will affect everything from treatment recommendations to a sense of agency. The many complexities attendant with good or ill health in later life, including medication side effects, fears about aging, the interplay between mental health and physical health, the expectations of peers and family, and so forth, can make it difficult to understand what is contributing to a set of symptoms or a particular clinical presentation. Specifically, the patient's and the clinician's positive and negative views and knowledge of the aging process affect how specific challenges (eg, life transitions) are seen, and how symptoms are presented and interpreted. This then also argues for an explicit addressing of potential ageist views (either conscious or unconscious) within training models for mental health professionals. (Of course, one could argue that such training, across all forms of bias, should be undertaken for all health professionals.)

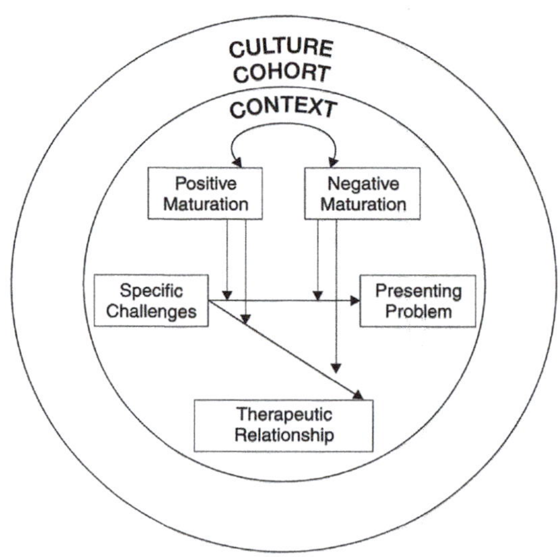

FIG. 2 Contextual Adult Lifespan Theory for Adapting Psychotherapy (CALTAP) model

Understanding how views of aging and specific challenges within the individual's environment or life circumstances may affect health and also the experience of health echoes the WHO emphasis on intrinsic capacity and its interaction with the environment. Such interactions may then influence how symptoms are presented and experienced. These factors are influenced by both culture and cohort, which can in turn affect assessment, diagnosis, and intervention choices. A solid understanding of later-life contexts and their influence on the experience of health and well-being can benefit both therapeutic outcomes and the therapeutic relationship [33].

Late Life Well-being Case Study: "If I cannot drive, life is not worth living"

Case *Presentation*. Mrs. K., aged 75, presented to the outpatient memory clinic, referred by her primary care physician after an accident in which Mrs. K. drove her car into the wall of her neighbor's home; no persons were injured. This was not the first time Mrs. K. had been in a motor vehicle accident; over the preceding 2 years she had dented her car several times and was involved in two minor instances of scraping her car against other parked vehicles in the local shopping mall.

Mrs. K. was a widow of just over 3 years; she was a retired high school teacher, as was her deceased spouse. Of their two children, their older son lived abroad and was not close to his parents; his younger sister lived with her husband in the same small town as her parents. The daughter had been suggesting for at least 18 months that her mother give up driving; her mother pointed to the lack of public transportation in their small town and the desire not to be a burden and "to live my own life."

The memory clinic assessment proved equivocal on whether cognitive impairment was present to such a degree that driving should cease. The psychologist on the team also noted that although Mrs. K. denied feelings of anxiety and depression, her conversation was peppered with statements suggesting a degree of unresolved bereavement for the deceased spouse, lack of connection with the couple's previously robust social network, and the fact that Mrs. K. often drove "just for the sake of something to do, to keep my mind away from dark thoughts."

Clinical Questions. The memory clinic's interdisciplinary treatment team felt that many potentially interrelated issues underlay Mrs. K.'s issues with cognition, social isolation, and driving concerns. Depression could impact negatively on cognition; poor cognition due to depression could impact driving ability; social isolation could exacerbate depressive symptoms. Given Mrs. K.'s lack of any previous psychiatric history, the close and positive relationship with her daughter and her daughter's husband, and Mrs. K.'s openness to intervention suggestions made the team lean toward treating the *contextual issues* potentially impacting on Mrs. K.'s well-being.

Proposed Treatment Plan. When the lack of social connection was discussed with Mrs. K., she admitted that she had taken her husband's sudden and unexpected death poorly, turning away from friends in whose company they had spent much time. Birdwatching, playing bridge, and volunteering at the local animal shelter had all been activities that the couple pursued together; being with those groups brought painful memories of her spouse. In using a tool to measure an individual's personally meaningful contributors to quality of life, the schedule for the evaluation of individual quality of life [34], it was clear that Mrs. K. had let a variety of sources of joy and companionship fall away.

She admitted at that point to sleeping poorly and often drinking excessively in the evening although she adamantly denied ever driving while intoxicated. It was clear that she felt unprepared to resume activities that she had previously pursued with her husband due to the pain of memories invoked.

An option to see a clinical geropsychologist to address potential unresolved bereavement was greeted with some hesitancy but was not rejected. For the moment, the issues around driving were considered not as pressing as Mrs. K.'s car had been deemed beyond repair, and so for the moment she could not drive. Mrs. K. also expressed dissatisfaction with the increase in her alcohol intake and was willing to examine this as part of engaging with the psychologist.

The psychologist and Mrs. K. explored options for increasing social connections, parallel to exploring issues of grief and bereavement. After a few sessions, Mrs. K. reported that she had made contact with former birdwatching friends, who had suggested an outing. When they had heard that she had no way of driving, they assured her that their club had the use of a van to take members on outings. With the psychologist's encouragement and support, an outing was arranged and Mrs. K. reported the positive effects of a day out in nature: "It brought back memories–some sad, but mostly it felt good to be walking and seeing birds."

Discussions of ways to rebuild social connections were fruitful. Although Mrs. K. had felt that her friends would "never forgive her" for rejecting their solicitations after her husband's death, the birdwatching outing was a chance to see that these relationships were resilient to time and distance. Mrs. K. decided to focus on the birdwatching social group given that it came with an option for transportation. The bridge meetings were rejected given the close nature of her and her husband's bridge partnership (they had won several minor competitions together). And while the animal shelter was appealing in terms of a feeling of accomplishment, Mrs. K. felt she wanted to instead volunteer at their local nature center, which was within walking distance and involved less physical labor.

Clinical Outcomes. The meetings with the clinical geropsychologist ended after 10 sessions. Mrs. K. felt that over that time she had felt the need to drink or to distract her mind from "dark thoughts" recede. In 6 months' time, after reassessment at the memory clinic, she was found to still have some equivocal results on neuropsychological testing, but her mood, sleep, and sense of well-being were much improved. She had also come to the decision that she could get by without a car given the offer of some help getting about by her daughter, as well as friends from the nature center and the birdwatching club. The final deciding factor regarding driving was the fact that the money saved by not having a car could pay for an interstate birdwatching excursion periodically.

Discussion. Although the issue of driving might have needed to be the immediate focus, having the chance to address unresolved grief issues and rebuild Mrs. K.'s social support network and social identity in the absence of her husband ultimately proved fruitful. With increased social support and social activities in place, the issues with driving resolved more naturally. An individual's circumstances, the presence of dementia, and a lack of family support can all contribute to less satisfactory outcomes. Here formal enrollment in a driving cessation intervention or a structured means to improve social connectivity, such as a GROUPS 4 HEALTH model, can be worthwhile. In some jurisdictions, social prescribing schemes may also facilitate establishment or re-establishment of social connections within the community [35].

INTERVENTIONS TO PREVENT PSYCHOLOGICAL DISORDERS IN LATER LIFE

Recognition of the benefits of prevention of mental disorders in later life has resulted from increasing research on, and interest in, such programs and their implementation in communities. These programs are varied and have originated in many parts of the globe, serving different community needs and responsive to varied economic, workforce, and operational constraints.

Problem-solving therapy (PST) is an intervention focused on training in constructive problem-solving attitudes and skills; it has been widely used in older populations [36]. PST has been used in several studies to prevent post-stroke depression, both on its own [37] as well as in combination with pharmaceutical intervention [38]. Developed initially for use in treating depression, PST has also been found to be effective in preventing depression relapse in older patients [39]. It has also been trialed in suicide prevention in veteran [40] and depressed older adults [41]. Although both patient satisfaction and effectiveness of PST is high [40], also echoed in meta-analyses of PST in older persons [36], a specific review or meta-analysis of PST in a preventative role is to date lacking.

Reminiscence and life review therapies have potential in preventing psychological distress in older persons not simply through ameliorating psychiatric symptoms such as depression but also through a mechanism of improving attitudes toward aging and older age itself [42]. Reminiscence group therapy has also been shown to reduce loneliness and improve life satisfaction within a community sample [43].

However, efforts to ensure preservation or recovery of psychological well-being in the community are not confined to more traditional one-on-one or group psychological interventions. Community-based prevention and intervention services may include telephone helplines, digital support services, and group social activities, and these activities have been shown to improve physical and mental health, social connectedness, and coping skills (in terms of managing caregiving responsibilities, for example), although as pointed out in a recent review [44], efficacy and benefits over time have been harder to judge due to a large variety of methodologies outcome measures employed. Social prescribing, where people using primary care services are linked with community-based organizations that can service specific needs such as social isolation, have been increasingly implemented, most notably within the National Health System in England [45]. Despite generally positive outcomes being reported, researchers have pointed to poor quality within the extant literature that must be addressed before the purported benefits of social prescribing can be better understood [46]. Deconstructing the processes of referral and uptake in a recent review [47], both clarified learnings from prior research (for example, that activities must be accessible and meaningful to be useful) while pointing out the need for higher-quality trials with improved patient follow-up.

Finally, ageism itself has been shown in a large number of studies internationally to undermine positive aging and, particularly with internalized ageism, to result in physical, cognitive, and emotional decline [48]. The Positive Education about Aging and Contact Experiences model [49] brings together evidence on two of the strongest means of combating the effects of ageism, namely psychoeducation and positive intergenerational contact. Becca Levy, whose research on ageism and its effects spans three decades, rightly points out that while individuals and health professionals may initiate practices to combat ageism, the continuation of structural or institutional ageism and ageist practices must also be tackled to advance widespread progress on the issue [50].

SUMMARY

The proactive prevention of mental ill-health is increasingly recognized as a priority in later life. A lifespan perspective on mental health emphasizes the many contributions of an individual's biology, historical and cultural context, and their interpersonal relationships and life events to mental well-being. Effective clinical practice, from initial assessment to diagnosis and treatment recommendations, must recognize this holistic picture of the individual to be effective and valid. Moreover, shared understandings of this lifespan context and the influence of aging is also vital between clinicians and their patients. Both an individual as well as a systems approach is required to combat the deleterious effects of ageism, which undermine positive well-being and health in later life.

CLINICS CARE POINTS

- Careful attention should be paid to making sure a patient's language and cultural background are taken into consideration at every step of treatment; supervision or expert advice should be sought if relevant experience or expertise are lacking.
- A patient should be asked about their individual goals in care, particularly in the face of life transitions (eg, driving cessation) as relying on age stereotypes or assumptions does not lead to psychological well-being.
- The clinician should be alert to ageist or stereotypical views which may be largely unconscious yet damaging to rapport and treatment outcomes.

REFERENCES

[1] Dixon A. The United Nations decade of healthy ageing requires concerted global action. Nat Aging 2021;1:2.

[2] World Health Organization (WHO). World report on ageing and health. Geneva: World Health Organization; 2015.

[3] D'cruz M, Banerjee D. 'An invisible human rights crisis': the marginalization of older adults during the COVID-19 pandemic–an advocacy review. Psychiatry Res 2020; 292:113369.

[4] Pachana NA, Beattie E, Byrne GJ, et al. Covid-19 and psychogeriatrics: the view from Australia. Int Psychogeriatr 2020;32:1135–41.

[5] Vahia IV, Jeste DV, Reynolds CF. Older adults and the mental health effects of COVID-19. J Am Med Assoc 2020;324:2253–4.

[6] Pachana NA, Wahl H-W. Healthy aging: current and future frameworks and developments. In: Asmundson G, editor. Comprehensive clinical psychology, vol. 7. Oxford (England): Elsevier; 2022. p. 1–20.

[7] Baltes PB, Baltes MM. Psychological perspectives on successful aging: the model of selective optimization with compensation. In: Baltes PB, Baltes MM, editors. Successful aging: perspectives from the behavioral sciences. New York: Cambridge University Press; 1990. p. 1–34.

[8] Ungar M, Theron L. Resilience and mental health: how multisystemic processes contribute to positive outcomes. Lancet Psychiatr 2020;7:441–8.

[9] Gopalkrishnan N. Cultural diversity and mental health: considerations for policy and practice. Front Public Health 2018;6:179.

[10] Knepper TC, McLeod HL. When will clinical trials finally reflect diversity? Nat 2018;557:157–9.

[11] Heim E, Mewes R, Abi Ramia J, et al. Reporting cultural adaptation in psychological trials–the RECAPT criteria. Clin Psychol Eur 2021;3:e6351.

[12] Pachankis JE. The scientific pursuit of sexual and gender minority mental health treatments: toward evidence-based affirmative practice. Am Psychol 2018; 73:1207.

[13] Freedman DM. Assessment of cognition in African American older adults. In: Asmundson G, editor. APA handbook of dementia. Washington, DC: American Psychological Association; 2018. p. 107–23.

[14] Lavin R, Park J. A characterization of pain in racially and ethnically diverse older adults: a review of the literature. J Appl Gerontol 2014;33:258–90.

[15] Muzacz A, Akinsulure-Smith A. Older adults and sexuality: implications for counseling ethnic and sexual minority clients. J Ment Health Couns 2013; 35:1–14.

[16] Haralambous B, Dow B, Goh A, et al. "Depression is not an illness. It's up to you to make yourself happy". Perceptions of health professionals and community workers about older Chinese immigrants' experiences

of depression and anxiety. Aust J Ageing 2016;35: 249–54.
[17] UNDP. 10. Things to Know about Indigenous Peoples. 2022. Available at: https://stories.undp.org/10-things-we-all-should-know-about-indigenous-people. Accessed March 7, 2022.
[18] Pachana NA. International trends in clinical geropsychology. In: Lichtenberg P, Mast B, editors. APA handbook of clinical geropsychology. Washington, DC: American Psychological Association; 2015. p. 421–41.
[19] Durie MH. A Māori perspective of health. J Soc Sci 1985; 20:483–6.
[20] Menzies O, Dudley M, Garrett N, et al. He Tūhononga Whaiaro: a Kaupapa Māori approach to Mate Wareware (dementia) and cognitive assessment of older Māori. J Appl Gerontol 2021;41(4):1066–73.
[21] Bisconti TL, Bergeman CS, Boker SM. Social support as a predictor of variability: an examination of the adjustment trajectories of recent widows. Psychol Aging 2006;21:590–9.
[22] Perissinotto CM, Covinsky KE. Living alone, socially isolated or lonely—What are we measuring? J Gen Intern Med 2014;29:1429–31.
[23] Chihuri S, Mielenz TJ, DiMaggio CJ, et al. Driving cessation and health outcomes in older adults. J Am Geriatr Soc 2016;64:332–41.
[24] Pachana NA, Jetten J, Gustafsson L, et al. To be or not to be (an older driver): social identity theory and driving cessation in later life. Ageing Soc 2017;37: 1597–608.
[25] Jetten J, Pachana NA. Not wanting to grow old: a Social Identity Model of Identity Change (SIMIC) analysis of driving cessation among older adults. In: Jetten J, Haslam C, Haslam SA, editors. The social cure: identity, health and well-being. East Sussex: Psychology Press; 2012. p. 97–113.
[26] Liddle J, Allen S, Tan A, et al. "The biggest problem we've ever had to face": how families manage driving cessation with people with dementia. Int Psychogeriatr 2016;28: 109–22.
[27] Liddle J, Reaston T, Pachana N, et al. Is planning for driving cessation critical for the well-being and lifestyle of older drivers? Int Psychogeriatr 2014;26: 1111–20.
[28] Wang M. Profiling retirees in the retirement transition and adjustment process: examining the longitudinal change patterns of retirees' psychological well-being. J Appl Psychol 2007;92:455–74.
[29] Haslam C, Steffens NK, Branscombe NR, et al. The importance of social groups for retirement adjustment: evidence, application, and policy implications of the social identity model of identity change. Soc Issues Policy Rev 2019;13:93–124.
[30] Haslam C, Lam BC, Branscombe NR, et al. Adjusting to life in retirement: the protective role of new group memberships and identification as a retiree. Eur J Work Organ 2018;27:822–39.
[31] Haslam SA, Haslam C, Cruwys T, et al. Social identity makes group-based social connection possible: implications for loneliness and mental health. Curr Opin Psychol 2022;43:161–5.
[32] Knight BG, Poon CYM. Contextual adult lifespan theory for adapting psychotherapy with older adults. J Rat Emot Cogn Behav Ther 2008;26:232–49.
[33] Pachana NA, Mitchell LK, Knight B. Using the CALTAP lifespan developmental framework with older adults. Gero Psych J 2015;28:77–86.
[34] O'Boyle CA. The schedule for the evaluation of individual quality of life (SEIQoL). (SEIQoL). Int J Ment Health 1994;23:3–23.
[35] Hamilton-West K, Milne A, Hotham S. New horizons in supporting older people's health and wellbeing: is social prescribing a way forward? Age Ageing 2020;49: 319–26.
[36] Kirkham JG, Choi N, Seitz DP. Meta-analysis of problem solving therapy for the treatment of major depressive disorder in older adults. Int J Geriatr Psychiatry 2016;31: 526–35.
[37] Mikami K, Jorge RE, Moser DJ, et al. Prevention of post-stroke apathy using escitalopram or problem-solving therapy. Am J Geriatr Psychiatry 2013;21:855–62.
[38] Robinson RG, Jorge RE, Moser DJ, et al. Escitalopram and problem-solving therapy for prevention of post-stroke depression: a randomized controlled trial. JAMA 2008;299:2391–400.
[39] Nezu AM, Nezu CM. Problem-solving therapy for relapse prevention in depression. In: Richards CS, Perri MG, editors. Relapse Prevention for Depression. Washington, DC: American Psychological Association; 2010. p. 99–130.
[40] Barnes SM, Monteith LL, Gerard GR, et al. Problem-solving therapy for suicide prevention in veterans with moderate-to-severe traumatic brain injury. Rehabil Psychol 2017;62:600.
[41] Gustavson KA, Alexopoulos GS, Niu GC, et al. Problem-solving therapy reduces suicidal ideation in depressed older adults with executive dysfunction. Am J Geriatr Psychiatry 2016;24:11–7.
[42] Siverová J, Bužgová R. The effect of reminiscence therapy on quality of life, attitudes to ageing, and depressive symptoms in institutionalized elderly adults with cognitive impairment: a quasi-experimental study. Inter J Ment Health Nurs 2018;27:1430–9.
[43] Liu SJ, Lin CJ, Chen YM, et al. The effects of reminiscence group therapy on self-esteem, depression, loneliness and life satisfaction of elderly people living alone. Mid Taiwan J Med 2007;12:133–42.
[44] Lee C, Kuhn I, McGrath M, et al. A systematic scoping review of community-based interventions for the prevention of mental ill-health and the promotion of mental health in older adults in the UK. Health Soc Care Community 2022;30:27–57.
[45] Drinkwater C, Wildman J, Moffatt S. Social prescribing. BMJ 2019;364.

[46] Bickerdike L, Booth A, Wilson PM, et al. Social prescribing: less rhetoric and more reality. A systematic review of the evidence. BMJ Open 2017;7: e013384.

[47] Husk K, Blockley K, Lovell R, et al. What approaches to social prescribing work, for whom, and in what circumstances? A realist review. Health Soc Care Community 2020;28:309–24.

[48] Chang ES, Kannoth S, Levy S, et al. Global reach of ageism on older persons' health: a systematic review. PLoS One 2020;15:e0220857.

[49] Levy SR. Toward reducing ageism: PEACE (positive education about aging and contact experiences) model. Gerontologist 2018;58:226–32.

[50] Levy BR. The role of structural ageism in age beliefs and health of older persons. JAMA Netw Open 2022;5: e2147802.

Advances in Psychiatry and Behavioral Health 2 (2022) 183–191

ADVANCES IN PSYCHIATRY AND BEHAVIORAL HEALTH

Addressing Mental Health in Aged Care Residents

A Review of Evidence-Based Psychological Interventions and Emerging Practices

Sunil Bhar, PhD[a,*], Deborah Koder, PhD[a], Hemalatha Jayaram, DPsych (Clinical)[b], Mark Silver, MSW[a], Tanya Davison, DPsych (Clinical)[c]

[a]Department of Psychological Sciences, School of Health Sciences, Swinburne University of Technology, H99 PO BOX 218, Hawthorn, VIC 3122, Australia; [b]Peter James Centre, Aged Persons Mental Health Service, Eastern Health, 321-345 Burwood Hwy, Burwood East, VIC 3151, Australia; [c]Research and Innovation, Silverchain, Silverchain House, 6 Sundercombe Street, Osborne Park, Perth, WA 6017, Australia

KEYWORDS

- Aged care residents • Aging • Anxiety • Cognitive behavioral therapy • Dementia • Depression
- Health care utilization • Long-term care settings

KEY POINTS

- Mental health difficulties are highly prevalent in residential aged care facilities, with up to 60% of residents having at least one mental health diagnosis.
- Psychological treatments are effective for addressing late life mental health difficulties and can be applied in residential aged care facilities.
- Treatments are most effective when they are applied systemically, that is when mental health clinicians collaborate with residents and their staff and/or family.

Residential aged care facilities (RACFs) provide a supported housing environment for individuals who require prolonged nursing care. Worldwide, 4% to 7% of older adults live in such facilities [1]. In Australia, more than 250,000 older adults live permanently in RACFs [2]. With longer life spans, 30% to 50% of older adults are estimated to enter into such care arrangements at some point in their lives [3].

The prevalence of mental health conditions in RACFs is high; yet psychological treatments are not easily accessible to aged care residents. In Australia, less than 14% of such facilities use psychologists or social workers [4]. Similarly, in the United States, mental health clinicians are rarely employed by such facilities. Research on effectiveness of psychological treatments for late life mental health conditions typically focus on community-dwelling populations. Hence, clinicians may not be as familiar with the literature on evidence-based treatment of residential aged care populations. They may also not be familiar with how to deliver psychological treatments to older adults with multiple physical and cognitive comorbidities.

For publication in: Advances in Psychiatry and Behavioral Health.

*Corresponding author. Swinburne University of Technology, H99, PO Box 218, Hawthorn, Victoria 3122, Australia. sbhar@swin.edu.au *E-mail address:* sbhar@swin.edu.au

https://doi.org/10.1016/j.ypsc.2022.06.002
2667-3827/22/

The aim of this article is to provide an overview of evidence-based psychological interventions and emerging practices for supporting the mental health of aged care residents. It reviews the evidence for these interventions and practices. The article also provides recommendations of how clinicians can deliver such strategies to residents who are living with cognitive impairment and physical health comorbidities.

MENTAL HEALTH CONDITIONS IN RESIDENTIAL AGED CARE FACILITIES

The prevalence of mental health conditions in RACFs is significant. In a review of the records of 430,862 aged care residents aged 65 years or older living in Australia, nearly 60% of residents were found to have significant mental health difficulties such as depressive, anxiety, or psychotic disorders [5], with the most common being depressive conditions. The prevalence of such conditions is typically higher in such settings than in the community. A study in the United Kingdom indicated that the rate of depressive symptoms among aged care residents was twice as high as that among community-dwelling older adults [6]. Similarly, up to one-third of aged care residents report suicidal ideation: a rate 4 times that of community-dwelling older adults [7]. Rates of anxiety disorders and symptoms are also higher in RACFs than in the community. For example, in their systematic review, Creighton and colleagues found that anxiety disorders in RACFs ranged from 3.2% to 20%, compared with estimates of 1.4% to 17% in the community [8].

The high rates of mental health conditions in RACFs are related to several factors: comorbid medical conditions, poor health, and poor engagement in meaningful activities [9]. For example, depression may be related to the sudden nature of residents' transition into such facilities [10,11] and to residents' perception of not being in control of the transition [9]. Many older adults move into RACFs when in crisis, such as following a fall, an acute hospitalization, or death of a spouse [12]. There can be limited control over the decision to relocate to the facility, and such relocation is often associated with losses in autonomy, independence, relationships, dignity, privacy, meaningful activities, valued routines, roles, and self-identity [13]. The first 12 months of living in the facility seem to be associated with significant mental health difficulties. In one study, 52% of residents who died by suicide had lived in the facility for less than 12 months [14].

INTERVENTIONS FOR SUPPORTING MENTAL HEALTH OF AGED CARE RESIDENTS

There are fewer high-quality clinical trials of psychological interventions focusing on people living in RACFs than in the community. Of research conducted in RACFs, studies have been underpowered and mostly focused on addressing depressive symptoms [15]. Wells and colleagues [16] reviewed the research evidence for more than 41 nonpharmacological interventions for late life depressive symptoms and anxiety in RACFs. They found that the following interventions were supported by at least "2 good studies": physical exercise, massage, aromatherapy, music and singing, animal-assisted therapy, cognitive behavioral therapy (CBT), and reminiscence therapy. Similarly, in their systematic review of 32 randomized controlled trials (RCTs) of nonpharmacological interventions for depression in aged care residents, Simning and Simons found that CBT and reminiscence therapy were effective for reducing depression in cognitively intact residents.

We provide a summary of research relating to the effectiveness of 2 *evidence-based psychological interventions* in RACFs: CBT and reminiscence therapy. We also review evidence for *emerging practices* such as intergenerational programs and technology-assisted treatments that are popular and seem promising for supporting mental health of aged care residents. Finally, we offer suggestions about how such interventions and practices can be delivered in RACFs to residents with cognitive impairments and/or physical comorbidities.

Cognitive Behavioral Therapy

CBT is the most widely researched psychological treatment [17] and is readily adaptable across diverse populations including older adults living in RACFs [15,18]. Several CBT protocols have been implemented in RACFs [15,18]. In a systematic review of 18 studies of CBT for RACFs, Chan and colleagues [15] summarized the characteristics and effectiveness of CBT for older people experiencing significant depressive or anxiety symptoms living in residential aged care. Of the 12 RCTs reviewed, 8 reported statistically significant reductions in depressive or anxiety symptoms, suggesting that CBT is an effective approach for aged care residents with such symptoms. Further, Chan and colleagues found that CBT was acceptable to aged care residents: uptake to treatment was high (averaged 73% over 14 studies) and attrition was low (averaged 19.9% over 9 studies). They also noted that CBT protocols involved a diverse range of strategies, most commonly behavioral activation, cognitive restructuring, and structured problem solving. Each of these common CBT strategies are described later, along with a summary of research on their effectiveness when used in RACFs.

Behavioral activation involves the scheduling of activities that help the individual feel pleasure, achievement, and purpose. Behavioral activation is one of the most research supported strategies for aged care residents. Examples of such programs are Behavioral Activities Intervention (BE-ACTIV) [19] and Positive Mood and Active Life Program (PMAL) [20].

The BE-ACTIV program involved 10 weekly sessions between the resident and therapist (psychology doctoral students). The goal of the program was to increase pleasant activities that were feasible within the RACF. Staff and family were involved in helping to identify and facilitate such activities. In a cluster RCT involving 23 RACFs and 82 aged care residents with major depressive episodes, Meeks and colleagues found that participants who received this program showed better diagnostic recovery following treatment, than participants receiving usual care [21]. Residents were included in this study if they were at least 55 years old, scored 14 or higher on the Mini-Mental State Examination (MMSE) [22], scored 11 or higher on the Geriatric Depression Scale-30, and met criteria for DSM-IV depressive disorder. Residents who were under the care of, or referred to, hospice for a terminal condition or who were physically unable to participate in study activities were not included in the study. The participants (65.4% women) had average age of 75.16 years (SD = 12.11), had lived in the facility an average of 37.70 months (SD = 74.56), and had multiple medical diagnosis (on average 9.31 diagnoses, SD = 4.2). The mean level of cognitive impairment in the sample was not reported.

The PMAL program has also been shown to be effective at reducing depressive symptoms of "at-risk" aged care residents. This program was delivered over 12 weeks. It aimed to facilitate residents' engagement with pleasant activities. Similar to BE-ACTIV, the PMAL program emphasized ongoing collaborations with staff. Lists of activities were developed in consultation with staff and residents. Staff helped residents engage in these activities at least 3 times per week, over a 6-week period. Then, over the next 6 weeks, residents were encouraged to self-initiate such activities. A cluster RCT involving 7 RACFs and 68 residents with depressive symptoms showed that depressive symptoms reduced significantly greater in the intervention condition than in usual care. Residents were eligible to participate in this study if they had a mood problem and scored 0 or 1 on the Cognitive Performance Scale [23] (indicating intact or borderline intact cognitive functioning). The participants (80.6% women) had an average age of 85.9 (SD = 7.14) in the PMAL intervention group and 84.4 (SD = 9.51) in the usual care control group. The mean level of cognitive impairment in each group, as measured by the MMSE, was 21.87 (*SD* = 4.38) and 21.50 (*SD* = 4.49), respectively, suggesting the presence of mild cognitive impairment in participants [24].

Cognitive restructuring involves a discussion between a clinician and client about the client's automatic thoughts (eg, thoughts or images that spontaneously are activated in specific situations), rules and assumptions, and core beliefs. Clients are encouraged to examine beliefs that may maintain depression or anxiety. The clinician helps clients examine the extent to which these beliefs are accurate or helpful. Research findings are mixed for the effectiveness of this strategy for depressed residents. In a small RCT of 8 depressed residents aged between 85 and 93 years without cognitive impairment, Sales and colleagues [25] found that depressive symptoms improved significantly in the treatment condition (4 weeks of group treatment) but not in the control condition. However, no differences were found between groups on posttest scores of depression. Similarly, Abraham and colleagues [26] randomly allocated 70 aged care residents without major cognitive impairments to 1 of 3 treatment groups lasting 24 weeks: cognitive restructuring, focused visual imagery, or education discussion. They did not find significant between-group differences in severity of depressive symptoms.

In contrast, in their RCT of 60 depressed residents, Zerhussen and colleagues [27] found that depressive symptoms significantly improved during a 10-week group program of cognitive restructuring, compared with music therapy and routine nursing care. Residents participating in this study were aged between 70 and 82 years, ambulatory and free of organic brain syndromes. Collectively, the evidence for the effectiveness of cognitive restructuring for reducing depressive symptoms in aged care residents remains equivocal; more research is needed to examine the applicability of cognitive restructuring for residents with and without cognitive impairment.

Structured problem-solving exercises involve defining problems and goals and brainstorming and testing solutions, all of which can be done in a structured and sequential manner. Clients can feel distressed because of the presence of problems that are part of living in institutionalized care. For example, they may have impaired sleep due to loud noises at night, resent substandard nursing care practices, feel threatened by other residents who enter their room, or become agitated when prevented from returning home. Often clients can feel helpless and disempowered to manage such problems. Clinicians can assist clients to define the problem, articulate a goal, brainstorm potential solutions, and experiment with solutions that are considered feasible and potentially effective. The outcomes of such an exercise can be a greater level of validation, a greater sense of self-efficacy, and the emergence of practical strategies for achieving a goal.

Evidence from a recent meta-analysis is strong for the effectiveness for such strategies for reducing late-life depressive symptoms [28], including for older people living in the community with medical comorbidities [29]. Further, problem solving interventions are embedded within effective CBT protocols to help residents overcome barriers to engaging in pleasant activities [15]. However, the effectiveness of such problem-solving strategies when used relatively exclusively as therapy (ie, as problem-solving therapy) is less well established in RACF settings. Reinhardt and colleagues [30] randomized 37 aged care residents with depressive symptoms to receive 6 sessions of problem-solving exercises or friendly visits (control). Most participants (76%) rated their health as very poor to fair. Participants had intact or mildly impaired cognitive status (MMSE average total score of 24.4 in the control condition and 25.0 in the intervention condition). Depressive symptoms reduced to a greater extent in the problem-solving condition, compared with the control condition, although due to the small sample size, the difference was nonsignificant. More research is needed to support the effectiveness of such therapy for aged care residents with depression or anxiety.

Reminiscence Therapy

Robert Butler proposed that memories, conversations, and reflections about the past can be helpful, not only for maintaining mental health but also for enhancing one's capacity to address current problems [31]. There are more than a hundred clinical trials showing that reminiscence as therapy is an effective intervention for depression, life satisfaction, and quality of life in older adults [32,33], including for aged care residents [34–37]. Reminiscence therapy has been delivered in 1 of 3 ways to older adults: simple reminiscence, life review, and life review therapy [38].

Simple reminiscence aims to improve aged care residents' feelings of enjoyment and connection with others. The resident is encouraged to talk about memories that are "light-hearted" or that allow for a joint discussion about shared experiences (eg, client and clinician talk about the "old days"). Music, photographs, and sensory experiences (eg, smells) are sometimes used to prompt memories and discussion [39]. In RACFs, simple reminiscence has been conducted one-on-one [40] or in groups where participants are asked to share personal memories relating to particular topics, developmental stages, music, or memorabilia. An example of group-based simple reminiscence is where participants are asked to reflect on memories related to festivals, daily routines (eg, walking to school), or important family occasions (eg, birth of a child) [36]. The primary aim of simple reminiscence in such groups is to assist individuals to engage more deeply with other group members, gain a sense of belonging in a community, and enjoy telling stories about the past.

Life review involves a more elaborate discussion about residents' past experiences, with a view to understand the residents' values, pivotal experiences, and identity. In such an approach, clients are prompted to review the significance of their positive and negative experiences and to consolidate these into a coherent narrative about their lives. Life review is more structured than simple reminiscence in that it guides the resident to answer a series of questions about various stages of life (eg, childhood, adolescence, adulthood) in chronologic order [41]. Life review can help the resident arrive at insights into how they developed throughout their lives, to clarify the meaning of life, and to identify their values and personal identity, as reflected by past experiences.

Karimi and colleagues [42] conducted an RCT to evaluate the effectiveness of integrative reminiscence (life review), instrumental reminiscence (life review therapy), and social discussion (control) for reducing depressive symptoms. The reminiscence and social discussion activities were conducted in a group format comprising 6 weekly 90-minute sessions. The sample comprised 29 aged care residents (59% women; age mean 70.5 years, range 64–87 years) with depressive symptoms (scored 5 or higher on the Iranian version of the Geriatric Depressive Scale-15 [43]) and intact cognitive functioning (scored 21 or higher on the Iranian version of the MMSE [44]). The participants were also physically well enough to participate in the study. There was no statistical difference in the severity of post-treatment depressive symptoms between the 2 reminiscence groups. However, participants in the life review group were significantly less depressed at postintervention than participants attending social discussion meetings.

Life review therapy focuses the resident's attention on specific positive memories. The goal of this intervention is to help residents construct a sense of self as efficacious and resourceful. In this form of reminiscence therapy, individuals are encouraged to reflect on past problem-solving successes and challenges, with the aim of emphasizing their agency and resilience. In a large systematic review of 128 studies on reminiscence, Pinquart and Forstmeier [37] observed that life review therapy was more effective than the other forms of reminiscence therapy in addressing symptoms of depression and positive well-being. However, life review therapy has not yet been widely researched in RACFs. Karimi and colleagues found that when applied in group format with a small number of residents, as described earlier, life review therapy reduced depression symptoms but not to a greater extent than social discussion. Hence, more research is needed to examine the effectiveness of this form of reminiscence therapy in residential settings.

Intergenerational Programs

Intergenerational programs are defined as activities or services that foster cooperation, interaction, and exchange between 2 or more generations [45]. Such programs have become more valued and more common in community and residential settings [46]. Some programs focus on pairing preschool children (up to 5 years old) with aged care residents [47,48]. Others encourage sharing of experiences between school aged children and older adults collaborating on activities such as school subjects, gardening, music, craft, and storytelling [49]. There are also mentoring programs where older adults assist students with homework, reading, or math. Conversely, some programs involve students assisting older adults with digital literacy and the use of technology [45,46].

As shown through 2 large reviews on the impact of intergenerational programs, such programs can be associated with multiple benefits [45,46]. Intergenerational programs have the potential to motivate and energize older adults, provide them with a sense of meaning and purpose, reduce their feelings of stress and isolation, improve their self-reported health, increase enjoyment, generate new skills, and improve mood [45,46]. They can also help change stereotypes about age held by both younger and older participants by fostering greater understanding and strengthening relationships across age groups [49,50]. Such programs have also been found to improve effect in aged care residents with cognitive impairments [51].

Research on such programs has been criticized as being methodologically weak; some studies rely on anecdotal evidence [48,52]; others make limited use of standardized measures [53] or assess the impact on only the younger generation [54], whereas other studies fail to evaluate longer term outcomes [46]. Gualano and colleagues [46] rated 26 of the 27 studies in their review of intergenerational programs as having a high risk of bias due to poor study designs. Further, of 50 studies reviewed by Canedo-Garcia and colleagues [45], only one [55] investigated the impact of such programs on aged care residents, and, of 27 studies on the impact of such programs on older adults, reviewed by Gualano and colleagues [46], only 5 were in RACFs. More empirical research is needed to further investigate the impact of such programs in an RACF environment to add to the growing body of anecdotal evidence suggesting that such programs positively affect participants.

TECHNOLOGY-ASSISTED TREATMENTS

Innovative interventions using technologies have been introduced in RACFs. Technology has been used to facilitate engagement and social connections as well as to facilitate psychological treatments. Such technologies have included electronic documentation, clinical decision support systems, safety technologies (eg, monitoring systems), virtual reality, Internet and touchscreens, robotics, and video conferencing [56]. As an example, in reminiscence sessions with residents, we have found that technology and the Internet are valuable resources for prompting memories and for engaging residents to talk about their past. For example, we have used applications such as "google maps" to assist residents recollect past experiences and contexts (eg, where they lived) or have streamed music on a tablet to enrich reminiscence about early experiences [57].

Telehealth is emerging health care delivery mechanism into RACF, where psychological services are provided by telephone or video conferencing. Telehealth enables the delivery of speciality services to aged care residents who do not have easy access to such face-to-face psychological services. Because of the COVID-19 social distancing requirements, a range of clinical and psychosocial services have been delivered via telehealth to aged care residents [58]. A recent systematic review found that telehealth had a significant impact on health outcomes in community-based older adults: reduced emergency visits, hospital admissions, cognitive functioning, and depressive symptoms [59]. The feasibility, acceptability, and effectiveness of telehealth counseling services for individuals living in RACFs remain to be empirically researched.

DELIVERING PSYCHOLOGY SERVICES IN RESIDENTIAL AGED CARE SETTINGS

RACFs are structured around the management of chronic conditions and disabilities and have not attended sufficiently to the mental health and psychosocial needs of residents. Despite advances in adapting evidence-based treatments to accommodate older adults, there remains a dearth of evidence for how best to adapt such treatments to aged care residents, particularly when such adults are also living with major physical and cognitive difficulties. Over the last decade we have delivered and supervised thousands of hours of counseling within RACFs [60–63]. We offer 3 suggestions for delivering such interventions in these settings: focus on engagement as an early therapeutic goal, be creative in individualizing treatment, and adopt a systemic model of care.

Focus on Engagement as an Early Therapeutic Goal

The engagement process in RACFs may take longer than that experienced in outpatient settings. Residents do not typically self-refer but instead are usually referred by staff, a family member, or a medical practitioner. In our experience, many residents who are referred to psychological services do not readily identify as having specific problems or needing assistance. Hence, the initial focus of the clinician is on developing an effective therapeutic relationship with the resident. Normally, such rapport can be built by engaging the residents in normalized discussion (eg, while going for a walk), self-disclosure (ie, the clinician discloses information about self), and an authentic demonstration of interest in the resident as a person (eg, asking resident about the contents of a photograph hanging on a wall). We have also found it helpful for the clinician to be introduced to the resident by facility staff. Early sessions with the resident typically do not focus on pathology but rather on understanding the specific life circumstances of the resident. Goals and presenting problems can be unclear at this early stage of treatment. Such initial sessions may feel more like "friendly chats" rather than structured treatment sessions.

Be creative in Individualizing Treatment

Once therapeutic trust is established, customize treatment approaches to suit the residents' conceptualization, language, and abilities. The psychological conceptualization of an aged care resident reflects the clinician's understanding of the resident's problem/s, treatment goal/s, and factors that maintain the problem. Treatment can be considered a method for helping residents overcome obstacles to reach goals. Use language that is simple and aligned with the residents' understanding of mental state and preferred terminology. For example, a resident may prefer the term "Wobblies" instead of anxiety; they may refer to depression as "the blues." Tailor interventions to accommodate physical frailty and cognitive impairment. For clients who are frail and tire easily, treatment sessions are likely to be shorter. For residents with cognitive impairments, treatments are likely to involve strategies to compensate for memory and cognitive impairments (eg, using memory aids, involving others in the treatment and using simpler and more concrete strategies) [64]. For example, a resident with memory difficulties may benefit from a therapy book, handouts, or cue-cards, where key messages and strategies from each session are written down for the resident to review.

Adopt a Systemic Model of Care

Shift the therapeutic focus from an individual level to an organizational level. A systemic approach shifts the structure of treatment from a one-to-one model (clinician and resident) to one that also involves the resident's family and health care staff and specialists. Family members and staff can provide clinicians with background information about the resident or day-to-day updates. Family and staff can help residents practice treatment strategies between sessions (eg, deep breathing exercises). Clinicians can also support families by normalizing their responses, providing education, and facilitating communication between families and staff. Examples of such models of support are Quall's Caregiver Family Therapy [65], Gaugler's Residential Care Transition Module [66], and the Swinburne Wellbeing Clinic model [61].

SUMMARY

CBT and reminiscence therapy are evidence-based interventions for reducing symptoms of depression and anxiety in RACFs. Intergenerational programs and technology-assisted treatments are also commonly used, although more research is needed to establish their effectiveness in residential aged care settings. Mental health clinicians can collaborate with family and aged care staff to offer a systemic and tailored approach to older adults living in RACFs. Clinicians can play a significant role in supporting the mental health of such residents including those with cognitive impairments and physical comorbidities.

CLINICS CARE POINTS

- CBT and reminiscence therapy are evidence-based interventions for reducing symptoms of depression and anxiety in residential aged care settings.
- Intergenerational programs and technology-assisted treatments such as telehealth are emerging approaches that can also support the mental health of aged care residents.
- Clinicians should collaborate with residential care staff and families to offer a systemic and integrated approach to care to residents.

DISCLOSURE

The authors have nothing to disclose.

REFERENCES

[1] Encyclopedia of Aging. Long-Term Care Around the Globe. 2020. 2020. Available at: https://www.encyclopedia.com/education/encyclopedias-almanacs-transcripts-and-maps/long-term-care-around-globe. Accessed October 16, 2020.
[2] Australian institute of Health and Welfare. Aged care. 2019. Available at: https://www.aihw.gov.au/reports/australias-welfare/aged-care. Accessed September 7, 2020.
[3] Department of Health and Ageing. Technical paper on the changing dynamics of residential aged care. Canberra: Author; 2011. Available at: http://www.pc.gov.au/inquiries/completed/aged-care/residential-care-dynamics/residential-caredynamics.pdf.
[4] Stargatt J, Bhar SS, Davison TE, et al. The Availability of Psychological Services for Aged Care Residents in Australia: A Survey of Facility Staff. Aust Psychol 2017;52(6):406–13.
[5] Amare AT, Caughey GE, Whitehead C, et al. The prevalence, trends and determinants of mental health disorders in older Australians living in permanent residential aged care: Implications for policy and quality of aged care services. Aust N Z J Psychiatry 2020;54(12):1200–11.
[6] Matthews FE, Bennett H, Wittenberg R, et al. Who lives where and does it matter? Changes in the health profiles of older people living in long term care and the community over two decades in a high income country. PLoS One 2016;11(9):e0161705.
[7] Mezuk B, Rock A, Lohman MC, et al. Suicide risk in long-term care facilities: A systematic review. Int J Geriatr Psychiatry 2014;29(12):1198–211.
[8] Creighton AS, Davison TE, Kissane DW. The prevalence of anxiety among older adults in nursing homes and other res aged care facilities. Int J Geriatr Psychiatry 2016;31(6):555–66.
[9] Davison TE, McCabe MP, Busija L, et al. Trajectory and Predictors of Mental Health Symptoms and Wellbeing in Newly Admitted Nursing Home Residents. Clin Gerontol 2021;1–14.
[10] Anstey KJ, von Sanden C, Sargent-Cox K, et al. Prevalence and risk factors for depression in a longitudinal, population-based study including individuals in the community and residential care. Am J Geriatr Psychiatry 2007;15(6):497–505.
[11] Pot AM, Deeg DJH, Twisk JWR, et al. The longitudinal relationship between the use of long-term care and depressive symptoms in older adults. Gerontologist 2005;45(3):359–69.
[12] Fraher A, Coffey A. Older people's experiences of relocation to long-term care. Nurs Old People 2011;23(10):23–7.
[13] Lee DTF, Woo J, Mackenzie AE. A review of older people's experiences with residential care placement. J Adv Nurs 2002;37(1):19–27.
[14] Murphy B, Bugeja L, Pilgrim J, et al. Completed suicide among nursing home residents: A systematic review. Int J Geriatr Psychiatry 2015;30(8):802–14.
[15] Chan P, Bhar S, Davison TE, et al. Characteristics and effectiveness of cognitive behavioral therapy for older adults living in residential care: a systematic review. Aging Ment Health 2021;25(2):187–205.
[16] Wells Y, Bhar SS, Kinsella G, et al. What works to promote emotional wellbeing in older people. Melbourne: BeyondBlue; 2014.
[17] David D, Cristea I, Hofmann SG. Why Cognitive Behavioral Therapy Is the Current Gold Standard of Psychotherapy. Front Psychiatry 2018;9:4.
[18] Simning A, Simons KV. Treatment of depression in nursing home residents without significant cognitive impairment: a systematic review. Int Psychogeriatr 2017;29(2):209–26.
[19] Meeks S, Looney SW, Van Haitsma K, et al. BE-ACTIV: a staff-assisted behavioral intervention for depression in nursing homes. Gerontologist 2008;48(1):105–14.
[20] Luo H, Lou VWQ, Chen C, et al. The Effectiveness of the Positive Mood and Active Life Program on Reducing Depressive Symptoms in Long-Term Care Facilities. Gerontologist 2020;60(1):193–204.
[21] Meeks S, Haitsma KV, Schoenbachler B, et al. BE-ACTIV for depression in nursing homes: Primary outcomes of a randomized clinical trial. J Gerontol Ser B Psychol Sci Soc Sci 2015;70(1):13–23.
[22] Folstein MF, Folstein SE, McHugh PR. Mini-mental state: A practical method for grading the cognitive state of patients for the clinician. J Psychiatr Res 1975;12(3):189–98.
[23] Morris JN, Fries BE, Mehr DR, et al. MDS Cognitive Performance Scale. J Gerontol 1994;49(4):M174–82.
[24] Tombaugh TN, McIntyre NJ. The mini-mental state examination: a comprehensive review. J Am Geriatr Soc 1992;40(9):922–35.
[25] Sales A, Atiénzar AP, Mayordomo T, et al. Effects of cognitive behavioral therapy on depression in

institutionalized elderly. Rev Psicopatol Psicol Clin 2015;20(2):165–72.

[26] Abraham IL, Neundorfer MM, Currie LJ. Effects of group interventions on cognition and depression in nursing home residents. Nurs Res 1992;41(4):196–202.

[27] Zerhusen JD, Boyle K, Wilson W. Out of the darkness: group cognitive therapy for depressed elderly. J Psychosoc Nurs Ment Health Serv 1991;29(9):16–21.

[28] Shang P, Cao X, You S, et al. Problem-solving therapy for major depressive disorders in older adults: an updated systematic review and meta-analysis of randomized controlled trials. Aging Clin Exp Res 2021;33(6): 1465–75.

[29] Frost R, Bauernfreund Y, Walters K. Non-pharmacological interventions for depression/anxiety in older adults with physical comorbidities affecting functioning: systematic review and meta-analysis. Int Psychogeriatr 2019;31(8):1121–36.

[30] Reinhardt JP, Horowitz A, Cimarolli VR, et al. Addressing depression in a long-term care setting: A Phase II pilot of problem-solving treatment. Clin Ther 2014;36(11): 1531–7.

[31] Butler RN. Successful aging and the role of the life review. J Am Geriatr Soc 1974;22(12):529–35.

[32] Bhar SS. Reminiscence therapy: A review. In: Pachana NA, Laidlaw K, editors. Oxford handbook of geropsychology. Oxford: Oxford University Press; 2014. p. 675–90.

[33] Chin AM. Clinical Effects of Reminiscence Therapy in Older Adults: A Meta-Analysis of Controlled Trials. Hong Kong J Occup Ther 2007;17(1):10–22.

[34] Chiang K-J, Chu H, Chang H-J, et al. The effects of reminiscence therapy on psychological well-being, depression, and loneliness among the institutionalized aged. Int J Geriatr Psychiatry 2009;25(25):380–8.

[35] Thomas JM, Sezgin D. Effectiveness of reminiscence therapy in reducing agitation and depression and improving quality of life and cognition in long-term care residents with dementia: A systematic review and meta-analysis. Geriatr Nurs 2021;42(6):1497–506.

[36] Syed Elias SM, Neville C, Scott T. The effectiveness of group reminiscence therapy for loneliness, anxiety and depression in older adults in long-term care: A systematic review. Geriatr Nurs 2015;36(5):372–80.

[37] Pinquart M, Forstmeier S. Effects of reminiscence interventions on psychosocial outcomes: A meta-analysis. Aging Ment Health 2012;16(5):541–58.

[38] Webster J, Bohlmeijer ET, Westerhof GJ. Mapping the Future of Reminiscence: A Conceptual Guide for Research and Practice. Res Aging 2010;32(4):527–64.

[39] Fu SR, Lee MF, Ou SJ. Effects of reminiscing about nostalgic smells on the physiological and psychological responses of older people in long-term care facilities. Ageing Soc 2020;40(3):501–11.

[40] Van Bogaert P, Tolson D, Eerlingen R, et al. SolCos model-based individual reminiscence for older adults with mild to moderate dementia in nursing homes: a randomized controlled intervention study. J Psychiatr Ment Health Nurs 2016;23(9–10):568–75.

[41] Haight BK, Haight BS. The handbook of structured life review. Baltimore: Health Professions Press; 2007.

[42] Karimi H, Dolatshahee B, Momeni K, et al. Effectiveness of integrative and instrumental reminiscence therapies on depression symptoms reduction in institutionalized older adults: An empirical study. Aging Ment Health 2010;14(7):881–7.

[43] Malakouti K, Fathollahi P, Mirabzadeh A, et al. Validation of Geriatric Depression Scale (GDS-15) in Iran. Pejouhesh dar Pezeshki (Research Medicine) 2006;30(4): 361–9.

[44] Foroughan M, Jafari Z, Shirin Bayan P, et al. Validation of Mini- Mental State Examination (MMSE) in The Elderly Population of Tehran. Adv Cogn Sci 2008;10(2):29–37.

[45] Canedo-García A, García-Sánchez J-N, Pacheco-Sanz D-I. A Systematic Review of the Effectiveness of Intergenerational Programs. Front Psychol 2017;8:1882.

[46] Gualano MR, Voglino G, Bert F, et al. The impact of intergenerational programs on children and older adults: a review. Int Psychogeriatr 2018;30(4):451–68.

[47] Kennedy-Behr A, Rosso E, McMullen-Roach S, et al. Intergenerational Virtual Program: Promoting Meaningful Connections Across the Lifespan During the COVID-19 Pandemic. Front Public Health 2021;9:768778.

[48] Rosa Hernandez GB, Murray CM, Stanley M. An intergenerational playgroup in an Australian residential aged-care setting: A qualitative case study. Health Soc Care Community 2022;30(2):488–97.

[49] Santini S, Tombolesi V, Baschiera B, et al. Intergenerational Programs Involving Adolescents, Institutionalized Elderly, and Older Volunteers: Results from a Pilot Research-Action in Italy. Biomed Res Int 2018;2018: 4360305.

[50] Heyman JC, Gutheil IA, White-Ryan L. Preschool Children's Attitudes Toward Older Adults: Comparison of Intergenerational and Traditional Day Care. J Intergenerational Relationships 2011;9(4):435–44.

[51] Baker JR, Webster L, Lynn N, et al. Intergenerational Programs May Be Especially Engaging for Aged Care Residents with Cognitive Impairment: Findings from the Avondale Intergenerational Design Challenge. Am J Alzheimers Dis Other Demen 2017;32(4):213–21.

[52] Mantie-Kozlowski A, Smythe H. Introducing an intergenerational relationship to improve engagement in aphasia therapy. Aphasiology 2014;28(1):49–61.

[53] Gallagher P, Carey K. Connecting with the Well-Elderly Through Reminiscence: Analysis of Lived Experience. Educ Gerontol 2012;38(8):576–82.

[54] Boswell SS. Old People are Cranky": Helping Professional Trainees' Knowledge, Attitudes, Aging Anxiety, and Interest in Working with Older Adults. Educ Gerontol 2012;38(7):465–72.

[55] Skropeta CM, Colvin A, Sladen S. An evaluative study of the benefits of participating in intergenerational

playgroups in aged care for older people. BMC Geriatr 2014;14(1):109.

[56] Kim DE, Kim H, Hyun J, et al. Interventions using technologies for older adults in long-term care facilities: A systematic review. J Korean Acad Community Health Nurs 2018;29(2):170–83.

[57] Rehm IC, Musić S, Carlsson A, et al. Integrating Web-Based Applications into Aged Care: Two Case Studies and Discussion. J Clin Psychol Med Settings 2016;23(3):285–97.

[58] Seifert A, Batsis JA, Smith AC. Telemedicine in Long-Term Care Facilities During and Beyond COVID-19: Challenges Caused by the Digital Divide. Front Public Health 2020;8:601595.

[59] Harerimana B, Forchuk C, O'Regan T. The use of technology for mental healthcare delivery among older adults with depressive symptoms: A systematic literature review. Int J Ment Health Nurs 2019;28(3):657–70.

[60] Bhar S, Koder D, Jayaram H, et al. Innovative approaches for long term care. In: Reference module in neuroscience and biobehavioral psychology. Elsevier; 2021.

[61] Bhar S, Silver M, Campbell J, et al. Counselling older adults living in residential aged care settings: Four illustrative case studies. Aust Psychol 2015;50:141–7.

[62] Bhar SS, Silver M. Introduction of a university-based counselling service for older adults. Australas J Ageing 2014;33(1):36–42.

[63] Davison TE, McCabe MP, Busija L, et al. A cluster randomised trial of the program to enhance adjustment to residential living (PEARL): A novel psychological intervention to reduce depression in newly admitted aged care residents. BMC Geriatr 2020;20(1):98.

[64] Koder D-A. Treatment of Anxiety in the Cognitively Impaired Elderly: Can Cognitive-Behavior Therapy Help? Int Psychogeriatr 1998;10(02):173–82.

[65] Qualls SH, Williams A. Caregiver family therapy. Washington, DC: American Psychological Association; 2013.

[66] Gaugler JE, Statz TL, Birkeland RW, et al. The Residential-Care Transition Module: A single-blinded randomized controlled evaluation of a telehealth support intervention for family caregivers of persons with dementia living in residential long-term care. BMC Geriatr 2020;20(1): 133.

Advances in Psychiatry and Behavioral Health 2 (2022) 193–210

ADVANCES IN PSYCHIATRY AND BEHAVIORAL HEALTH

Advances in the Psychological Management of Older Adult Mental Health

Viviana M. Wuthrich, MPsych (Clin), PhD*, Jessamine T-H. Chen, MPsych (Clin), PhD, Diana Matovic, PhD

School of Psychological Sciences, Centre for Emotional Health, Centre for Ageing, Cognition & Wellbeing, Macquarie University, Sydney, New South Wales, 2109 Australia

KEYWORDS

• Geriatric • Anxiety • Depression • Cognitive behavioral therapy • Clinical psychology

KEY POINTS

- Untreated anxiety, depressive, and substance use disorders in older adults are associated with poor physical health, disability, mortality, increased costs of service use, and medications.
- Accurate assessment of geriatric depression, anxiety, and substance abuse requires understanding of the nuance differences in symptom presentation.
- Practitioners should not dismiss symptoms of depression and anxiety as a normal part of aging.
- Research and practitioners need to address lower referral rates of older adults for treatment of common mental disorders and lower access to evidence-based treatments.
- When minor adaptations to the presentation of therapy skills are used to accommodate any reductions in cognitive ability, older adults can still benefit from psychological interventions.

INTRODUCTION

This review outlines the key information needed for the psychological management of common mental disorders in older adults. As the world's population is aging and people are living longer, soon there will be more older people with mental disorders than ever before. The most common mental disorders in later life are unipolar mood disorders, anxiety disorders, and substance use disorders. In later life, some differences in the prevalence of these disorders occurs, as well as differences in the way in which the disorders present clinically; this requires some modification to the way in which symptoms are assessed and treated. However, there are more similarities than differences in the overall assessment and treatment techniques needed to work with this population, and so with minor upskilling, practitioners can be confident to manage common mental disorders in later life. The key is that practitioners do not dismiss symptoms as a normal part of aging and aggressively treat these symptoms as they would in younger age groups.

Prevalence of Common Mental Disorders

Epidemiologic studies vary considerably in their estimates of common mental disorders in older adults with differences associated with variations in the measurement scale used, geographic location, and setting (eg, community-dwelling vs aged care). See Table 1

*Corresponding author, *E-mail address:* Viviana.Wuthrich@mq.edu.au
Twitter: @VivianaWuthrich; @ChenJessamine

https://doi.org/10.1016/j.ypsc.2022.05.008

TABLE 1
Twelve-Month and Lifetime Prevalence Rates of Common Mental Disorders Across Countries

Time Period	Country	Mood Disorders (%)	Anxiety (%)	Substance Use (%)
12-mo	Europe (CIDI65+) [67]	13.7	17.2	8.9
	Europe (CIDI) [68]	4.9	11.6	—
	Australia (CIDI) [69]	2.4	4.1	0.7
Lifetime	Europe (CIDI65+) [67]	14.3	25.6	18.2
	Australia (CIDI) [69]	8.0	10.2	11.8
	USA (CIDI) [70]	11.9	15.3	6.3
	China [71]	9.8	3.7	5.6

Note: CIDI, Composite International Diagnostic Interview [72]; CIDI65+ CIDI geriatric adaptation [73]. China used a Structured Clinical Interview for DSM-IV instead of the CIDI.

for differences in lifetime and 12-month prevalence rates across samples. Overall, prevalence rates are generally lower than for younger populations, although prevalence rates are more similar to younger samples when geriatric adaptations of diagnostic interviews are used. A meta-analysis on North American and European older adult populations found that lifetime major depression had the highest prevalence estimate (16.52%), with current major depression (3.29%) also relatively highly prevalent [1]. Similarly, lifetime alcohol use disorders (11.71%) had one of the highest prevalence rates. However, current alcohol use disorders (0.96%) and current and lifetime drug use disorders (0.34% and 0.19%, respectively) had relatively low prevalence estimates. The most prevalent geriatric anxiety disorders were lifetime and current specific phobia (6.66% and 4.52%, respectively), lifetime and current generalized anxiety disorder (6.36% and 2.30% respectively), and lifetime and current social phobia (5.07% and 1.31%, respectively).

As in younger samples, geriatric mental disorders are often comorbid. For instance, 47.5% of older adults with major depressive disorder also have anxiety disorders, whereas 26.1% of those with geriatric anxiety disorders also have major depressive disorder [2]. High-risk older adult alcohol users (>7 drinks/wk and alcohol use and dependence symptoms) have a higher prevalence of major depression compared with moderate- and low-risk alcohol users (24.90%, 3.18% and 3.22%, respectively) and anxiety disorders (8.78%, 2.28% and 1.37% 5.91%, 1.24% and 0.87%, respectively) [3]. Social anxiety disorder and specific phobias are also commonly comorbid with substance abuse or dependence among older adults [4].

Risk Factors

The risk factors for depression, anxiety, and substance abuse in later life are similar to the risk factors in younger samples. A meta-analysis [5] indicated that psychological risk factors for depression and anxiety included personality traits (eg, external locus of control and neuroticism), dysfunctional coping strategies, and psychopathology. Similar risks are reported for substance use in late life [6]. Biological risk factors for anxiety include cognitive impairment, hypertension, chronic health conditions, poor self-perceived health, and functional limitations. Biological risk factors for depression included chronic diseases, vascular factors, health status, medicine use, self-perceived health, disability, and severe alcohol use or smoking [5]. Ageing-related and disease-related processes, including arteriosclerosis and inflammatory, endocrine, and immune changes, can compromise the integrity of frontostriatal pathways, the amygdala, and the hippocampus, thus increasing vulnerability to depression [7]. Further, increased risk of problematic drinking is associated with male gender, older age, Caucasian versus African American and Asian American races, less high school education [3], and more pain [8].

Prognosis

Evidence indicates untreated geriatric anxiety is associated with depression [9], cardiovascular disease, respiratory problems, disability [10], and health service use [11]. Outcomes associated with untreated depression include all-cause mortality, coronary heart disease, increased physical health problems, functional disability, and suicide [12]. Geriatric depression is also a risk factor for dementia, as is middle-aged (45–65 years) alcohol overuse [13]. In addition, high-risk drinking is correlated with lower self-rated physical health [3,14].

A systematic review of longitudinal trials tracking the naturalistic course of anxiety disorders found relapse rates of 39% to 52% for anxiety disorders over a 3- to 6-year follow-up, with large progression to comorbid anxiety-depression and pure depression [9]. Moreover, comorbid anxiety-depression resulted in poorer prognosis than anxiety or depression alone, with higher relapse rates [9]. A systematic review of depression in primary care and community sample found that about 1 in 3 older patients developed a chronic course of depression, and poorer prognosis was associated with older age, chronic illnesses, and functional limitations [15].

Relapse rates for anxiety disorders and mood disorders following treatment are relatively high. In pharmacotherapy trials for anxiety disorders, placebo was associated with 36% relapse compared with 16% for antidepressants. Interestingly, discontinuation of antidepressants in recovered patients was associated with depression with an odds ratio of 3.11 compared with continuing antidepressants [16]. Longitudinal studies (>3.5 years follow-up) of hospitalized (in patient) older depressed patients suggested 30% were nondepressed, 24% had relapsing course with recovery, 22% had residual symptoms, 11% were depressed, and the presence of a personality disorder was associated with a worse prognosis [17]. In addition, following short-term treatment of alcohol use disorder, having one versus no residual alcohol use disorder symptoms at 6 months (independent of alcohol use at 6 months) predicts a 1-year "slip," including exceeding a blood alcohol concentration of 0.05% on at least one occasion, heavy episodic drinking, and hazardous use [14].

Age-Related Emotion Regulation Changes

Emotion regulation skills improve in later life such that older adults have higher levels of positive affect, and this might be somewhat protective for the onset of mental disorders in later life. There is a large body of evidence including a meta-analysis of 100 studies [18] showing older adults experience more positive affect as they age, including evidence from longitudinal experience sampling studies. There are 2 major developmental theories that outline the reasons for increased positive affect with age (termed the "positivity effect"): the Socioemotional Selectivity Theory (SST [19]) and the Strength and Vulnerability Integration (SAVI [20]) model.

The SST [19] posits systematic changes in personal goals as a result of changes in perceived time horizons with age. That is, expansive goals such as learning new information or exploring unfamiliar social connections are hypothesized to be prioritized in younger adults when time is perceived as open-ended and there is the potential long-term payoff. In contrast, the SST suggests that in later life goals shift to present-focused emotion-related goals, as time horizons shrink with an increased sense of impending death, such that older adults prioritize balancing emotional states, increasing satisfaction and savoring, and increasing emotional meaning. This age-dependent motivational prioritization is thus likely to influence attention and memory processes in older adults that underpin mental disorders.

The SAVI model develops SST by theorizing that the positivity effect in aging is due to increased strengths in the frequency and successful use of cognitive skills and behaviors. These strategies serve to avoid or limit exposure to negative stimuli, resulting in age-related improvements in affective well-being. However, the SAVI model predicts that if older adults are unable to avoid or limit their exposure to negative stimuli (eg, bereavement, caregiving, financial stress), they should experience *more* negative affect and greater difficulties returning to homeostasis than younger adults due to age-related vulnerabilities related to reduced physiologic flexibility in the cardiovascular and neuroendocrine systems causing prolonged physiologic arousal in distressing situations. Thus, prolonged emotional distress is likely to induce or maintain mental disorders in older adults by superseding their usual ability to redirect attention, change the situation, or reappraise situations to reduce the impact of less chronic negative events.

Consistent with the SST and SAVI models, older adults attend to and remember positive information more than negative information [21], including in short-term memory, working memory, long-term memory, and autobiographical memory. Moreover, the positivity effect persists in the face of prolonged stressors such the COVID-19 pandemic, with several studies reporting greater well-being in older adults compared with younger adults [22,23]. The exact mechanism associated with this general finding of better emotion regulation are still not clear, but there is some evidence that older adults are better at avoiding negative stimuli and therefore reducing the onset of distress [24]. Although avoidance is generally seen as an unhelpful emotion regulation strategy, it may have a protective role in later life. Once distress is activated in older adults, there is some evidence that in nonclinical samples, older adults are better able to recover from distress. There is some suggestion that emotion regulation strategies of reappraisal and avoidance might be particularly relevant [25]. However, for older adults who do suffer a clinical mood or anxiety disorder, the evidence suggests that the apparent better emotional regulation strategies in their older nonclinical counterparts might be weaker.

CLINICAL ASSESSMENT

Diagnostic Issues

Several issues can complicate the recognition and diagnosis of geriatric anxiety, depression, and substance use disorders. These pertain to medical comorbidities, changes in the way that symptoms present, age stereotypes that serve to dismiss and normalize symptoms, and the lack of use of age-appropriate symptom measurement tools. In substance use, age-related physiologic changes increase the effects of alcohol and other substances, yet impacts on social and vocational roles may be less obvious.

Medical comorbidity

Comorbid medical illnesses can complicate the recognition of depression [26] and anxiety [27] in later life due to overlapping symptoms. Older adults, or indeed health professionals, may disproportionally attribute somatic symptoms of anxiety (eg, muscle tension and sleep difficulties) or symptoms of depression (eg, fatigue and decreased appetite) to physical illnesses when other symptoms of these psychological disorders are present. Common medical conditions in later life that have overlapping symptoms with depression and anxiety include cardiovascular disease, respiratory diseases, hypertension, endocrine disorders, and diabetes. Substance use effects can be attributed to health or other causes for instance, poor nutrition, blackouts, headaches, poor hygiene, falls, bruises, and burns [6].

Differences in symptom presentation

There is some evidence that symptom presentation for depression and anxiety differs in later life [28]. See Table 2 for examples of the clinical manifestations of mood and anxiety disorder presentation in later life. For instance, older adults with anxiety commonly report reduced symptoms of muscle tension, headaches, worrying, and irritability compared with younger adults [29]. Thematically, older adults' worries are less focused on interpersonal relationships and work relative to younger adults, instead older adults are more likely to report worry about their health, and the health and welfare of loved ones [30], which in the presence of comorbid health conditions can be dismissed as being a normal response to health challenges [31]. For instance, excessive checking of blood pressure and frequent calls to family to check on their welfare can indicate anxiety. Relative to younger adults, older adults with social anxiety endorse fear in a smaller range of social situations, as well as less distress and interference [28]. It has also been reported that older adults endorse fear of situations that are not included on typical measures of social anxiety at high rates, such as asking for favors/help, attending medical appointments, using technology in front of others, and socialising as a single person with couples [32]. In specific phobia, fear of animals seems to decrease with age, whereas situational fears (eg, fear of lifts/falls) or fear of inanimate stimuli increases with age [33].

When it comes to reporting symptoms of anxiety, previous investigations comparing symptoms across the lifespan have indicated that older adults most commonly use words such as "stressed," "tense," and "concerned" to describe their anxiety symptoms, whereas younger adults most commonly use "anxious," "worried," and "nervous" [28]. There is also evidence to suggest that older adults avoid common anxiety-provoking situations and stimuli is often normalized, such as when older adults refuse to drive outside their local area, go out at night, attend new social situations, and avoid crowded places [34]. In terms of depression, although both older and younger age groups commonly endorse sadness as a symptom of major depressive disorder, older adults are more likely than younger adults to describe their low mood as "flat" or "not feeling myself," which can be perceived to be less severe mood dysregulation, whereas younger adults most frequently described their mood as being down, unhappy, or unmotivated [28]. Anhedonia is also particularly common in older adult presentations, in which older adults report feeling unmotivated and find it difficult to get on with things they usually do, which might be tasks or jobs around the house or engaging in social activities or recreational pursuits once enjoyed. Older adults' withdrawal from activities is likely to indicate depressed mood, but due to comorbid health conditions, can make differential diagnosis difficult. Suicidal thinking and self-harm are relatively common in older adult samples, and there is evidence globally of higher suicide rates in older men [35], highlighting the importance of careful detection of, and management of, depressed mood and suicidal intent.

Collectively, these findings on age group differences suggest that older adults might endorse different

TABLE 2
Examples of Clinical Manifestations of Diagnostic Criteria for Mood and Anxiety Disorders in Later Life

Disorder Diagnostic Criteria	Examples of Clinical Manifestations
Mood Disorder	
Depressed mood	Feeling depressed, flat, down, "blah," "not myself," hopeless, helpless, or observation of depressed mood by others.
Diminished interest or pleasure	Lack of motivation, stopped engaging in normal activities that are within their physical capabilities, not going out, stopped engaging in hobbies, struggling to complete tasks around the home. May be observed by others.
Insomnia or hypersomnia	Difficulty falling asleep, staying asleep, or early morning waking. Excessive sleepiness, for example, frequent daytime napping.
Generalized Anxiety Disorder	
Excessive anxiety and worry (apprehensive expectation) about several events or activities (such as work or school performance).	Worry tends not to be about work or school performance, but instead are reported as "concerns" related to their health or the health of others, welfare of family, friends, children, grandchildren, overwhelmed by tasks or events, excessive need for control, overplanning for outings, difficulty making decisions.
Worry is difficult to control	Worry is difficult to control, disrupts sleep and activities. Attempts to control the worry include frequent reassurance seeking, calling to check on family regularly, frequent checking of health indicators more than clinically required (eg, blood pressure), avoiding making decisions, avoiding ambiguous or new situations.
Social Anxiety Disorder	
Marked fear or anxiety about one or more social situations in which the individual is exposed to possible scrutiny by others. For example, social interactions, being observed, and performing in front of others (eg, giving a speech). The individual fears they will act in a way or show anxiety symptoms that will be negatively evaluated.	Social situations typically include talking to authority figures such as doctors, being assertive with others, or expressing their opinion. Excessive concerns about appearance and grooming and judgment related to using walking, hearing or other aids, or new technology in front of others.
The social situations are avoided or endured with intense fear or anxiety.	Avoidance of social situations and social groups, for example, social citizen clubs, avoidance of volunteer roles due to concerns of being judged.
Specific Phobia	
Marked fear or anxiety about a specific object or situation	Fear of animals less common, fear of situations more common. Fear of falling onset (avoidance of unfamiliar or uneven terrain, even with no history of falling).

symptom profiles for anxiety and mood disorders and that they describe their anxiety and depression symptoms using terms that downplay the severity of the problem. Older adults' preference for words that are more general, less specific to anxiety or depression, and might be seen to be less severe might result in underdetection of excessive worry, anxiety, or depression. Although the symptoms of substance abuse are not different in older adults, they have also been found to be downplayed by older adults, misattributed to other causes, and dismissed by professionals and family members [6]. These symptom presentation differences have implications for the clinical assessment using clinical interviews and self-report symptoms measures.

Best practice assessment

A combination of clinical interviews and self-report measures of symptomatology that are tailored to older adults is likely to inform the most effective case conceptualization and treatment planning. Depending on the person's functioning, assessment might include informants such as spouses or adult children. Accurate assessment of geriatric depression, anxiety, and substance abuse requires understanding of the nuance differences in symptom presentation (as discussed earlier) so that symptoms are not dismissed as being due to health or age. Symptom measures should only be used if they have been validated in older samples, as findings indicate that the psychometric properties and factor structure of general symptom measures differ in older samples particularly in medical or aged care populations. For example, many commonly used depression measures contain items assessing somatic symptoms (eg, decreased appetite or sleeping disturbance), which by and large overlap with physical conditions typically observed in older adult populations. As such, high scores on these depression measures can result in an overestimation of symptom severity in older adults or misattributing these symptoms to physical illnesses. See Table 3 for list of recommended self-report measures validated in older samples.

CLINICAL MANAGEMENT

Efficacy and Effectiveness

Pharmacology and psychological interventions are effective for the management of depression and anxiety in older adults. Psychological interventions are the treatment of choice, with the strongest evidence for cognitive behavioral therapy (CBT). Meta-analyses and systematic reviews of randomized controlled trials have found that CBT is efficacious for treating late-life depression compared with treatment as usual or being on a waiting list, although treatment effects are weaker in studies that use an active control group and in studies of physically ill or cognitively impaired patients [36]. Findings from meta-analyses and systematic reviews of randomized controlled trials also suggest that CBT is effective at reducing anxiety symptoms compared with treatment as usual or being on a waiting list, although the treatment effect size is smaller when compared with active control (ie, other treatments such as pharmacotherapy, supportive psychotherapy, or counseling) [37].

Research also indicates that co-occurring anxiety and mood disorders can be treated simultaneously with psychological interventions (CBT, mindfulness) in older adults with moderate effect sizes; however, more research is needed [38]. Given comorbidity is common and associated with worse clinical outcomes [39], more high-quality clinical trials using validated outcome measures are needed that target the treatment of co-occurring anxiety and depressive disorders. Research on the treatment of substance use disorder in older adults is very limited [40]. However, the most evidence exists for the use of CBT to reduce substance use [41].

Cognitive Behavioral Therapy Strategies

Specific CBT elements for treating geriatric anxiety and depressive disorders vary by disorder across different treatment manuals but generally include psychoeducation, cognitive restructuring, and behavior change, with an emphasis on graded exposure to feared situations/activities and relaxation for anxious older patients and/or increasing regular pleasant activities and problem solving for depressed older patients. The same skills are used for the treatment of substance abuse. Following are some recommendations for clinicians when conducting CBT with older patients:

Psychoeducation should focus on fostering an understanding of causal and maintaining factors in late-life anxiety and depressive disorders, as well as treatment rationale and strategies to be implemented. It is important for patients to understand the maladaptive nature of avoidance in maintaining anxiety and withdrawal for maintaining low mood. Given the misconception among many older adults themselves that anxiety and depression are normal consequences of aging [42], clinicians should encourage older patients to recognizing symptoms of anxiety and depression in later life. Education on normative levels of drinking in later life are recommended to motivate behavior change in substance abuse.

TABLE 3
Self-Report Measures of Anxiety, Depression, and Substance Misuse in Older Adults

Anxiety Measures	Description	Items	Psychometric Properties	Language
Geriatric Anxiety Scale (GAS) [74]	The GAS assesses the frequency of anxiety symptoms using a four-point scale ranging from 0 (not at all) to 3 (all of the time). The time frame of the scale covers the past week.	30 items [74] 10 items [75] An adapted 10-item GAS-LTC [76] is specifically tailored for long-term care settings.	Excellent psychometric properties, including reliability, convergent validity, and unidimensionality, have been reported [75]	English, Chinese, German, Italian, Arabic, Persian, and Turkish.
Geriatric Anxiety Inventory (GAI) [77]	The GAI utilizes a simple dichotomous response format (agree/disagree) and minimizes inclusion of somatic complaints that are likely to overlap with medical conditions. The time frame of the scale covers the past week.	20 items [78] 5 items [78]	The GAI has shown good to excellent internal consistency in a sample of community-dwelling older adult participants. Divergent validity has been demonstrated in a clinical sample from the Geriatric Depression Scale but not in a nonclinical sample.	English, Chinese, Persian, Hindi, Indonesian (Bahasa), Korean, Malay, Thai, Czech, Dutch, Finnish, French (France and Canada), Greek, German, Italian, Norwegian, Polish, Portuguese, Slovak, Spanish, Swedish, and Turkish.
Worry Scale [79]	The Worry Scale assesses worry about problems in the areas of finances, health, and social conditions, on a 5-point scale ranging from never and rarely (1–2 times a month) to often (1–2 times per day) and much of the time (<2 times per day).	35 items [79]	Although adequate internal consistency has been demonstrated among older adults with generalized anxiety disorder and nonclinical samples, the subscale scores need to be interpreted with caution.	English

(continued on next page)

TABLE 3
(continued)

Anxiety Measures	Description	Items	Psychometric Properties	Language
Hospital Anxiety and Depression Scale (HADS) [80]	The HADS assess depression and anxiety symptoms. Items are rated on a 4-point severity scale. The HADS produces 2 scales, one for anxiety (HADS–A) and one for depression (HADS–D), differentiating the 2 states. Scores of greater than or equal to 11 on either scale indicate a definitive case. The HADS can be administered repeatedly without affecting validity, but at least 1 wk should elapse between administrations.	14 items: 7 depression items, 7 anxiety items	The 2 HADS subscales (anxiety and depression) have shown excellent internal consistencies (Cronbach's α value 0.82–0.83), and factor analysis confirmed a 2-factor structure.	English, French, German, Dutch, Italian, Spanish, Croatian, Chinese, and Arabic.
Depression Measures	**Description**	**Items**	**Psychometric Properties**	**Language**
Geriatric Depression Scale (GDS) [81]	The GDS assesses depressive symptoms in cognitively intact or mildly impaired adults aged 65 y and older. None of the scale items concerns somatic symptoms, thus avoiding the confusion of somatic symptoms with	30 items [81] 15 items [82] 5 items [83]	The validity and reliability of the GDS have been supported through both clinical practice and research. In a validation study comparing the Long and Short Forms of the GDS for self-rating of symptoms of depression, both	Available in 27 languages, including English, Chinese, Japanese, Korean, Hindi, Turkish, Greek, Italian, Portuguese, and Persian.

	physical disturbances that were common in the elderly. The dichotomous response format (Yes/No) is also easier for the elderly to select an answer. The time frame of the scale covers the past week.		were successful in differentiating depressed from nondepressed adults with a high correlation ($r = .84$, $P < .001$).	
Beck depression inventory-II (BDI-II) [84]	The BDI-II measures depression symptom severity in adults, with responses range from 0 to 3 representing ascending levels of severity. Some overlap with somatic symptom items (exercise caution).	21 items [84]	The BDI-II has shown good internal scale consistency of 0.86 and a test–retest reliability coefficient of 0.93 among older adults.	English, Chinese, Korean, Dutch, Finnish, Spanish, French (Canadian), German, Polish, Swedish, Arabic, and Turkish.
Center for Epidemiologic Studies-Depression (CES-D) [85]	The CESD measures symptoms associated with depression (eg, restless sleep, poor appetite, and feeling lonely). Response options range from 0 (Rarely or None of the Time) to 3 (Most or Almost All the Time). Scores range from 0 to 60, with high scores indicating greater depressive symptoms. Some overlap with somatic symptom items (exercise caution).	20 items [85] 11 items 10 items 8 items	The CES-D has shown high internal consistency in community and clinical populations (Cronbach's αs 0.85 –0.90) [85]; convergent validity with other commonly used measures of depressive experiences such as the Patient Health Questionnaire-9 ($r = 0.85$) and the BDI-II; and divergent validity.	English, Korean

(continued on next page)

TABLE 3
(continued)

Depression Measures	Description	Items	Psychometric Properties	Language
Hospital Anxiety and Depression Scale (HADS) [80]	As discussed earlier in anxiety section	As discussed earlier in anxiety section	As discussed earlier in anxiety section	As discussed earlier in anxiety section
Substance Abuse	**Description**	**Items**	**Psychometric Properties**	**Language**
The Alcohol Use Disorders Identification Test (AUDIT) [86]	The AUDIT assesses amount of alcohol consumption, frequency of alcohol use, alcohol dependency, and the consequences of alcohol abuse. The AUDIT can be administered through an interview or self-administered. A cut-off threshold of 5 was identified to indicate alcohol use disorder among older adults	10 items	Five items on the AUDIT: items 1 (frequency), 2 (amount), 4 (difficulty resisting urge to drink), 5 (impact of alcohol use), and 10 (concerns by others about alcohol use) are particularly sensitive and specific to alcohol use disorder among older adults and together have outperformed the full AUDIT.	English, Chinese, Turkish, Greek, Hindi, German, Dutch, Polish, Japanese, French, Portuguese, Spanish, Danish, Flemish, Bulgarian, Italian, Russian, and Nigerian dialects.
The Michigan Alcohol Screening Test-Geriatric Version (MAST-G) [87]	The MAST-G identifies drinking problems in older adults using a simple dichotomous response format (yes/no). 5 or more positive responses indicate problematic use	24 items	The original MAST has shown a sensitivity of 98% and a specificity of 95% for identifying alcohol abuse or dependence in a primary care sample.	English, Portuguese

The Comorbidity-Alcohol Risk Evaluation Tool (CARET) [88]	The CARET identifies older adults who are at risk because of the quantity and frequency of their alcohol consumption, presence of comorbid diseases, high-risk behaviors (eg, drinking and driving), and concomitant use of medications whose efficacy may be diminished or that may interact negatively with alcohol. The time frame of the scale covers the past 12 mo.	27 items	The CARET has demonstrated good face, content, and criterion validity with older adults [88].	English

Cognitive therapy: during cognitive therapy, a patient is guided to shift their maladaptive or unrealistic thoughts and beliefs in a particular adaptive way through verbal and written investigations. Integral to this process is the patient's ability to consider diverse ideas and response alternatives, as well as modifying thinking and behaviors to manage changing circumstances. Older adults with poorer cognitive flexibility may not find cognitive therapy as useful to alleviate emotional distress as those with better cognitive flexibility, but given sufficient practice and repetition, even older adults with poor flexibility still benefit from standardized CBT [43]. Maladaptive cognitions that maintain substance abuse can be targeted, and these often relate to beliefs that they cannot cope without the substance.

Behavioral therapy: clinicians should encourage depressed older adults to engage in pleasant event scheduling or behavioral activation early in therapy, as these skills have been associated with large effect size benefits in a range of populations including community-dwelling and medical settings [44]. In addition, problem-solving therapy has been well established as an effective intervention for depression in older adults [36,45]. Graded exposure is an effective core behavioral skill for anxiety treatment that involves gradually facing feared situations/activities in order to learn that the situations/activities are not as threatening and/or that fear is tolerable. Progressive muscle relaxation has also been demonstrated to be effective in reducing anxiety in patients with generalized anxiety disorder [46]. Problem solving, relaxation, and activity scheduling toward activities not associated with substance use are useful for the management of substance use disorders.

Modifications to CBT delivery: research indicates that very minor adaptations, if any, are needed to deliver CBT effectively to anxious or depressed older adults despite normal age-related changes in cognitive ability [43,47]. See Box 1 for suggested modifications to CBT delivery to increase acceptability for older patients.

Complications of Medical and Other Mental Comorbidities and Management

Physical and/or other mental health complications are prevalent in late life [26,27], thus presenting challenges to psychological interventions. However, with minor modifications CBT skills can be implemented within the functional boundaries of the individual [47]. Clinicians need to be aware of their biased assumptions and be wary of accepting health limitations as inevitable and that older patient's distress cannot be reduced. Instead, clinicians should consider working creatively with older adults and their specialists to generate solutions in response to health or physical limitations or to find ways to engage in socially and mentally stimulating activities given these challenges. As in the case for medical populations, CBT has great benefit in assisting patients to manage illness-related distress and reduce catastrophic or unhelpful thinking [31]. Emerging research also suggests that nonpharmacological interventions, such as adapted CBT, are likely to provide an effective method for managing co-occurring anxiety and depression among people with Parkinson disease [48].

Advances in Psychological Therapies

There is emerging evidence for a range of other psychological therapies for the treatment of depression and anxiety in older adults, as well as novel methods of delivering CBT skills to older adults. The evidence for acceptance and commitment therapy for the treatment of geriatric anxiety disorder [49] and mindfulness-based therapies [38,50] in community-dwelling older adults is developing. There is also emerging evidence for the efficacy of Internet-based interventions that utilize CBT techniques to treat anxiety [51] and depression in older samples [52]. Although not a therapy itself, there is also interest in utilizing stepped-care interventions in older adult populations that focus on delivering CBT interventions via self-help, telephone, and Internet approaches in early therapy steps, before therapies that require more direct therapist inputs are offered [53]. These developments promise to offer some exciting new options over the next few years.

Cognitive Decline

In later life normal age-related changes in cognition occur, most notably reductions in processing speed, memory, and cognitive flexibility [54]. These cognitive changes can be confronting to practitioners and perhaps have contributed to the attitudes that older adults are less likely to benefit from psychological interventions. As discussed earlier, there is now evidence to the contrary, particularly when minor adaptations to the presentation of therapy skills are used to accommodate any reductions in cognitive ability. More challenging is the onset of abnormal cognitive decline; this can make differential diagnosis challenging, as the onset of depressed mood or anxiety in later life can be a prodrome to cognitive decline [55], but it can also occur for the first time in later life or be an exacerbation of previous emotional vulnerabilities triggered by current stressors. Whether depression or anxiety occurs as part

BOX 1
Basic Modifications to Conducting Cognitive Behavioral Therapy with Older Adults

General recommendations:

- Focus on recent history and *current* maintaining factors.
- Cap "story telling" in treatment.
- Look out for well-established avoidance behaviors.
- Accept that some older adults might show slower orientation to CBT and idea of changing thoughts/behaviors.
- Focus on repetition of skills if rigidity and/or cognitive deficits are evident.
- Use simplified forms and handouts as needed.
- Presenting skills via multiple formats (visual and auditory).
- Emphasize that skill practice between therapy sessions is critical for skill generalization.
- Be flexible and accept approximations of change initially.
- Work toward extending the patient's functioning.

For telehealth sessions:

- Send patients copies of materials that they can read and work on separately during the sessions.
- Ask patients to sit at a table during the telehealth session so they can take relevant notes.
- Record sessions so that patient can review contents later.
- Check sound quality: adjust sound volume for older patients with hearing issues.
- Keep sessions short to reduce fatigue especially in frail or much older patients.

of cognitive decline or not, it is important that it is still identified and treated promptly. Untreated depression in the context of early cognitive decline has been associated with an increase in later cognitive decline [55]. There is evidence that older people with early cognitive decline and even moderate dementia can benefit from a range of psychological strategies to address depression and anxiety with large effect sizes reported for CBT and music-based therapies [56]. The most evidence is for behavior therapy strategies such as activity scheduling and problem solving [57].

CHALLENGES IN THE FIELD

Several issues affect the recognition and treatment of mental disorders in later life. These issues include lower referral rates of older adults for treatment of common mental disorders and lower access to evidence-based treatments, especially when in aged care or in the presence of cognitive impairment. Challenges also include the lack of research in this population in general, with many gaps in our knowledge about how to best assess and treat these conditions.

Reduced Access to Treatment

Although good treatments are available for this age group, older adults are referred to receive psychological treatment at the lowest rates in the population [58]. Referral rates for older adults with dementia and/or living in aged care is particularly poor. The reasons for the lower referral rates particularly for community-dwelling older adults are unknown, but there seem to be several contributing factors. Older adult samples experience similar barriers to care as other age groups, such as the cost of treatment, lack of access to mental health services [59], and difficulties with transportation [60]. Simple strategies such as providing in-home services, telehealth services, and self-help services can overcome some of these barriers. However, additional barriers seem to relate to attitudinal barriers about symptoms being normal, given older adults' age or health conditions. Evidence indicates that older people themselves are more likely to attribute symptoms to their health conditions or to getting older, as well as their practitioners [14]. A common example is when an older person reports lethargy and loss of motivation to engage in activities; this is often attributed to poor health or to slowing down in aging, when it can also be a sign of anhedonia, one of the 2 criterion A symptoms for a diagnosis of major depressive disorder. There is also evidence that older adults have lower perceived need for help for their mental disorders [59], and practitioners are less optimistic that depression and anxiety can be treated in older patients, especially in those with medical comorbidities [42]. Left unaddressed, negative clinician attitudes toward older patients may create a vicious cycle, that is, when older patients are seen as having a poorer prognosis and are viewed with more hesitation, there will be little interest in working with older age groups. From this perspective, clinicians will need to be further upskilled in not only understanding age-related differences in the presentation of anxiety and depression but also challenge their own stereotyped thinking about older adults' ability to benefit from evidence-based psychological interventions [61].

Contributing to the lack of treatment of common mental disorders in this age group is the lack of access to evidence-based treatments available. In particular, access to psychological interventions is particularly low, with medications primarily used to treat symptoms [9]. Barriers related to the lack of training of clinicians in the assessment and treatment of common mental disorders in later life have been well documented in many countries, and there have been numerous calls to increase course content on working with older adults into the training programs for clinicians across a range of disciplines [62]. The lack of specialized training and willingness to treat older adults with dementia is particularly striking. However, as discussed earlier in the assessment and treatment sections, most clinicians can be easily upskilled to work in this age group, as the adaptations needed to apply psychological strategies to community-dwelling older adults and to those in aged care are relatively minor [47,61].

Telehealth Psychological Interventions

Before the COVID-19 pandemic, few studies had evaluated the effectiveness of telehealth interventions in older adults, but there was emerging evidence that psychological interventions can be effective when delivered to older adult populations via the telephone [48,63], the Internet [51], and video conferencing [64]. One fortunate outcome of the COVID-19 outbreak is there has been a global shift to utilizing telehealth services for routine delivery of health services including in older adults. However, this sudden move to telehealth services has also been associated with challenges for health services, as some telehealth modalities are more easily adopted and integrated than others. In an examination of the use of telehealth services during the pandemic, Meuldijk and colleagues [65] found that older patients preferred telephone-delivered psychological services over video conferencing and preferred using a telephone landline rather than their mobile telephone. Some of the challenges with video conferencing were noted for older adults living in rural and remote communities in which Internet connections were unreliable and difficulty accessing compatible devices. A recent systematic review of 7 studies found that older adults with cognitive issues experienced several barriers related to conducting telehealth video sessions due to technical issues or natural decreases in focus/attention; however, despite the barriers, telehealth was a feasible approach [66]. Collectively, these findings indicate promising feasibility and efficacy of telehealth psychological interventions for reducing anxiety and depressive symptoms in older adults. However, further research is needed to identify and address barriers related to support needed for older adults in engaging with psychological interventions via telehealth, and clinicians need to be aware of these barriers and prepare for these barriers ahead of time.

DISCUSSION

As the world's population is aging, more older adults require management of common mental disorders in the near future. Although there are many gaps in our knowledge about how these disorders present in later life, especially in the oldest of the old, as well as the most efficient methods to treat symptoms, there is already clear evidence that depression, anxiety, and substance abuse can be managed effectively in this age group including for those older adults with health conditions and cognitive impairments. The major challenges to care relate to barriers with older adults' ability to access services, attitudes by patients and practitioners that depression and anxiety are normal in later life, and that older people are unable to benefit from psychological therapies and telehealth approaches. Significant inroads to these challenges can be made by simple upskilling of existing practitioners, ensuring training programs include components related to older adult mental health, as well as taking care to ensure all older people are offered the opportunity to receive appropriate treatment.

SUMMARY

Older adult mental health has been largely neglected. However, recent advances have shown that common mental disorders can be readily identified and treated with similar effectiveness to younger age groups.

CLINICS CARE POINTS

- Practitioners should not dismiss symptoms of depression and anxiety as a normal part of aging. Instead, they should aggressively treat these symptoms as they would in younger age groups.
- Accurate assessment of geriatric depression, anxiety, and substance abuse requires understanding of the nuance differences in symptom presentation so that symptoms are not dismissed as being due to health or age. Symptom measures should only be used if they have been validated in older samples
- Pharmacology and psychological interventions are effective for the management of depression and anxiety in older adults. Psychological interventions are the treatment of choice, with the strongest evidence for cognitive behavioral therapy.
- When minor adaptations to the presentation of therapy skills (eg, simplified worksheets, repetition of skills) are used to accommodate any reductions in cognitive ability, older adults can still benefit from psychological interventions.
- Although further research is needed to identify and address barriers related to support needed for older adults in engaging with psychological interventions via telehealth, research findings indicate promising feasibility and efficacy of telehealth psychological interventions for reducing anxiety and depressive symptoms in older adults. Clinicians need to be aware of these barriers to engaging in telehealth and prepare for these barriers ahead of time.

DISCLOSURE

This research was funded by a Medical Research Future Fund Emerging Leadership II Fellowship to Viviana Wuthrich (APP1197846).

REFERENCES

[1] Volkert J, Schulz H, Härter M, et al. The prevalence of mental disorders in older people in Western countries – a meta-analysis. Ageing Res Rev 2013;12(1):339–53.

[2] Beekman AT, de Beurs E, van Balkom AJ, et al. Anxiety and depression in later life: Co-occurrence and communality of risk factors. Am J Psychiatry 2000;157(1): 89–95.

[3] Sacco P, Bucholz KK, Spitznagel EL. Alcohol use among older adults in the National Epidemiologic Survey on Alcohol and Related Conditions: a latent class analysis. J Stud Alcohol Drugs 2009;70(6):829–38.

[4] Chou KL. Social anxiety disorder in older adults: evidence from the National Epidemiologic Survey on alcohol and related conditions. J Affect Disord 2009; 119(1–3):76–83.

[5] Vink D, Aartsen MJ, Schoevers RA. Risk factors for anxiety and depression in the elderly: a review. J Affect Disord 2008;106(1–2):29–44.

[6] Kuerbis ALP, Sacco PPL, Blazer DGMDP, et al. Substance abuse among older adults. Clin Geriatr Med 2014;30(3): 629–54.

[7] Alexopoulos GS. Depression in the elderly. Lancet (London, England) 2005;365(9475):1961–70.

[8] Brennan PL, Schutte KK, Moos RH. Pain and use of alcohol to manage pain: prevalence and 3-year outcomes among older problem and non-problem drinkers. Addiction 2005;100(6):777–86.

[9] Sami MB, Nilforooshan R. The natural course of anxiety disorders in the elderly: a systematic review of longitudinal trials. Int Psychogeriatr 2015;27(7):1061–9.

[10] Wolitzky-Taylor KB, Castriotta N, Lenze EJ, et al. Anxiety disorders in older adults: a comprehensive review. Depress Anxiety 2010;27(2):190–211.

[11] de Beurs E, Beekman ATF, van Balkom AJLM, et al. Consequences of anxiety in older persons: its effect on disability, well-being and use of health services. Psychol Med 1999;29(3):583–93.

[12] Pickett YR, Bazelais KN, Bruce ML. Late-life depression in older African Americans: a comprehensive review of epidemiological and clinical data. Int J Geriatr Psychiatry 2013;28(9):903–13.

[13] Livingston G, Huntley J, Sommerlad A, et al. Dementia prevention, intervention, and care: 2020 report of the Lancet Commission. Lancet 2020;396(10248): 413–46.

[14] Behrendt S, Kuerbis A, Braun-Michl B, et al. Residual alcohol use disorder symptoms after treatment predict long-term drinking outcomes in seniors with DSM-5 alcohol use disorder. Alcohol Clin Exp Res 2021; 45(11):2396–405.

[15] Licht-Strunk E, van der Windt DAWM, van Marwijk HWJ, et al. The prognosis of depression in older patients in general practice and the community. a systematic review. Fam Pract 2007;24(2):168–80.

[16] Batelaan NM, Bosman RC, Muntingh A, et al. Risk of relapse after antidepressant discontinuation in anxiety disorders, obsessive-compulsive disorder, and post-traumatic stress disorder: systematic review and meta-analysis of relapse prevention trials. BMJ 2017;358: j3927.

[17] Stek ML, Van Exel E, Van Tilburg W, et al. The prognosis of depression in old age: outcome six to eight years after clinical treatment. Aging Ment Health 2002;6(3):282–5.

[18] Reed AE, Chan L, Mikels JA. Meta-analysis of the age-related positivity effect: age differences in preferences for positive over negative information. Psychol Aging 2014;29(1):1–15.

[19] Carstensen LL. Evidence for a life-span theory of socioemotional selectivity. Curr Dir Psychol Sci 1995;4(5): 151–6.

[20] Charles ST. Strength and vulnerability integration: a model of emotional well-being across adulthood. Psychol Bull 2010;136(6):1068–91.
[21] Carstensen LL, DeLiema M. The positivity effect: a negativity bias in youth fades with age. Curr Opin Behav Sci 2018;19:7–12.
[22] Carstensen LL, Shavit YZ, Barnes J T. Age Advantages in Emotional Experience Persist Even Under Threat From the COVID-19 Pandemic. Psychol Sci 2020;31(11):1374–85.
[23] Strutt PA, Johnco CJ, Chen J, et al. Stress and coping in older Australians during COVID-19: Health, service utilization, grandparenting, and technology use. Clin Gerontol 2022;45(1):106–19.
[24] Reed AE, Carstensen LL. The theory behind the age-related positivity effect. Front Psychol 2012;3:339.
[25] Mather M. The emotion paradox in the aging brain. Ann N Y Acad Sci 2012;1251(1):33–49.
[26] Krishnan KR, Delong M, Kraemer H, et al. Comorbidity of depression with other medical diseases in the elderly. Biol Psychiatry 2002;52(6):559–88.
[27] Yohannes AM, Willgoss TG, Baldwin RC, et al. Depression and anxiety in chronic heart failure and chronic obstructive pulmonary disease: prevalence, relevance, clinical implications and management principles. Int J Geriatr Psychiatry 2010;25(12):1209–21.
[28] Wuthrich VM, Johnco CJ, Wetherell JL. Differences in anxiety and depression symptoms: comparison between older and younger clinical samples. Int Psychogeriatr 2015;27(9):1523–32.
[29] Christensen H, Jorm AF, Mackinnon AJ, et al. Age differences in depression and anxiety symptoms: a structural equation modelling analysis of data from a general population sample. Psychol Med 1999;29(2):325–39.
[30] Gonçalves DC, Byrne GJ. Who worries most? Worry prevalence and patterns across the lifespan. Int J Geriatr Psychiatry 2013;28(1):41–9.
[31] Read JR, Sharpe L, Burton AL, et al. Preventing depression in older people with multimorbidity: 24-month follow-up of a trial of internet-delivered cognitive behaviour therapy. Age Ageing 2021;50(6):2254–8.
[32] Ciliberti C, Gould C, Smith M, et al. A preliminary investigation of developmentally sensitive items for the assessment of social anxiety in late life. J Anxiety Disord 2011; 25(5):686–9.
[33] Fredrikson M, Annas P, Fischer H, et al. Gender and age differences in the prevalence of specific fears and phobias. Behav Res Ther 1996;34(1):33–9.
[34] Mohlman J, Bryant C, Lenze EJ, et al. Improving recognition of late life anxiety disorders in Diagnostic and Statistical Manual of Mental Disorders, Fifth Edition: observations and recommendations of the Advisory Committee to the Lifespan Disorders Work Group. Int J Geriatr Psychiatry 2012;27(6):549–56.
[35] De Leo DDB, Krysinska K. Suicidal elderly people in clinical and community settings Risk factors, treatment, and suicide prevention. In: Wasserman DWC, editor. Oxford textbook of suicidology and suicide prevention. a global perspective. Oxford: Oxford University Press; 2009. p. 703–19.
[36] Cuijpers P, Karyotaki E, Pot AM, et al. Managing depression in older age: psychological interventions. Maturitas 2014;79(2):160–9.
[37] Gould RL, Coulson MC, Howard RJ. Efficacy of cognitive behavioral therapy for anxiety disorders in older people: a meta-analysis and meta-regression of randomized controlled trials. J Am Geriatr Soc 2012;60:218–29.
[38] Wuthrich VM, Meuldijk D, Jagiello T, et al. Efficacy and effectiveness of psychological interventions on co-occurring mood and anxiety disorders in older adults: a systematic review and meta-analysis. Int J Geriatr Psychiatry 2021;36(6):858–72.
[39] Prina AM, Ferri CP, Guerra M, et al. Co-occurrence of anxiety and depression amongst older adults in low- and middle-income countries: findings from the 10/66 study. Psychol Med 2011;41(10):2047–56.
[40] Kuerbis A, Sacco P. A review of existing treatments for substance abuse among the elderly and recommendations for future directions. Subst Abuse 2013;7:13–37.
[41] Schonfeld L, Dupree LW, Dickson-Euhrmann E, et al. Cognitive-behavioral treatment of older veterans with substance abuse problems. J Geriatr Psychiatry Neurol 2000;13(3):124–9.
[42] Wuthrich VM, Frei J. Barriers to treatment for older adults seeking psychological therapy. Int Psychogeriatr 2015; 27(7):1227–36.
[43] Johnco C, Wuthrich VM, Rapee RM. The influence of cognitive flexibility on treatment outcome and cognitive restructuring skill acquisition during cognitive behavioural treatment for anxiety and depression in older adults: Results of a pilot study. Behav Res Ther 2014;57:55–64.
[44] Orgeta V, Brede J, Livingston G. Behavioural activation for depression in older people: systematic review and meta-analysis. Br J Psychiatry 2017;211(5):274–9.
[45] Arean P, Hegel M, Vannoy S, et al. Effectiveness of problem-solving therapy for older, primary care patients with depression: results from the IMPACT project. Gerontologist 2008;48(3):311–23.
[46] Thorp SR, Ayers CR, Nuevo R, et al. Meta-analysis comparing different behavioral treatments for late-life anxiety. Am J Geriatr Psychiatry 2009;17(2):105–15.
[47] Wuthrich VM. Cognitive behavioral therapy for anxiety in cognitively intact older adults. J Cogn Psychother 2017;31(1):57–71.
[48] Wuthrich VM, Rapee RM. Telephone-delivered cognitive behavioural therapy for treating symptoms of anxiety and depression in parkinson's disease: a pilot trial. Clin Gerontol 2019;42(4):444–53.
[49] Gould RL, Wetherell JL, Kimona K, et al. Acceptance and commitment therapy for late-life treatment-resistant generalised anxiety disorder: a feasibility study. Age Ageing 2021;50(5):1751–61.
[50] Reangsing C, Rittiwong T, Schneider JK. Effects of mindfulness meditation interventions on depression in older adults: A meta-analysis. Aging Ment Health 2021;25(7):1181–90.

[51] Dear BF, Zou JB, Ali S, et al. Clinical and cost-effectiveness of therapist-guided internet-delivered cognitive behavior therapy for older adults with symptoms of anxiety: a randomized controlled trial. Behav Ther 2015; 46(2):206–17.
[52] Titov N, Fogliati VJ, Staples LG, et al. Treating anxiety and depression in older adults: randomised controlled trial comparing guided v. self-guided internet-delivered cognitive-behavioural therapy. BJPsych Open 2016; 2(1):50–8.
[53] Meuldijk D, Wuthrich VM, Rapee RM, et al. Translating evidence-based psychological interventions for older adults with depression and anxiety into public and private mental health settings using a stepped care framework: Study protocol. Contemp Clin Trials 2021;104: 106360.
[54] Christensen H. What cognitive changes can be expected with normal ageing? Aust N Z J Psychiatry 2001;35(6): 768–75.
[55] Potter GG, Steffens DC. Contribution of depression to cognitive impairment and dementia in older adults. Neurologist 2007;13(3):105–17.
[56] Kishita N, Backhouse T, Mioshi E. Nonpharmacological interventions to improve depression, anxiety, and quality of life (QoL) in people with dementia: an overview of systematic reviews. J Geriatr Psychiatry Neurol 2020; 33(1):28–41.
[57] Chan P, Bhar S, Davison TE, et al. Characteristics and effectiveness of cognitive behavioral therapy for older adults living in residential care: a systematic review. Aging Ment Health 2021;25(2):187–205.
[58] Prina AM, Marioni RE, Hammond GC, et al. Improving access to psychological therapies and older people: findings from the Eastern Region. Behav Res Ther 2014; 56(100):75–81.
[59] Robb C, Haley WE, Becker MA, et al. Attitudes towards mental health care in younger and older adults: Similarities and differences. Aging Ment Health 2003;7(2):142–52.
[60] Pepin R, Segal DL, Coolidge FL. Intrinsic and extrinsic barriers to mental health care among community-dwelling younger and older adults. Aging Ment Health 2009;13(5):769–77.
[61] Wuthrich VM. Changing our thinking about changing their thinking in older adulthood. Int Psychogeriatr 2017;29(9):1405–7.
[62] Pachana NA. Special issue on training in psychogeriatrics. Int Psychogeriatr 2010;22(6):851–3.
[63] Brenes GA, Miller ME, Williamson JD, et al. A randomized controlled trial of telephone-delivered cognitive-behavioral therapy for late-life anxiety disorders. Am J Geriatr Psychiatry 2012;20(8):707–16.
[64] Gould CE, Kok BC, Ma VK, et al. Video-delivered relaxation intervention reduces late-life anxiety: a pilot randomized controlled trial. Am J Geriatr Psychiatry 2019; 27(5):514–25.
[65] Meuldijk D, Wuthrich VM, Johnco J, et al. Telehealth in older adult mental healthcare: A key weapon in the fight against the COVID 19 pandemic. Int Psychiatr Assoc Bull 2020;(August):13–7.
[66] Elbaz S, Cinalioglu K, Sekhon K, et al. A systematic review of telemedicine for older adults with dementia during COVID-19: an alternative to in-person health services? Front Neurol 2021;12:761965.
[67] Andreas S, Schulz H, Volkert J, et al. Prevalence of mental disorders in elderly people: The European MentDis_ICF65+ study. Br J Psychiatry 2017;210(2):125–31.
[68] Byers AL, Yaffe K, Covinsky KE, et al. High occurrence of mood and anxiety disorders among older adults: the national comorbidity survey replication. Arch Gen Psychiatry 2010;67(5):489–96.
[69] Sunderland M, Anderson TM, Sachdev PS, et al. Lifetime and current prevalence of common DSM-IV mental disorders, their demographic correlates, and association with service utilisation and disability in older Australian adults. The Aust New Zealand J Psychiatry 2015;49(2): 145–55.
[70] Kessler RC, Berglund P, Demler O, et al. Lifetime prevalence and age-of-onset distributions of DSM-IV disorders in the National comorbidity survey replication. Arch Gen Psychiatry 2005;62(6):593–602.
[71] Xu G, Chen G, Zhou Q, et al. Prevalence of mental disorders among older chinese people in Tianjin city. Can J Psychiatry 2017;62(11):778–86.
[72] Kessler RC, Ustün TB. The world mental health (WMH) survey initiative version of the world health organization (WHO) composite international diagnostic interview (CIDI). Int J Methods Psychiatr Res 2004;13(2):93–121.
[73] Wittchen HU, Strehle J, Gerschler A, et al. Measuring symptoms and diagnosing mental disorders in the elderly community: the test-retest reliability of the CIDI65. Int J Methods Psychiatr Res 2015;24(2):116–29.
[74] Segal DL, June A, Coolidge FL, et al. Development and initial validation of a self-report assessment tool for anxiety among older adults: the Geriatric Anxiety Scale. J Anxiety Disord 2010;24(7):709–14.
[75] Mueller AE, Segal DL, Gavett B, et al. Geriatric Anxiety Scale: item response theory analysis, differential item functioning, and creation of a ten-item short form (GAS-10). Int Psychogeriatrics 2015;27(7):1099–111.
[76] Pifer MA, Segal DL. Geriatric anxiety scale: development and preliminary validation of a long-term care anxiety assessment measure. Clin Gerontologist 2020;43(3): 295–307.
[77] Pachana NA, Byrne GJ, Siddle H, et al. Development and validation of the Geriatric Anxiety Inventory. Int Psychogeriatrics 2007;19(1):103–14.
[78] Byrne GJ, Pachana NA. Development and validation of a short form of the Geriatric Anxiety Inventory–the GAI-SF. Int Psychogeriatr 2011;23(1):125–31.
[79] Wisocki PA, Handen B, Morse CK. The Worry Scale as a measure of anxiety among homebound and community active elderly. Behav Therapist 1986;9(5):91–5.
[80] Zigmond AS, Snaith RP. The hospital anxiety and depression scale. Acta Psychiatrica Scand 1983;67(6):361–70.

[81] Yesavage JA, Brink TL, Rose TL, et al. Development and validation of a geriatric depression screening scale: a preliminary report. J Psychiatr Res 1983; 17(1):37–49.

[82] Sheikh J. Geriatric depression scale (GDS): recent evidence and development of a shorter version. Clin Gerontologist 1986;5:165–73.

[83] Hoyl MT, Alessi CA, Harker JO, et al. Development and testing of a five-item version of the geriatric depression scale. J Am Geriatr Soc 1999;47(7):873–8.

[84] Beck AT, Steer RA, Brown GK. Manual for the beck depression inventory-II. San Antonio, TX: Psychological Corporation; 1996.

[85] Radloff LS. The CES-D scale: a self-report depression scale for research in the general population. Appl Psychol Meas 1977;1(3):385–401.

[86] Saunders JB, Aasland OG, Babor TF, et al. Development of the alcohol use disorders identification test (AUDIT): WHO collaborative project on early detection of persons with harmful alcohol consumption–II. Addiction (Abingdon, England) 1993;88(6):791–804.

[87] Blow FC, Brower KJ, Schulenberg JE, et al. The Michigan alcoholism screening test-geriatric version (MAST-G): a new elderly-specific screening instrument. Alcohol Clin Exp Res 1992;16:372.

[88] Moore AA, Beck JC, Babor TF, et al. Beyond alcoholism: identifying older, at-risk drinkers in primary care. J Stud Alcohol 2002;63(3):316–24.

Education and Clinical Practice

Advances in Psychiatry and Behavioral Health 2 (2022) 211–219

ADVANCES IN PSYCHIATRY AND BEHAVIORAL HEALTH

Training and Education Related to Suicide Prevention

Zheala Qayyum, MD, MMSc[a,*], Samantha M. Taylor, MD[b], Marguerite Reid Schneider, MD, PhD[b]

[a]Child & Adolescent Psychiatry Fellowship Program, Department of Psychiatry and Behavioral Sciences, Boston Children's Hospital, Harvard Medical School, 300 Longwood Avenue, Hunnewell Administrative Offices – Mailstop 3022, Boston, MA 02115, USA; [b]Department of Psychiatry and Behavioral Sciences, Boston Children's Hospital, Harvard Medical School, 300 Longwood Avenue, Hunnewell Administrative Offices – Mailstop 3022, Boston, MA 02115, USA

KEYWORDS

• Suicide • Prevention • Postvention • Education • Training • Screening • Assessment

KEY POINTS

- Appropriate training of clinicians around patient suicide includes education about suicide prevention, preparedness, and postvention.
- Suicide prevention training requires knowledge of core risk and protective factors associated with suicidality.
- Clinicians should know how to screen for suicidality using an age-appropriate evidence-based suicide-screening tool and how to complete a full suicide risk assessment in the event of a positive screen for suicidality.
- Clinicians should be educated about triaging suicidality risk and direct individuals to the most appropriate next level of supportive medical care along with completing an evidence-based suicide safety plan.
- The experience of losing a patient to suicide can have a profound effect on clinicians, and it is essential that institutions develop comprehensive programming for responding to patient suicide.

INTRODUCTION

Suicide is a large and growing public health issue in the United States and around the world. In recent decades, the problem has become increasingly urgent, as the total age-adjusted suicide rate in the United States increased by approximately 32% between 1999 and 2019 [1]. In the United States, suicide is now the 10th leading cause of death overall [2], and the second leading cause of death for people ages 10 to 34 [3]. However, suicide deaths reveal only a small number of the people affected by suicidality. For example, a 2019 national survey in the United States found that while 1.8 million adults had attempted suicide in the past year, during that same period 3.5 million had made a suicidal plan, and a staggering 4.8% of adults, or 12 million people, had serious thoughts of suicide [4]. Recent data suggest that the situation has only worsened since the outset of the coronavirus disease 2019 (COVID-19) pandemic, as during the first months of the pandemic, hospital presentations for suicidality among children, adolescents, and adults, were significantly higher than prepandemic rates [5].

Suicide is often thought of as primarily a problem for mental health providers. While it is true that the vast majority of people that die by suicide have a psychiatric illness [6], a recent meta-analysis showed that only 25% of suicide decedents had contact with inpatient or outpatient mental health care in the year before their death [7]. However, those that die by suicide very often have contact with other components of the health care system in the period shortly before their death. According to a recent meta-analysis, 80% had interactions

*Corresponding author, *E-mail address:* Zheala.Qayyum@childrens.harvard.edu
Twitter: @ZhealaQayyum(Z.Q)

https://doi.org/10.1016/j.ypsc.2022.03.005
2667-3827/22/

with primary care in the year before their death, and 44% in the month before death [8]. Furthermore, a recent French study found that 60.9% of suicide deaths had contact with a physician or emergency room in the month before death [9]. Therefore, training and education related to suicide prevention are essential for all health care professionals regardless of specialty or practice environment.

Effective suicide prevention is multi-factorial. For health care professionals, a core awareness of risk and protective factors associated with suicidality is essential knowledge. However, suicide prevention education must also impart practical skills. Specifically, providers need to learn to use tools to allow them to screen patients for suicidality, perform further risk assessment in those that screen positive, and engage in treatment and safety planning for those found to be at acutely elevated risk. Beyond the role of health care professionals, other community members can also play a key role in suicide prevention and the identification of those at risk.

Another important topic to consider in education related to suicidality is the consequences for providers, survivors, and the community at-large following a death by suicide. Losing a patient to suicide can have profound effects on the personal and professional lives of the providers involved in the patient's care [10,11]. In addition to the profound effects that losing a patient to suicide can have on providers, suicide deaths can also have harmful effects on the community at large, including increasing the risk of other suicide deaths in the affected community [12]. Therefore, guidelines and educational programs for suicide prevention often include recommendations for actions to be taken to limit the negative consequences of a suicide death, also known as postvention [13].

In the following pages, we will identify core knowledge elements regarding risk and protective factors that are associated with suicide. We will then discuss validated suicidality screening tools, as well as tools for the more detailed assessment of risk, and for safety and treatment planning for those found to be at elevated risk. We will provide a summary of several training programs and educational resources that have been developed and studied in the field both for health care providers and for other members of the community. Finally, we will discuss community response and postvention following a death by suicide, including recent data on how providers, training programs, institutions, and communities can respond effectively to limit further adverse outcomes in the event of a suicide death.

CORE KNOWLEDGE: RISK AND PROTECTIVE FACTORS FOR SUICIDALITY

It is critical that those who seek to prevent suicide have familiarity with the risk and protective factors for suicidality and be able to recognize behaviors that are associated with increased risk for suicide. These areas represent the core knowledge that is a part of most suicide prevention education programs including training targeted toward nurses [14], pharmacists [15], and medical students [16]. However, recent review suggests that knowledge about suicide risk and prevention in various groups of health care workers varies widely [17].

Suicide affects American individuals of all demographics. However, certain populations within the United States do show higher rates of suicide compared with the general American population. These more vulnerable groups include veterans, people who live in rural areas, identified sexual and gender minorities, middle-age adults, and tribal populations [3]. The annual rate of suicide is approximately four times higher in men than women; however, the annual rate of nonfatal suicide attempts and suicidal ideation are comparable for men and women [4]. Common among all United States demographics are the 2 suicide methods with highest rates of death: firearms and suffocation [3]. In 2019, firearms were the most common method used in suicide deaths in the United States, accounting for a little more than half of all suicide deaths (50.3%) [3].

Nondemographic risk factors for suicide are multifactorial and are often grouped into modifiable and nonmodifiable categories. Some of these risk factors include prior suicide attempt, psychiatric illness, social isolation, legal problems, financial problems, job problems, serious illness, substance use disorder, adverse childhood experiences, bullying, family history of suicide, relationship problems, intimate partner violence, barriers to accessing health care, discordant cultural and religious beliefs, mental health stigma, easy access to lethal means. Important risk factors from a community perspective include suicide clustering and unsafe media portrayal of suicide [18–20].

Protective factors against suicide are also complex. Some of these protective factors include supportive medical and psychiatric health care providers in the community, good medication compliance, developed coping and problem-solving skills, cultural or religious beliefs which discourage suicide, supportive relationships (friends, family, and community), access to available medical and psychiatric care, and limited access to lethal means [18,19].

Fortunately, a recent review concluded suicide prevention training for health care providers is effective; both face-to-face and digital training modules of varying length and content were associated with improvement in knowledge outcomes, although a poster campaign was not successful [17]. Importantly, improving knowledge about topics related to suicide tends to increase both providers' willingness to care for patients with suicide risk and their confidence in their ability to do so [21]. Awareness of risk and protective factors varies widely in the community, but the 2021 *Surgeon General's Call to Action to Implement the National Strategy for Suicide Prevention* (2021 Call to Action) encourages broad awareness of warning signs and risk and protective factors among all community members [22].

IDENTIFYING THOSE AT HIGHEST RISK: SUICIDE SCREENING

Suicide screening is an essential component of suicide prevention. Most individuals with suicidal ideation are willing to disclose it if asked. A 2020 Harris Poll found that 73% of Americans said they would disclose suicidal thoughts if they were directly asked about having them. However, whom they would tell varied, with most people stating they would tell either a mental health provider, family member, spouse, or friend [23]. Effective suicide screening is now a mandated part of behavioral health treatment. Effective July 2019, the Joint Commission set forth new suicide screening and risk assessment standards to reduce suicide risk. Patient Safety Goal 15.01.01 mandates the screening of all behavioral health patients for suicidal ideation using an appropriate validated screening tool [24].

Several evidence-based, validated tools exist to screen individuals for suicidality. Perhaps the most generalizable of these is the triage version of the Columbia-Suicide Severity Rating Scale (C-SSRS) [25]. The C-SSRS 6-question triage screening tool is validated to be used for suicide risk assessment in both adults and children. Several versions of the tool have been developed for use across various clinical and nonclinical settings. Thus, the C-SSRS is largely accessible to individuals in the community interested in supporting suicide screening.

For children and adolescents, another evidence-based suicide screening tool is the Ask Suicide-Screening Questions (ASQ) screening questionnaire, a component of the ASQ Toolkit created by the National Institute of Mental Health [26]. The ASQ screening questionnaire is a 4-question suicide screener designed exclusively for health care providers to administer to youth aged 10 to 24 in emergency departments, inpatient units, or primary care facilities. The ASQ screening tool has both high sensitivity and high negative predictive value which demonstrates the strength of this tool in ruling in children and adolescents at risk for suicide.

The Patient Health Questionnaire-9 (PHQ-9) Depression Scale, particularly item 9, which has become largely incorporated into many health care systems, is an evidence-based screening tool for depression and suicidality in individuals aged 12 and older [27–29]. However, for children and adolescents younger than 12 years of age, the PHQ-9 is not sufficient alone for suicidality screening. The PHQ-9 is intended to be administered by health care providers in a medical setting.

Other validated, evidence-based suicide screening tools include the Suicide Behavior Questionnaire-Revised [30] and The Patient Safety Screener (PSS-3) [31].

FURTHER ASSESSMENT OF ACUTE RISK: TOOLS FOR FOLLOWING UP ON A POSITIVE SCREEN

While the implementation of screening protocols is an essential step, training and education must also include specific guidelines for the appropriate response in the event of a positive screen. Evidence suggests that provider confidence in this area is lower than confidence with screening. For example, in a recent survey of pediatric chief residents, more than 80% reported that they were at least somewhat comfortable conducting screening, and only 58% reported the same level of comfort with conducting a further risk assessment [32]. The lack of knowledge on how to respond in the event of a positive screen has been cited by providers as a reason for not deploying screening [33]. Indeed, even in programs whereby suicide screening was relatively well established, such as the Veterans Health Administration (VHA), a lack of knowledge regarding the next steps for patients screening positive in telehealth visits early in the COVID-19 pandemic led to decreased screening at some sites [34].

Several validated, evidence-based suicide risk assessment tools currently exist to help triage risk and guide disposition planning for those that screen positive for possible suicidality.

The most generalizable tool is the C-SSRS Risk Assessment tool which was designed for use by both health care and nonhealth care providers to assess adults and children of all ages. The C-SSRS Risk Assessment tool combines the C-SSRS triage questionnaire with a thoroughly outlined suicide risk assessment called the Colombia Protocol. The C-SSRS Risk Assessment tool was the first tool ever developed to assess the full range of suicidal ideation and behavior in individuals by evaluating suicidal ideation severity, ideation intensity, suicidal behavior, and suicide lethality. The C-SSRS Risk Assessment tool also comes with a checklist of suicide risk factors and protective factors which is intended to be used alongside the C-SSRS Risk Assessment tool for completeness.

Conveniently, the ASQ toolkit comes with a Brief Suicide Safety Assessment (BSSA), which providers are prompted to use if a patient screens positive for suicide risk on the ASQ. The BSSA is not a validated comprehensive suicide risk assessment tool. However, it is intended to help guide health care providers in further triaging suicide safety risks to help determine the appropriate disposition.

A second validated, evidence-based suicide risk assessment tool designed for health care providers is the Suicide Assessment Five-Step Evaluation and Triage (SAFE-T) pocket card developed by SAMHSA. The SAFE-T card incorporates the C-SSRS risk assessment questions into the SAFE-T card design and provides recommended triage categories for suicide risk on completion. Of note, the SAFE-T pocket card was intentionally designed for use only by health care providers who have been trained to work with those at risk for suicide. Thus, other nonhealth care providers should use the C-SSRS Risk Assessment tool.

Other validated suicide risk assessment tools included the Scale for Suicide Ideation—Worst and Beck Scale for Suicide Ideation [35].

INTERVENTIONS FOR SUICIDALITY

While many suicidal patients will require acute inpatient care for safety and stabilization, less acute suicidality can often be managed in the community. A key strategy that supports outpatient treatment of those that are found to be at elevated risk for suicide following screening and further assessment is the safety-planning type intervention. In this type of intervention, a provider works with the suicidal patient (as well as sometimes with their family and other supports) to create a predetermined strategy for coping with suicidal ideation, including identifying specific coping skills, sources of support, and plans for help-seeking if these are ineffective. One well-validated and structured example of safety-planning intervention is the Stanley-Brown Safety Plan Tool [36]. This type of intervention is recommended for patients who demonstrate suicidality by the Suicide Prevention Resource Center (www.sprc.org/.) A recent meta-analysis supports the effectiveness of this type of intervention: across 6 studies, the safety-planning intervention condition was associated with a 43% reduction in suicidal behavior, although there was some evidence of publication bias [37].

Another intervention that can be an essential part of safety planning is what's known as lethal means restriction, which involves preventing the suicidal individual from having access to potentially fatal means of ending their life, including firearms and potentially toxic substances. Lethal means restriction has been found to be effective at preventing suicide [38], and the reducing access to lethal means is often not associated with the substitution of other means of suicide [39]. Given the efficacy of lethal means restriction in the prevention of suicide, the 2021 Call to Action identifies ensuring lethal means safety as one of the 6 key actions to reduce the trend of increasing suicide deaths in the US [22].

Unfortunately, knowledge of these types of intervention is not universal among health care providers. For example, in a recent study more than half of pediatric chief residents reported that they had only some knowledge of how to construct a safety plan with a patient, and 44% reported being uncomfortable with counseling about means restriction [32]. Similarly, a survey of Canadian emergency physicians found that while 64% were confident regarding their skills for suicide screening, less than 1/3 had the same confidence about safety planning. Educational efforts targeted at improving awareness of these key interventions are critical to overall suicide prevention, as a lack of knowledge about the next steps or a lack of comfort with safety planning is often cited by providers as a reason not to conduct suicide screening or assessments.

POSTVENTION AND ITS ROLE IN PREVENTION

Impact of Suicide Death on Treating Clinicians

The death of a patient by suicide has been described as an occupational hazard and designated as "the *trauma* for the mental health professional" by Sudak and the "ultimate narcissistic injury" to the clinician by Gabbard [40]. Many clinicians including, psychiatrists, psychologists, social workers as well as nursing and other health care staff will experience the death of a patient due to suicide in their professional lives.

The suicide of a patient has significant implications in the professional lives of clinicians. Very commonly there is a jarring emotional impact on the clinician. These emotional responses can range from shock, sadness and grief reactions to guilt, shame, and anger [10,11]. Many clinicians also experience trauma- and stress-related responses after a patient suicide. These traumatic responses include avoidance, hypervigilance, intrusive thoughts, sleep disturbance, or nightmares [41,42]. Experienced clinicians may have lower rates of these trauma-related responses and changes in self-esteem compared with younger clinicians and trainees [10].

The suicide of a patient also impacts the professional identity and sense of competence of the clinician. Many clinicians feel a sense of responsibility for this adverse outcome or a sense of failure in carrying out their duty toward the patient. Clinicians can also experience the death of a patient by suicide as a blow to their sense of competence and their confidence in their clinical decision making. As a result, many find themselves tentative around patient care especially for high-risk patients in the immediate aftermath, spending a lot more time reviewing their clinical documentation and focusing on risk assessments [11].

Some trainees and clinicians find themselves subject to blame from others, doubting their effectiveness as clinicians or losing faith in the treatment process, at times even questioning if this was the right career choice for them. They also describe feeling judged by peers or feeling isolated in their grief because this adverse outcome happened to them and their patient, not other clinicians [11].

At times administrative processes such as formal peer reviews or mortality morbidity conferences can allow for an objective analysis of the care and treatment provided, but if not supportively conducted these can result in certain individuals feeling blamed. It is important to note that formal debriefing processes and meetings with risk management are analytically focused, whereas the clinical team responsible for the care of the patient who died by suicide experiences a deeply emotional response to the event, and the 2 may not be aligned [11].

Therefore, the suicide of a patient effect the clinician's relationships—with themselves, with other peers and supervisors, and with their subsequent patients. At times a conversation with the deceased patient's family can provide support and closure but there are instances whereby the family is grieving and angry, and this may be displaced onto the clinician which further complicates how this loss is experienced [11,41].

Many clinicians, especially trainees feel torn between the need to care for themselves and the obligation toward caring for their other patients. In high volume, high acuity practices or in places whereby there is a culture of stoicism, it may prove to be challenging for clinicians to take a moment for themselves to grieve or find appropriate supervision and support within which they can process this loss and what it means to them [11]. Hence these professional relationships with peers and supervisors are important for support during this challenging and vulnerable time.

Fear of litigation is a cause of great worry and distress for clinicians. Clinicians in medical institutions have access to risk management, patient relations, and legal services but clinicians in private practice must reach out to their malpractice carriers at a time when they are grieving and need time and space to process the event. Many clinicians are advised to refrain from contacting the family or discussing the case with anyone [11,41]. It is helpful for the clinicians to know their state laws pertaining to patient suicide and statute of limitations which is the prescribed period within which legal proceedings can be initiated. It is also important to note that even though the clinicians may be instructed not to discuss the details of the case, this does not preclude them from seeking out support to process their emotional response to the patient suicide which can at times be intense and devastating [43].

Legal procedures in the event of patient suicide both in inpatient and outpatient settings center around the issues of foreseeability and causation [44]. The experience of patient suicide for the clinician often involves the tension between the societal expectation that clinicians should be able to predict and prevent all suicide and realistically the ability to do so. Therefore, foreseeability relates more to assessing elevated levels of risk of suicide for the patient.

Common reasons for malpractice lawsuits usually pertain to concerns of negligence especially in failing to properly diagnose or assess the risk of suicide, or failure to take adequate protective measures to keep the patient safe. In the inpatient setting, this can relate to failing to commit the patient or negligent release of the patient from the inpatient setting [45]. Training clinicians in thorough risk assessments, comprehensive documentation, and thoughtfully consulting colleagues who have expertise in this area for high-risk patients is critical in building their confidence in caring for patients at risk for suicidality.

Postvention: response after a suicide death

Optimal training and education of clinicians around patient suicide should focus on prevention, enhancing preparedness, and postvention. However, only about

1 in 5 psychiatry residency-training programs have formal postvention and suicide response protocols in place [46]. These protocols should be more widely disseminated and adapted according to feasibility for each institution. Whatever form these protocols take, broadly they should aim to streamline the notification and communication process, support the clinical team and health care providers involved, and guide the clinician through the formal case review and risk management process [47].

Notification Process

Guidelines should delineate the chain of communication especially if trainees are involved. It is ideal that trainees hear from their supervisor directly and in-person as much as possible, so they have support and guidance available immediately. Other trainees, clinicians, and team members should also be notified once the primary team has been informed, while maintaining the confidentiality of the patient [47]. In the immediate aftermath, the clinician should have support in notifying the family or any initial communication with them with guidance from supervisors and consultation with risk management [48].

Support

If there are crisis support teams available within the institution, they can be used within the first 72 hours or week of the event to create a safe space for the team and affected clinicians to debrief and reflect [43,47]. Clinical teams can also set aside time to debrief among themselves informally. Support should focus on validating the emotional response and identifying personal and institutional supports for the clinical team. Process groups are also helpful in bringing the team together; however, some individuals may not feel comfortable participating in a group process. Connecting trainees and clinicians to peers or supervisors who have experienced patient suicide can be beneficial and minimize the sense of isolation created as a result of this loss. Additionally, supervisors and training directors should continue to check in with the clinicians and trainees intermittently after the event for on-going support [43,48].

In particular, trainees may be hesitant to request explicit accommodations in their workload, call schedule, or time-off. It is incumbent on the training program and chief residents to proactively offer these accommodations which the trainees can then use based on what would be most helpful to them [43].

Formal Debriefings

Preparing clinicians for the formal peer-review process, meetings with risk management, and supporting them in presenting at department morbidity and mortality conferences is critical in minimizing the sense of isolation and blame. As mentioned earlier, these proceedings are analytically focused and removed from the emotional impact experienced by the clinicians. Trainees should be allowed to decide if they would like to participate in these formal meetings and be allowed flexibility in their level of involvement [43,47].

Role in Prevention

Postvention support in the patient suicide and processing in the event not only allows for grieving but also helps reduce the risk and stress such an incident places on the clinician. Coordinating efforts to support clinicians who are impacted and having open and frank conversations can help reduce stigma and mitigate the sense of isolation due to patient suicide. It also allows clinicians to work through this traumatic experience and feel empowered to improve suicide prevention efforts [49].

RECOMMENDATIONS AND GUIDELINES

Suicide prevention training for health care professionals should lead to competence in the following areas.

1. Knowledge of core risk and protective factors associated with suicidality
2. How to screen for suicidality using an age-appropriate evidence-based suicide screening tool
3. How to complete a full suicide risk assessment in the event of a positive screen for suicidality
4. How to triage suicidality risk and direct individuals to the most appropriate next level of supportive medical care
5. How to complete an evidence-based suicide safety plan with an individual, including consideration of means restriction
6. How to provide evidence-based psychoeducation on harm reduction and suicide prevention strategies with individuals and, if appropriate, their living partners and/or family members

DISCUSSION

Suicide is a large and growing public health problem [1]. While mental health providers certainly have a key role to play in suicide prevention, the data support more universal screening for potential suicidality, and basic interventions are often needed in other health care settings, including urgent care centers and emergency rooms, primary care visits, and other ambulatory practices. Therefore, we need to educate health care professionals broadly to create a health care system that can more universally deliver compassionate preventative care and treatment of suicidal patient.

While training in suicide prevention frequently includes the key knowledge base of risk and protective factors for suicide, and screening is becoming increasingly common, it is key that education programs for health care providers move beyond these basics into more thorough assessment and treatment planning, as a lack of resources and knowledge about what to do following a positive screen is often cited as a barrier to more universal screening. Therefore, comprehensive suicide prevention education must include practical skills for using evidence-based tools for a complete assessment, triage, and treatment planning following a positive screen, and skills for basic brief interventions for those individuals with suicidality not requiring urgent inpatient care, including safety planning and lethal means restriction.

While such programs are likely to be effective in reducing the number of suicides, prevention is not the same as prediction, and the death of a patient by suicide is an occupational hazard that will be faced by many health care professionals during their career. This experience of losing a patient to suicide can have a profound effect on providers, especially when it occurs during training. Therefore, it is essential that institutions develop comprehensive programming for responding to suicide when one takes place. Such programming is essential to the mental health and professional wellbeing of the health care workforce, and therefore should be widely disseminated and implemented.

CLINICS CARE POINTS

- Screening tools such as Columbia-Suicide Severity Rating Scale (C-SSRS) should be included in the training curriculum.
- Triaging and disposition planning specific to suicide risk should be included in the training curriculum.
- Education related to the impact on suicide on trainees and its adverse effects on patient care should be factored in clinical teaching environments.
- Issues related to risk management should be addressed and included in clinical case discussions.

DISCLOSURE

The authors have nothing to disclose.

REFERENCES

[1] Hedegaard H, Curtin SC, Warner M. Increase in Suicide Mortality in the United States, 1999-2018. NCHS Data Brief 2020;(362):1–8.

[2] Kochanek KD, Xu J, Arias E. Mortality in the United States, 2019. NCHS Data Brief 2020;(395):1–8.

[3] CDC. Web-based Injury Statistics Query and Reporting System. Centers for Disease Control and Prevention, National Center for Injury Prevention and Control. 2021. Available at: https://www.cdc.gov/injury/wisqars/index.html.

[4] SAMHSA. Key substance use and mental health indicators in the United States: Results from the 2019 National Survey on Drug Use and Health (HHS Publication No. PEP20-07-01-001, NSDUH Series H-55). Cent Behav Health Stat Qual 2022. Available at: https://www.samhsa.gov/data/.

[5] Holland KM, Jones C, Vivolo-Kantor AM, et al. Trends in US Emergency Department Visits for Mental Health, Overdose, and Violence Outcomes Before and During the COVID-19 Pandemic. JAMA Psychiatry 2021;78(4): 372–9.

[6] Cavanagh JT, Carson AJ, Sharpe M, et al. Psychological autopsy studies of suicide: a systematic review. Psychol Med 2003;33(3):395–405.

[7] Walby FA, Myhre MO, Kildahl AT. Contact With Mental Health Services Prior to Suicide: A Systematic Review and Meta-Analysis. Psychiatr Serv 2018;69(7):751–9.

[8] Stene-Larsen K, Reneflot A. Contact with primary and mental health care prior to suicide: A systematic review of the literature from 2000 to 2017. Scand J Public Health 2019;47(1):9–17.

[9] Laanani M, Imbaud C, Tuppin P, et al. Contacts with Health Services During the Year Prior to Suicide Death and Prevalent Conditions A Nationwide Study. J Affect Disord 2020;274:174–82.

[10] Chemtob CM, Hamada RS, Bauer G, et al. Patients' suicides: frequency and impact on psychiatrists. Am J Psychiatry 1988;145(2):224–8.

[11] Qayyum Z, AhnAllen CG, Van Schalkwyk GI, et al. You Really Never Forget It!" Psychiatry Trainee Supervision Needs and Supervisor Experiences Following the Suicide of a Patient. Acad Psychiatry 2021;45(3):279–87.

[12] Hill NTM, Robinson J, Pirkis J, et al. Association of suicidal behavior with exposure to suicide and suicide attempt: A systematic review and multilevel meta-analysis. Plos Med 2020;17(3):e1003074.

[13] Andriessen K, Krysinska K, Kolves K, et al. Suicide Postvention Service Models and Guidelines 2014-2019: A Systematic Review. Front Psychol 2019;10:2677. https://doi.org/10.3389/fpsyg.2019.02677.

[14] Ferguson M, Reis J, Rabbetts L, et al. The impact of suicide prevention education programmes for nursing

students: A systematic review. Int J Ment Health Nurs 2020;29(5):756–71.
[15] Stover AN, Lavigne JE, Carpenter DM. A Scoping Review of Suicide Prevention Training Programs for Pharmacists and Student Pharmacists. Am J Pharm Educ 2022;10: 8917. https://doi.org/10.5688/ajpe8917.
[16] Chuop M, Michel Z, Shah R, et al. From Screening to Interventions: Teaching Clinical Suicide Prevention Skills to Medical Students. Acad Psychiatry 2021;45(3):292–6.
[17] Dillon CB, Saab MM, Meehan E, et al. Staff awareness of suicide and self-harm risk in healthcare settings: A mixed-methods systematic review. J Affect Disord 2020; 276:898–906.
[18] Wasserman D, Carli V, Iosue M, et al. Suicide prevention in childhood and adolescence: a narrative review of current knowledge on risk and protective factors and effectiveness of interventions. Asia Pac Psychiatry 2021; 13(3):e12452.
[19] Steele IH, Thrower N, Noroian P, et al. Understanding Suicide Across the Lifespan: A United States Perspective of Suicide Risk Factors, Assessment & Management. J Forensic Sci 2018;63(1):162–71.
[20] McClatchey K, Murray J, Rowat A, et al. Risk Factors for Suicide and Suicidal Behavior Relevant to Emergency Health Care Settings: A Systematic Review of Post-2007 Reviews. Suicide Life Threat Behav 2017;47(6):729–45.
[21] Boukouvalas E, El-Den S, Murphy AL, et al. Exploring Health Care Professionals' Knowledge of, Attitudes Towards, and Confidence in Caring for People at Risk of Suicide: a Systematic Review. Arch Suicide Res 2020; 24(sup2):S1–31.
[22] HHS O. The Surgeon General's Call to Action to Implement the National Strategy for Suicide Prevention. United States Department of Health and Human Services, Office of the Surgeon General. 2022. Available at: https://www.hhs.gov/sites/default/files/sprc-call-to-action.pdf.
[23] Poll H. Public Perception of Mental Health and Suicide Prevention survey Results. American Foundation for Suicide Prevention and National Action Alliance for Suicide Prevention. Available at: https://www.sprc.org/resources-programs/public-perception-mental-health-suicide-prevention-survey-results.
[24] Comission TJ. R3 Report: Requirement, Rationale, Reference. The Joint Comission. Available at: https://www.jointcommission.org/-/media/tjc/documents/resources/patient-safety-topics/suicide-prevention/r3_18_suicide_prevention_hap_bhc_5_6_19_rev5.pdf?db=web&hash=887186D9530F7BB8E30C28FE352B5B8C.
[25] Posner K, Brown GK, Stanley B, et al. The Columbia-Suicide Severity Rating Scale: initial validity and internal consistency findings from three multisite studies with adolescents and adults. Am J Psychiatry 2011;168(12): 1266–77.
[26] Horowitz LM, Bridge JA, Teach SJ, et al. Ask Suicide-Screening Questions (ASQ): a brief instrument for the pediatric emergency department. Arch Pediatr Adolesc Med 2012;166(12):1170–6.
[27] Simon GE, Rutter CM, Peterson D, et al. Does response on the PHQ-9 Depression Questionnaire predict subsequent suicide attempt or suicide death? Psychiatr Serv 2013;64(12):1195–202.
[28] Rossom RC, Coleman KJ, Ahmedani BK, et al. Suicidal ideation reported on the PHQ9 and risk of suicidal behavior across age groups. J Affect Disord 2017;215:77–84.
[29] Louzon SA, Bossarte R, McCarthy JF, et al. Does Suicidal Ideation as Measured by the PHQ-9 Predict Suicide Among VA Patients? Psychiatr Serv 2016;67(5):517–22.
[30] Osman A, Bagge CL, Gutierrez PM, et al. The Suicidal Behaviors Questionnaire-Revised (SBQ-R): validation with clinical and nonclinical samples. Assessment 2001;8(4): 443–54.
[31] Boudreaux ED, Jaques ML, Brady KM, et al. The patient safety screener: validation of a brief suicide risk screener for emergency department settings. Arch Suicide Res 2015;19(2):151–60.
[32] Shahidullah JD, Forman SG, Lekwa AJ. Assessment and management of depression and suicidality: Pediatric resident perspectives on training and practice. Fam Syst Health 2020;38(2):172–83.
[33] LeCloux M, Aguinaldo LD, Lanzillo EC, et al. PCP Opinions of Universal Suicide Risk Screening in Rural Primary Care: Current Challenges and Strategies for Successful Implementation. J Rural Health 2021;37(3):554–64.
[34] Newell S, Denneson L, Rynerson A, et al. Veterans Health Administration staff experiences with suicidal ideation screening and risk assessment in the context of COVID-19. PLoS One 2021;16(12):e0261921.
[35] Beck AT, Brown GK, Steer RA. Psychometric characteristics of the Scale for Suicide Ideation with psychiatric outpatients. Behav Res Ther 1997;35(11):1039–46.
[36] Stanley B, Brown GK. Safety planning intervention: A brief intervention to mitigate suicide risk. Cogn Behav Pract 2012;19:256–64.
[37] Nuij C, van Ballegooijen W, de Beurs D, et al. Safety planning-type interventions for suicide prevention: meta-analysis. Br J Psychiatry 2021;219(2):419–26.
[38] Zalsman G, Hawton K, Wasserman D, et al. Suicide prevention strategies revisited: 10-year systematic review. Lancet Psychiatry 2016;3(7):646–59.
[39] Daigle MS. Suicide prevention through means restriction: assessing the risk of substitution. A critical review and synthesis. Accid Anal Prev 2005;37(4):625–32.
[40] Gabbard GO. Miscarriages of psychoanalytic treatment with suicidal patients. Int J Psychoanal 2003;84(Pt 2): 249–61.
[41] Tillman JG. When a patient commits suicide: an empirical study of psychoanalytic clinicians. Int J Psychoanal 2006;87(Pt 1):159–77.
[42] Barman R, Kablinger A. Prevalence of trauma- and stress-related symptoms in psychiatrists and trainees following patient suicide in the United States. Soc Psychiatry Psychiatr Epidemiol 2021;56(7):1283–8.
[43] Qayyum Z, Luff D, Van Schalkwyk GI, et al. Recommendations for Effectively Supporting Psychiatry Trainees

Following a Patient Suicide. Acad Psychiatry 2021;45(3): 301–5.

[44] Simon RI. Psychiatrists awake! Suicide risk assessments are all about a good night's sleep. Psychiatr Ann 1998; 28(9):479–85.

[45] Packman WL, Pennuto TO, Bongar B, et al. Legal issues of professional negligence in suicide cases. Behav Sci Law 2004;22(5):697–713.

[46] Tsai A, Moran S, Shoemaker R, et al. Patient suicides in psychiatric residencies and post-vention responses: a national survey of psychiatry chief residents and program directors. Acad Psychiatry 2012;36(1):34–8.

[47] Cazares PT, Santiago P, Moulton D, et al. Suicide Response Guidelines for Residency Trainees: A Novel Postvention Response for the Care and Teaching of Psychiatry Residents who Encounter Suicide in Their Patients. Acad Psychiatry 2015;39(4):393–7.

[48] Agrawal A, Gitlin M, Melancon SNT, et al. Responding to a Tragedy: Evaluation of a Postvention Protocol Among Adult Psychiatry Residents. Acad Psychiatry 2021;45(3): 262–71.

[49] Moutier CY. Innovative and Timely Approaches to Suicide Prevention in Medical Education. Acad Psychiatry 2021;45(3):252–6.

Advances in Psychiatry and Behavioral Health 2 (2022) 221–230

ADVANCES IN PSYCHIATRY AND BEHAVIORAL HEALTH

Neurostimulation and Women's Health

Deval Zaveri, MD[a,*], Monica Rettenmier, MD[b], Patricia Carlson, MD[c]

[a]Department of Psychiatry, Sheppard Pratt Health Systems, 6501 N Charles Street, Towson, MD 21204, USA; [b]Electroconvulsive Therapy, Department of Psychiatry, Sheppard Pratt Health Systems, 6501 N Charles Street, Towson, MD 21204, USA; [c]TMS Program, Department of Psychiatry, Sheppard Pratt Health Systems, 6501 N Charles Street, Towson, MD 21204, USA

KEYWORDS

• Neuromodulation • Neurostimulation • ECT • TMS • DBS • VNS • Pregnant/postpartum • Menopausal women

KEY POINTS

- There is a need to better understand mental health issues specific to women across all phases of life.
- Further research is needed to understand these issues, particularly mental health issues related to hormonal changes surrounding menstruation, pregnancy, and menopause, as well as effective and safe treatment options during these reproductive phases.
- Neurostimulation is often an underutilized treatment option for men and women alike for a variety of psychiatric conditions.
- Pregnant women are generally excluded from randomized clinical trials for neurostimulation, yet open-label studies have found some forms of neurostimulation to be safe and effective during pregnancy and postpartum periods.

INTRODUCTION

Psychotherapy and medication management have been the mainstay of treatment of a variety of psychiatric disorders. These treatment options can be used alone or in combination. Some patients, however, do not necessarily respond to these individual or combination treatments in the desired way. In clinical situations like this, also referred as treatment-resistant conditions, alternative modalities like neurostimulation techniques have been used. Neuromodulation techniques have been studied and researched and are known to produce benefits.

Neuromodulation and neurostimulation are often used interchangeably in scientific literature. In simple terms "neurostimulation" can be described as stimulating the brain by using a stimulus-electric or magnetic. The stimulus modulates dysfunctional neuronal circuits, which in turn helps improve symptoms in various psychiatric conditions. In contrast to popular belief, it is not simply stimulating a specific area of the brain. It is hypothesized that stimulating the neuronal circuitry pathways in addition to specific areas of the brain, is what helps in treatment-refractory conditions, whereas psychopharmacology is directed toward only specific receptors and/or neurotransmitters.

Neurostimulation techniques have been widely used and have gained popularity for the management of treatment-resistant depression. They have also been used in other psychiatric disorders like obsessive-compulsive disorders, addiction, Alzheimer's disease (AD), Tourette's syndrome, autism spectrum disorder, schizophrenia, and attention-deficit hyperactive syndrome [1].

Electroconvulsive therapy (ECT) is the oldest of the neurostimulation treatments and has been widely used for many years in the management of treatment-resistant depression. Other newer techniques available include transcranial magnetic stimulation (TMS), vagal nerve stimulation (VNS), and deep brain stimulation (DBS).

*Corresponding author, *E-mail addresses:* Deval.zaveri@sheppardpratt.org; mrettenmier@sheppardpratt.org; PACarlson@sheppardpratt.org

https://doi.org/10.1016/j.ypsc.2022.03.006

DISCREPANCIES BETWEEN OVERALL MENTAL HEALTH DIAGNOSIS, TREATMENTS, AND OUTCOMES BETWEEN MEN AND WOMEN

Reproductive cycle and related changes impact the mental health of women. Certain psychiatric disorders like premenstrual dysphoric mood disorder, depression, and other psychiatric diagnoses in the perinatal period and postmenopausal syndrome are unique to women. Hormonal changes as well changes in usual life routines, during these reproductive phases do make women predisposed to develop psychiatric disorders. Paying special attention to hormonal changes often helps guide treatment approaches.

In this article, we intend to review the above-mentioned neurostimulation treatments, specifically looking at any gender-based differences or special considerations in women.

ELECTROCONVULSIVE THERAPY

ECT, previously known as "shock therapy," is an FDA-approved medical treatment prescribed to treat severe and treatment-resistant unipolar and bipolar depression, as well as catatonia. It also has the potential to be used off-label for other treatment-refractory cases, such as aggression in autism spectrum disorder (ASD), treatment-refractory suicidality, primary psychotic disorders such as schizophrenia, and bipolar mania not responding to pharmacotherapy alone. In this article, its ability to improve women's mental health is the predominant focus, specifically the use of ECT in the childbearing and geriatric phases of life.

ECT is a medical treatment that uses a brief electrical stimulus to invoke a controlled seizure while under anesthesia [2]. It is the first of the neurostimulation treatments developed for mental illness, introduce as far back as 1937 when physicians noted that patients would have an improvement in their psychiatric symptoms after a "seizure." Treatment approaches have significantly changed over the years; however, new advances in how the energy is administered to the patient have improved side effect profiles and overall functionality compared with previous methods.

Though its initial focus was the treatment of patients suffering from chronic schizophrenia [3], over the years its use has changed and at present, it is currently FDA approved for the treatment of refractory unipolar and bipolar depression as well as for catatonia [2]. It is often thought of as the "last option" for patients suffering from treatment depression; however, ECT does not necessarily need to be used only when a patient has suffered through years of failed medication trials. According to the American Psychiatric Association, ECT can be considered a first-line treatment when:

1. The severity of the psychiatric illness requires a rapid and definitive response,
2. When the risks of other treatments outweigh the risks of ECT,
3. A patient's history of poor medication response or good response to ECT in a previous episode, and
4. A patient is particularly focused on using ECT above other forms of treatment [4].

Efficacy in Depression

Through multiple clinical trials comparing the treatment response of ECT to that of sham ECT (where a patient underwent anesthesia but didn't receive an ECT treatment). Recovery rate of 80% to 90% was seen in individuals who received ECT for unipolar depression [5,6]. In bipolar depression, the ECT response rate was nearly equivocal to that of unipolar depression [6]. For postpartum depression and postpartum psychosis, ECT has been found to be between 80% and 87% effective, respectively [7].

Delivery of Treatment

Traditionally an index course of ECT for depression involves anywhere between 8 and 14 treatments though there really is no set "number" of treatments required to complete a full course of ECT. Rather it is based on an individualized plan determined by the ECT team and patient based on symptom resolution. With technological advances to the way in which ECT is administered, specifically the advent of right unilateral electrode placement as well as ultra-brief energy settings, providers are now able to administer a therapeutic treatment while reducing the overall memory and cognitive side effect burden that previously occurred.

A typical series will start with treatments three times per week, usually Monday, Wednesday, and Friday for a period of 2 to 3 weeks or until symptoms of depression resolve. Once the targeted symptoms have resolved, a further 2 to 3 treatments spaced out over a few weeks may be recommended to ensure a patient doesn't relapse abruptly with worsening depressive symptoms.

An anesthesiologist or CRNA under the supervision of an anesthesiologist is part of the treatment team and is responsible for administering all medication during an ECT treatment. Multiple medications are usually given before a treatment including a short-acting sedative that allows the patient to "sleep" through the treatment and a muscle relaxant to ensure the individual does not have any excessive motor movement which could lead to injury. This individual is also responsible for maintaining a patient's health and safety during the ECT treatment.

ECT is effective as monotherapy but as it does not have the ability to "cure" depression, rather it helps to resolve the current episode of depression, coadministration of pharmacotherapy and psychotherapy is recommended in conjunction with the completion of the series [8]. For medications that have antiepileptic properties, a discussion before ECT is initiated must occur.

Adverse Effects and Management

The most commonly reported side effects include headaches (45%), fatigue (73%), muscle pain/aches (15%), and nausea (23%). Cognitively the most common side effect is anterograde memory impairment which can affect roughly 41% of patients during their ECT series [5]. However, it is important to also note that most patients report cognitive functioning and various aspects of memory and recall actually improve beyond their pre-ECT baseline once the series is completed [9,10].

Special Considerations

Elderly patients

Though it is well documented that elderly patients tend to respond more robustly to ECT interventions, they also traditionally have greater medical comorbidities and thus have a higher inherent risk of complications with ECT. Generally, a full medical evaluation including physical examination, EKG (electrocardiogram), and laboratory work (CBC, CMP, TSH/Free T4, urine drug screen, and pregnancy test) are required for any medical clearance before initiating a series of ECT. Additionally, further evaluation of a patient's cardiac and/or respiratory function may be needed if an individual has comorbid illnesses. It is known that women classically will have a dramatic rise in their cardiac risk after menopause and currently heart disease is still the number cause of death in women [11]. Further, with normal aging and brain atrophy, geriatric patients are more at risk for prolonged confusion, greater memory deficits, and higher risk for delirium after an ECT treatment compared with their younger counterparts. Though this does not mean that ECT is not an option, as a majority of ECT is performed on individuals more than the age of 65 [8], detailed screening and monitoring of the patient as well as education of both patient and family are recommended to reduce risk.

Pregnancy

ECT is an efficacious treatment of women in all trimesters of pregnancy. Though it is not often considered a first-line treatment in pregnancy, it can be an effective tool for the treatment of acute illnesses including depression, bipolar disorder, and psychosis when the medication needed to treat the mother will harm the fetus or when a patient does not want to use medications that may impact their baby. Additionally, depending on the level of illness that the mother to be is experiencing, at times ECT is required to maintain the safety of both the mother and the child. All women should have an Obstetric consultation before the initiation of ECT to review risks/other medical concerns. Additionally, a robust consent process is required to ensure that the mother is aware of the risks/benefits/side effects that can happen to both her and the baby.

The risk of aspiration is higher with pregnancy due to the ever-growing space needed in the abdomen for the pregnancy. Other important aspects of treatment in this population include fetal heart monitoring beginning between 14 and 16 weeks as well as ensuring that services for the management of any obstetric and/or neonatal emergencies are available [8,11].

Postpartum

ECT is efficacious treatment of women during the period leading up to and following the delivery of a child. Postpartum depression can present between 1 and 4 weeks postdelivery, especially with the rapid changes in both hormone levels as well as significant changes to their usual routines. Postpartum psychosis can also manifest, though less common (prevalence of 0.089%–0.5% [12]). Women with a previous diagnosis of bipolar disorder are also at higher risk for decompensation, both from the changes listed above but also if they required a medication holiday to reduce the risk of harm to the infant while in utero.

Though most medications are safe when breastfeeding and will not cross-over in breast milk to a nursing infant, there are certain pharmacotherapeutic agents that can negatively impact a growing infant and a decision to use ECT can mitigate these risks. The anesthetic agents administered during ECT pose little risk to an infant at baseline [8]. There is some potential certain anesthetic agents crossing over into breast milk, but typically these agents are very short-acting and are excreted out of the mother's body within a short period of time. Pumping and storing breast milk to be used immediately following treatment can reduce the risk of infant exposure.

REPETITIVE TRANSCRANIAL MAGNETIC STIMULATION

rTMS is a noninvasive, nonpharmacological treatment of major depression that was FDA cleared in 2008, also gained FDA approval for the indications of obsessive-compulsive disorder in 2018 and smoking cessation in 2020. rTMS devices create repetitive, time-varying magnetic fields, resulting in an electric field that induces neural action potentials in the brain, in effect, causing stimulation to occur [13]. Unlike ECT, no seizure is induced with TMS. There is no need for anesthesia and no downtime associated with TMS treatments.

Indications

Major depression

rTMS is a well-tolerated treatment of major depression in adults who have not achieved satisfactory improvement from prior antidepressant medications in the current episode [14]. rTMS is not FDA cleared for major depression with psychosis or bipolar depression.

A meta-analysis of 29 randomized controlled trials found that treatment with rTMS yields a clinically significant pooled odds ratio for a response of 3.3 (95% confidence interval [CI, 2.35–4.64) with an NNT of 8 (95% CI, 5.8–10.5) [15] Another study noted significant improvement in the Clinician Global Impressions-Severity of Illness (CGI-S) with 58.0% response rate and remission rate of 37.1%. Patient-reported responses ranged from 56.4% to 41.5% and remission rate ranged from 28.7% to 26.5%, (PHQ-9 and IDS-SR scales, respectively) [16].

In patients followed over 12 months, response rate was 45% to 60% and remission rate was 30% to 40%, with durable clinical response over the follow-up period of 12 months [17].

The typical treatment course involves 5 treatments per week for 4 to 6 weeks, with a taper down in frequency for several weeks thereafter. One daily treatment takes roughly 19 to 40 minutes depending on the device used, patient comfort, and other factors. The amount of energy used is found by determining a *motor threshold* which is the minimum amount of stimulation needed to induce a thumb or finger twitch > or = 50% of the time on the side contralateral to the stimulus [18]. TMS can be used effectively as monotherapy or as an adjunct to medications [19] and adjusting the adjunct medications as needed [18].

Obsessive compulsive disorder

In 2018, FDA clearance was granted for the treatment of obsessive compulsive disorder (OCD), targeting various areas of the brain including the medial prefrontal cortex and the anterior cingulate cortex as well as the supplementary motor area (SMA) [20,21].

In 2020, a retrospective study examined pharmaco-resistant OCD outpatients. 46.2% of all patients responded, with a 30% reduction in Y-BOCS (Yale-Brown Obsessive-Compulsive Scale) scores. There was no significant difference between response rates of patients in dorsolateral prefrontal cortex and SMA groups [22].

Smoking cessation

In 2020, the manufacturer BrainsWay gained FDA approval for its device designed to induce short-term smoking cessation. The protocol involves treatment 5 days a week for 3 weeks, followed by 3 times a week for 3 weeks, for a total of 18 treatment sessions [23]. This is a new treatment indication in the United States through many TMS studies have shown some efficacy in reducing cravings for various substances [24].

Safety and side effect profile

The most common side effect of TMS treatment is head or scalp pain in the area of the stimulation. Headache is another common side effect that gradually improves.

Seizures are a rare side effect, with a risk of 0.02 seizures per 1000 treatment sessions in individuals with no risk factors. 75% of seizures occurred within the first 3 exposures to TMS. Higher incidence of seizure occurred in those with elevated risk for seizures such as epilepsy, brain lesions, and on certain medications [25].

Contraindications and cautions

Nonremovable ferromagnetic or magnetic sensitive metal in the head or neck area is contraindicated. Biologically driven devices such as pacemakers, ICDs, and vagal nerve stimulators may be contraindicated. Any recent head injury or other neurologic conditions should be thoroughly considered before recommendation for treatment with rTMS. History of seizures is not an absolute contraindication, but the risk and benefits of treatment in this population must be thoroughly examined.

Special Consideration for Women

Depression in pregnancy

As TMS is a nonpharmacologic treatment, it can be an advantageous option for pregnant women. However, clinical trials for all indications excluded participants who were pregnant.

In 2011, Dr Deborah Kim and colleagues conducted an open-label study of 10 pregnant women with TMS, low frequency (1 Hz) over the right dorsolateral prefrontal cortex at 100% of motor threshold level, for a total of 20 treatment sessions. 7/10 responded achieving at least a 50% reduction in scores on the Hamilton Depression Rating Scale (HDRS-17). Mild headaches were reported in 4 women. There were no adverse effects on the pregnancy or fetal outcomes [26].

Another study in 2014 of 30 pregnant women with depression found that rTMS over the left prefrontal cortex, 6 days a week for 3 weeks, was effective in reducing depressive symptoms. 41.4% of the study group demonstrated significant mood improvements as indicated by a decrease in HAMD (17-item Hamilton depression rating scale) by 50% or more. 20.7% attained remission (HAMD score < 8), 34.5% achieved a partial response, and 3.4% had worsening HAMD scores at the end of treatment. No significant adverse effects were reported [27].

A 2019 randomized controlled trial studied 22 women with major depressive disorder in their second or third trimesters, treated with 20 sessions of TMS at 1 Hz as a single train of 900 pulses per session at 100% of motor threshold. Results found a significant decrease in HAMD score over the sham group ($P = .003$), remission rate of 27.27% versus 18.18%. Response rates were 81.82% for the active rTMS group and 45.45% for the sham rTMS group ($P = .088$) [28]. Late preterm birth occurred in 3 subjects in the active arm. Other maternal and labor outcomes were normal, concluding that rTMS was effective and low risk during pregnancy [28].

Postpartum depression

In 2010, a study of 10 women with postpartum depression found significant improvement in symptoms by week 2 of treatment. At week 4, 8 patients achieved remission and 7 patients remained in remission at 6 months out [29]. A randomized double-blind pilot study treated 14 women with postpartum depression. Women received 20 sessions of 5 Hz TMS over the left dorsolateral prefrontal cortex at 120% motor threshold versus sham procedure. The active arm group showed statistically significant improvement in depressive symptoms. Subjects reported no significant side effects during the study except 2 reported minor scalp discomfort and/or headache immediately after their rTMS sessions [30].

Menopause

Few studies specifically examine menopausal depression and neurostimulation. A 2008 study examined the antidepressant efficacy of rTMS on 31 women (17 premenopausal, 14 postmenopausal), and 16 men, also examining the role of female reproductive hormones. No difference in the rTMS response was observed between male and premenopausal female patients (68.8% and 70.6%, respectively), but postmenopausal women responded least (0%). There was a greater improvement with a higher estradiol/progesterone ratio in premenopausal women ($P<.05$), suggesting an important role of hormones in the therapeutic response. A small sample size and a shorter duration of treatment influence the generalization of this data [31].

Summary

Pregnant women were not included in the initial clinical trials for rTMS for the treatment of depression but there is some evidence that rTMS can be a safe and effective option for women with perinatal depression.

For recent OCD and smoking cessation indications, no studies conducted included pregnant women.

rTMS and other transcranial stimulation modalities are rapidly advancing with new protocols and indications for use. More specialized studies targeting mental health issues in women are needed to gain evidence for safety and efficacy in this special population.

VAGAL NERVE STIMULATION

VNS was introduced initially in the 19th century for seizure control. Initially, animal models demonstrated antiepileptic properties with VNS. Following this numerous human studies also showed the effectiveness of VNS in causing significant seizure reduction in intractable epilepsy [32,33]. Subsequently, the US Food and Drug Administration (FDA) approved VNS for the management of treatment-refractory epilepsy.

Vagus nerve is mixed sensory motor nerve. The motor (visceromotor) fibers originate in the dorsal motor nucleus of the medulla oblongata. Sensory fibers terminate in the nucleus tractus solitarius (NTS). And NTS eventually sends projections to the hindbrain, midbrain, and forebrain structures, which directly or indirectly connected to the limbic system and areas of the brain pertinent in depression. Connections to the medullary motor nuclei, mid-brain (locus coeruleus, dorsal raphe nucleus), and brain stem nuclei including the reticular formation and parabrachial nucleus, forebrain connections include-hypothalamus, amygdala, stria terminalis, and insular cortex [34–36].

Delivery of Treatment

VNS placement is a day outpatient procedure, whereby a stimulation device is placed around the left vagus nerve. The device consists of bipolar electrodes which when stimulated, activates the AV node of the heart generating action potential which then spreads to the central nervous system. After surgical placement, the device is externally activated via telemetry and is then set to desired parameters (also referred the dose of VNS stimulation), preferably at the lowest setting to begin with. The dose of stimulation can be then gradually increased based on clinical response [37].

VNS device needs to be turned off for procedures like MRI, ECT, and defibrillation.

Noninvasive VNS (n VNS) is now gaining popularity in the treatment of depression, PTSD, and other stress-related psychiatric conditions [38]. Two type of noninvasive VNS devices are now available-trans auricular (taVNS) and transcervical (tcVNS) [39]. The taVNS device stimulates the auricular branch of the vagus nerve and tcVNS device stimulates both the sensory and motor fibers of the vagal nerve in the carotid sheath [39].

Indications

Treatment-resistant depression (TRD): The US FDA-approved VNS for the treatment of TRD in 2005. It was approved as adjunctive treatment of the long-term management of chronic recurrent depression at ages 18 and over.

Cognitive disorders: There is growing evidence through clinical trials of VNS use in the improvement of cognitive disorders, emerging as a promising tool in the treatment of cognitive disorders [40].

Safety and side effect profile

Common complications include intraoperative cardiac issues-bradycardia, asystole due to collateral current spread or electrode placement on the vagal nerve branches. Delayed arrhythmias and syncope can also occur. Complications secondary to trauma to the neighboring anatomic structures-damage to the trachea-hematoma, vocal cord damage-cough, pain, dyspnea, voice alteration, airway obstruction. No significant risk of mortality is noted.

Special considerations in women

Theoretically, brain stimulation especially stimulating the areas of brain involved with the endocrine function can affect the uterus and the reproductive function. VNS activates the hypothalamus, which is the center for the regulation of gonadal hormones, estrogen, and progesterone. Through animal studies, we know that vagal stimulation can impact progesterone levels in mice [41]. Vagal nerve fibers innervate the uterus, which regulates the contraction of uterine muscles and affects blood flow to the uterus [42].

Through the stimulation of the various brain stem nuclei like NTS, locus coeruleus, reticular structures and parabrachial nucleus, can activate the secretion and release of norepinephrine which can potentially cause uterine smooth muscle contraction increasing the risk of abortion or preterm labor [43,44].

VNS procedure has been used for more than 32 years now. But only a small sample size is available when specially looking at its use in pregnant women.

Data gathered from the International Registry of Antiepileptic Drugs and Pregnancy (EURAP) reviewing the outcomes of pregnancy in women with epilepsy receiving VNS during their pregnancy, 25 out of 26 pregnant women who received VNS for refractory epilepsy showed no clear teratogenic effects or additional risks for congenital malformations on fetal outcome. There may be an increased need for obstetric interventions [45]. Another prospective study reviewed and followed 26 pregnancies in 25 women with epilepsy and receiving VNS treatment, reaffirmed these findings, of no clear evidence of fetal teratogenicity. However, there may be a slightly increased rate of obstetric interventions during delivery needing cesarean sections, vacuum extractions, or induced deliveries [46].

Another study of 48 pregnancies studied the effect of VNS on maternal and fetal outcomes. This review included studies whereby VNS was used either for the treatment of refractory epilepsy or TRD. With regards to maternal outcomes, 2 out of 44 pregnancies had a miscarriage, both early in the first trimester of pregnancy, attributed to refractory seizure and comorbid use of antiepileptic drugs along with VNS treatment. There was no correlation between the risk of spontaneous abortion and VNS. Overall the risk of spontaneous abortion in VNS remains comparable or even lower than the risk in the general population. Other obstetric complications included—preeclampsia, but both of younger age and being on multiple antiepileptic drugs. 1 out of 42 fetuses, was born with severe malformations, which also was in a 22-year-old mother with epilepsy and was treated on multiple antiepileptic drugs—clonazepam, levetiracetam, phenobarbital, and carbamazepine at the same time. In conclusion, the adverse maternal or fetal outcomes noted, though low incidence, were noted in pregnant women receiving VNS for refractory epilepsy, and adverse outcomes attributed to perinatal exposure to multiple antiepileptic drugs [47].

No specific gender-based differences in treatment-related information are available for use of VNS in postmenopausal women.

Summary

VNS is a rapidly merging treatment and advancing its scope for practice for various psychiatric conditions. Overall, noted to be safe for use in pregnant and postpartum populations. More research is needed to study and identify if there are any gender-specific differences in treatment approaches needed in women at different reproductive stages of life.

DEEP BRAIN STIMULATION

DBS is a neurosurgical technique in which specific target areas of the brain are stimulated through surgically placed electrodes. It was first used in 1980s for the treatment of essential tremors, using electrical stimulation of the midbrain and basal ganglia. The introduction and use of DBS paved the way for the development of newer techniques like TMS, magnetic seizure therapy.

Delivery of Treatment

Exact mechanism of action is still not clearly understood. In literal sense, the procedure involves placing electrodes around the axons in specific target areas of the brain, causing changes in the voltage of the neuronal cell, generating action potential sequences, which then control the release of neurotransmitters.

Four mechanisms of action have been and are believed that multiple mechanisms work together. (1) direct inhibition of neural activity as is noted in surgical procedures like thalamotomy, pallidotomy, and cingulotomy-suppression of neuronal activity by direct suppression or by the activation of inhibitory neurons in specific brain areas; (2) direct excitation of neural activity; (3) Disruption of the flow of information through the neurons in the targeted areas and (4) synaptic filtering-filtering between the high and low-frequency stimulation. Long-term effect of DBS can lead to neurogenesis, synaptogenesis increasing neuronal plasticity.

Indications

1. Parkinson's disease (PD)- FDA approval in 2002, targeting the subthalamic nuclei [48] globus pallidus intermedius (GPI) [49] ventral intermediate thalamic nucleus (VIM) [50].
2. Essential tremors-targeting the VIM, ventrolateral thalamus, and adjacent white matter tracts. The other areas of target include posterior subthalamic area/caudal zona incerta (PSA/cZI) [51].
3. Dystonia-targeting the GPI [52].
4. OCD: FDA-approved indication for DBS. The brain areas targeted in OCD include—primarily the ventral capsule/ventral striatum (VC/VS) for medically refractory OCD. Less often other areas of target are the nucleus accumbens (NAc), bed nucleus of the stria terminalis (BNST), STN, anterior limb of the internal capsule (ALIC), and inferior thalamic peduncle (ITP) [53].
5. Epilepsy-medically refractory seizures, which cannot be resected by surgery. The specific areas targeted here are the anterior nucleus of the thalamus as well the cerebellum [54,55].
6. Tourette's syndrome-targeting areas are either the dorsomedial thalamus and CMPfc separately or in combination with the GP [56].
7. Major depressive disorder - not very promising efficacy results targeting the subcallosal cingulate gyrus [57].
8. Eating Disorders and Obesity- Inconclusive results for anorexia nervosa targeting the subgenual cingulate cortex [58], NAc [59], VC/VS. [60].
9. Addiction and substance use: NAc and the STN [61,62].
10. Alzheimer's disease-forniceal DBS or activation of the nbM and the VC/VS. [63].
11. PTSD-targeting the basolateral amygdala [64] and the subgenual cingulate gyrus [65].

Safety and side effect profile

Risks with DBS include-risks of surgery-most common one is intracranial hemorrhage seen in 1% to 2% of cases [66], followed by the risk of seizures (1%) [67]. Complications can occur secondary to the DBS device implanted; these may include-device migration, fracture, nerve impingement, or infection.

Risks of infection, Deep Vein Thrombosis, and Pulmonary Embolism like any other medical procedure.

Special Considerations in Women

A retrospective case series of DBS cases followed during pregnancy, who received DBS for either movement disorder or a psychiatric disorder by Scelzo and colleagues found DBS to be safe in pregnant women. Continuing DBS during pregnancy helped reduction in both movement disorder as well reduction of behavioral symptoms. In patients with PD, DBS also allowed reduction in medication doses needed during pregnancy. No notable adverse effects on pregnancy or fetal outcomes were noted [68].

In another small sample ($n = 6$), a series of dystonia patients who became pregnant showed no adverse effects on their pregnancy, fetal outcomes, or breastfeeding with the use of DBS [69].

Safety of DBS in pregnant epileptic patients was also noted in other case reports by Bone and colleagues [70].

No other gender-specific or special treatment recommendations-related research is available for menopausal women.

Summary

DBS has significantly evolved over the last 4 to 5 decades, with newer indications added than what it started it, with a considerable expansion in the scope of practice. Though its safety and efficacy are established in a wide age group, including pregnant and postpartum women, more research is needed about its use especially regarding any specific treatment modifications or special considerations in women.

CLINICS CARE POINTS

- Neurostimulation techniques like ECT, VNS, TMS, and DBS offer different rates of efficacy in the treatment and management of various psychiatric disorders. They are particularly valuable and often underutilized for treatment-resistant conditions.
- Neurostimulation can be a safe and effective treatment option for use in pregnant and postpartum women.
- ECT shows robust results in older and postmenopausal women. However, with medical comorbidities there may be a higher inherent risk of complications with ECT.
- A thorough discussion with patients, careful informed consent, weighing risks, potential side effects, and benefits must be completed before any neurostimulation technique is recommended or initiated. This discussion should be meticulously documented in patient clinical records.

DISCLOSURE

The authors have nothing to disclose.

REFERENCES

[1] Temel Y, Hescham SA, Jahanshahi A, et al. Neuromodulation in psychiatric disorders. Int Rev Neurobiol 2012; 107:283–314.

[2] McDonal W, Fochtmann L. What is Electroconvulsive therapy (ECT)? In: American Psychiatric Association. 2019. Available at: https://www.psychiatry.org/patients-families/ect. Accessed November 23, 2021.

[3] Mankad MV, Beyer JL, Weiner RD, et al. Indications for use. In: Clinical manual of electroconvulsive therapy. Arlington: APA Publishing; 2010. p. 76–7, 139-141, 81-91.

[4] Walsh S. FDA In Brief: FDA takes action to ensure regulation of electroconvulsive therapy devices better protects patients, reflects current understanding of safety and effectiveness. 2018. Available at: https://www.fda.gov/news-events/fda-brief/fda-brief-fda-takes-action-ensure-regulation-electroconvulsive-therapy-devices-better-protects. Accessed November 20, 2021.

[5] UK ECT Review Group. Efficacy and safety of electroconvulsive therapy in depressive disorders: a systematic review and meta-analysis. Lancet 2003;361(9360): 799–808.

[6] Dierckx B, Heijnen WT, van den Broek WW, et al. Efficacy of electroconvulsive therapy in bipolar versus unipolar major depression: a meta-analysis. Bipolar Disord 2012;14(2):146–50.

[7] Rundgren S, Brus O, Båve U, et al. Improvement of postpartum depression and psychosis after electroconvulsive therapy: A population-based study with a matched comparison group. J Affect Disord 2018;235:258–64.

[8] Weiner Richard. Use of medications during the ECT course. In: Committee on The practice of ECT. 2nd edition. Arlington: APA; 2001. p. 16, 23, 44, 56-57,81-91.

[9] Semkovska M, McLoughlin DM. Objective cognitive performance associated with electroconvulsive therapy for depression: a systematic review and meta-analysis. Biol Psychiatry 2010;68(6):568–77.

[10] Coleman EA, Sackeim HA, Prudic J, et al. Subjective memory complaints prior to and following electroconvulsive therapy. Biol Psychiatry 1996;39(5):346–56.

[11] Benjamin EJ, Muntner P, Alonso A, et al. Heart Disease and Stroke Statistics-2019 Update: A Report From the American Heart Association. Circulation 2019;139(10): e56–528 [published correction appears in Circulation. 2020 Jan 14;141(2):e33].

[12] VanderKruik R, Barreix M, Chou D, et al. The global prevalence of postpartum psychosis: a systematic review. BMC Psychiatry 2017;17(1):272.

[13] Costello AH. Repetitive Transcranial Magnetic Stimulation (rTMS) Systems - Class II Special Controls Guidance for Industry and FDA Staff. In: US Food & Drug Administration, Medical Devices. 2011. Available at: https://www.fda.gov/medical-devices/guidance-documents-medical-devices-and-radiation-emitting-products/repetitive-transcranial-magnetic-stimulation-rtms-systems-class-ii-special-controls-guidance. Accessed November 11,2021.

[14] Janicak PG, O'Reardon JP, Sampson SM, et al. Transcranial magnetic stimulation in the treatment of major depressive disorder: a comprehensive summary of safety experience from acute exposure, extended exposure, and during reintroduction treatment. J Clin Psychiatry 2008; 69(2):222–32.

[15] Berlim MT, van den Eynde F, Tovar-Perdomo S, et al. Response, remission and drop-out rates following high-frequency repetitive transcranial magnetic stimulation (rTMS) for treating major depression: a systematic review and meta-analysis of randomized, double-blind and sham-controlled trials. Psychol Med 2014;44(2):225–39.

[16] Carpenter LL, Janicak PG, Aaronson ST, et al. Transcranial magnetic stimulation (TMS) for major depression: a multisite, naturalistic, observational study of acute treatment outcomes in clinical practice. Depress Anxiety 2012;29(7):587–96.

[17] Dunner DL, Aaronson ST, Sackeim HA, et al. A multisite, naturalistic, observational study of transcranial magnetic stimulation for patients with pharmacoresistant major depressive disorder: durability of benefit over a 1-year follow-up period. J Clin Psychiatry 2014;75(12): 1394–401.

[18] McClintock SM, Reti IM, Carpenter LL, et al. Consensus Recommendations for the Clinical Application of Repetitive Transcranial Magnetic Stimulation (rTMS) in the Treatment of Depression. J Clin Psychiatry 2018;79(1): 16cs10905.

[19] Berlim MT, Van den Eynde F, Daskalakis ZJ. High-frequency repetitive transcranial magnetic stimulation accelerates and enhances the clinical response to antidepressants in major depression: a meta-analysis of randomized, double-blind, and sham-controlled trials. J Clin Psychiatry 2013;74(2):e122–9.

[20] Carmi L, Alyagon U, Barnea-Ygael N, et al. Clinical and electrophysiological outcomes of deep TMS over the medial prefrontal and anterior cingulate cortices in OCD patients. Brain Stimul 2018;11(1):158–65.

[21] Rehn S, Eslick GD, Brakoulias V. A Meta-Analysis of the Effectiveness of Different Cortical Targets Used in Repetitive Transcranial Magnetic Stimulation (rTMS) for the Treatment of Obsessive-Compulsive Disorder (OCD). Psychiatr Q 2018;89(3):645–65.

[22] Rostami R, Kazemi R, Jabbari A, et al. Efficacy and clinical predictors of response to rTMS treatment in pharmacoresistant obsessive-compulsive disorder (OCD): a retrospective study. BMC Psychiatry 2020;20(1):372.

[23] Huber J. BrainsWay Receives FDA Clearance for Smoking Addiction in Adults. In Brainsway News. 2020. Available at: https://www.brainsway.com/news_events/brainsway-receives-fda-clearance-for-smoking-addiction-in-adults/. Accessed November 11,2021.

[24] Ekhtiari H, Tavakoli H, Addolorato G, et al. Transcranial electrical and magnetic stimulation (tES and TMS) for addiction medicine: A consensus paper on the present state of the science and the road ahead. Neurosci Biobehav Rev 2019;104:118–40.

[25] Lerner AJ, Wassermann EM, Tamir DI. Seizures from transcranial magnetic stimulation 2012-2016: Results of a survey of active laboratories and clinics. Clin Neurophysiol 2019;130(8):1409–16.

[26] Kim DR, Epperson N, Paré E, et al. An open label pilot study of transcranial magnetic stimulation for pregnant women with major depressive disorder. J Womens Health (Larchmt) 2011;20(2):255–61.

[27] Hızlı Sayar G, Ozten E, Tufan E, et al. Transcranial magnetic stimulation during pregnancy. Arch Womens Ment Health 2014;17(4):311–5.

[28] Kim DR, Wang E, McGeehan B, et al. Randomized controlled trial of transcranial magnetic stimulation in pregnant women with major depressive disorder. Brain Stimul 2019;12(1):96–102.

[29] Garcia KS, Flynn P, Pierce KJ, et al. Repetitive transcranial magnetic stimulation treats postpartum depression. Brain Stimul 2010;3(1):36–41.

[30] Myczkowski ML, Dias AM, Luvisotto T, et al. Effects of repetitive transcranial magnetic stimulation on clinical, social, and cognitive performance in postpartum depression. Neuropsychiatr Dis Treat 2012;8:491–500.

[31] Huang CC, Wei IH, Chou YH, et al. Effect of age, gender, menopausal status, and ovarian hormonal level on rTMS in treatment-resistant depression. Psychoneuroendocrinology 2008;33(6):821–31.

[32] Uthman BM, Wilder BJ, Penry JK, et al. Treatment of epilepsy by stimulation of the vagus nerve. Neurology 1993;43(7):1338–45.

[33] Penry JK, Dean JC. Prevention of intractable partial seizures by intermittent vagal stimulation in humans: preliminary results. Epilepsia 1990;31(Suppl 2):S40–3.

[34] Berthoud HR, Neuhuber WL. Functional and chemical anatomy of the afferent vagal system. Auton Neurosci 2000;85(1–3):1–17.

[35] George MS, Aston-Jones G. Noninvasive techniques for probing neurocircuitry and treating illness: vagus nerve stimulation (VNS), transcranial magnetic stimulation (TMS) and transcranial direct current stimulation (tDCS). Neuropsychopharmacology 2010;35(1): 301–16.

[36] Yuan H, Silberstein SD. Vagus Nerve and Vagus Nerve Stimulation, a Comprehensive Review: Part I. Headache 2016;56(1):71–8.

[37] Yuan H, Silberstein SD. Vagus Nerve and Vagus Nerve Stimulation, a Comprehensive Review: Part II. Headache 2016;56(2):259–66.

[38] Bremner JD, Gurel NZ, Wittbrodt MT, et al. Application of Noninvasive Vagal Nerve Stimulation to Stress-Related Psychiatric Disorders. J Pers Med 2020;10(3): 119.

[39] Ben-Menachem E, Revesz D, Simon BJ, et al. Surgically implanted and non-invasive vagus nerve stimulation: a review of efficacy, safety and tolerability. Eur J Neurol 2015;22(9):1260–8.

[40] Broncel A, Bocian R, Kłos-Wojtczak P, et al. Vagal nerve stimulation as a promising tool in the improvement of cognitive disorders. Brain Res Bull 2020;155:37–47.

[41] Morales-Ledesma L, Betanzos-García R, Domínguez-Casalá R. Unilateral or bilateral vagotomy performed on prepubertal rats at puberty onset of female rat deregulates ovarian function. Arch Med Res 2004;35(4): 279–83.

[42] Ortega-Villalobos M, García-Bazán M, Solano-Flores LP, et al. Vagus nerve afferent and efferent innervation of the rat uterus: an electrophysiological and HRP study. Brain Res Bull 1990;25(3):365–71.

[43] Manta S, El Mansari M, Debonnel G, et al. Electrophysiological and neurochemical effects of long-term vagus nerve stimulation on the rat monoaminergic systems. Int J Neuropsychopharmacol 2013;16(2):459–70.

[44] Raedt R, Clinckers R, Mollet L, et al. Increased hippocampal noradrenaline is a biomarker for efficacy of vagus nerve stimulation in a limbic seizure model. J Neurochem 2011;117(3):461–9.

[45] Tomson T, Battino D, Bonizzoni E, et al. Dose-dependent risk of malformations with antiepileptic drugs: an analysis of data from the EURAP epilepsy and pregnancy registry. Lancet Neurol 2011;10(7):609–17.

[46] Sabers A, Battino D, Bonizzoni E, et al. Maternal and fetal outcomes associated with vagus nerve stimulation during pregnancy. Epilepsy Res 2017;137:159–62.

[47] Ding J, Wang L, Wang C, et al. Is vagal-nerve stimulation safe during pregnancy? A mini review. Epilepsy Res 2021; 174:106671.

[48] Castrioto A, Lozano AM, Poon YY, et al. Ten-year outcome of subthalamic stimulation in Parkinson disease: a blinded evaluation. Arch Neurol 2011;68(12): 1550–6.

[49] Follett KA, Weaver FM, Stern M, et al. Pallidal versus subthalamic deep-brain stimulation for Parkinson's disease. N Engl J Med 2010;362(22):2077–91.

[50] Lee DJ, Lozano CS, Dallapiazza RF, et al. Current and future directions of deep brain stimulation for neurological and psychiatric disorders. J Neurosurg 2019;131(2): 333–42.

[51] Zesiewicz TA, Elble R, Louis ED, et al. Practice parameter: therapies for essential tremor: report of the Quality Standards Subcommittee of the American Academy of Neurology. Neurology 2005;64(12):2008–20.

[52] Moro E, LeReun C, Krauss JK, et al. Efficacy of pallidal stimulation in isolated dystonia: a systematic review and meta-analysis. Eur J Neurol 2017;24(4):552–60.

[53] Naesström M, Blomstedt P, Bodlund O. A systematic review of psychiatric indications for deep brain stimulation, with focus on major depressive and obsessive-compulsive disorder. Nord J Psychiatry 2016;70(7): 483–91.

[54] Fisher R, Salanova V, Witt T, et al. Electrical stimulation of the anterior nucleus of thalamus for treatment of refractory epilepsy. Epilepsia 2010;51(5):899–908.

[55] Cooper IS, Amin I, Gilman S. The effect of chronic cerebellar stimulation upon epilepsy in man. Trans Am Neurol Assoc 1973;98:192–6.

[56] Baldermann JC, Schüller T, Huys D, et al. Deep Brain Stimulation for Tourette-Syndrome: A Systematic Review and Meta-Analysis. Brain Stimul 2016;9(2):296–304.

[57] Holtzheimer PE, Husain MM, Lisanby SH, et al. Subcallosal cingulate deep brain stimulation for treatment-resistant depression: a multisite, randomised, sham-controlled trial. Lancet Psychiatry 2017;4(11):839–49.

[58] Lipsman N, Lam E, Volpini M, et al. Deep brain stimulation of the subcallosal cingulate for treatment-refractory anorexia nervosa: 1 year follow-up of an open-label trial. Lancet Psychiatry 2017;4(4):285–94.

[59] Wang J, Chang C, Geng N, et al. Treatment of intractable anorexia nervosa with inactivation of the nucleus accumbens using stereotactic surgery. Stereotact Funct Neurosurg 2013;91(6):364–72.

[60] McLaughlin NC, Didie ER, Machado AG, et al. Improvements in anorexia symptoms after deep brain stimulation for intractable obsessive-compulsive disorder. Biol Psychiatry 2013;73(9):e29–31.

[61] Chen L, Li N, Ge S, et al. Long-term results after deep brain stimulation of nucleus accumbens and the anterior limb of the internal capsule for preventing heroin relapse: An open-label pilot study. Brain Stimul 2019; 12(1):175–83.

[62] Kuhn J, Gründler TO, Bauer R, et al. Successful deep brain stimulation of the nucleus accumbens in severe alcohol dependence is associated with changed performance monitoring. Addict Biol 2011;16(4):620–3.

[63] Luo Y, Sun Y, Tian X, et al. Deep Brain Stimulation for Alzheimer's Disease: Stimulation Parameters and Potential Mechanisms of Action. Front Aging Neurosci 2021; 13:619543.

[64] Koek RJ, Langevin JP, Krahl SE, et al. Deep brain stimulation of the basolateral amygdala for treatment-refractory combat post-traumatic stress disorder (PTSD): study protocol for a pilot randomized controlled trial with blinded, staggered onset of stimulation. Trials 2014;15:356.

[65] Lavano A, Guzzi G, Della Torre A, et al. DBS in Treatment of Post-Traumatic Stress Disorder. Brain Sci 2018;8(1): 18.

[66] Videnovic A, Metman LV. Deep brain stimulation for Parkinson's disease: prevalence of adverse events and need for standardized reporting. Mov Disord 2008; 23(3):343–9.

[67] Hamani C, Richter E, Schwalb JM, et al. Bilateral subthalamic nucleus stimulation for Parkinson's disease: a systematic review of the clinical literature. Neurosurgery 2005;56(6):1313–24.

[68] Scelzo E, Mehrkens JH, Bötzel K, et al. Deep Brain Stimulation during Pregnancy and Delivery: Experience from a Series of "DBS Babies. Front Neurol 2015;6:191.

[69] Ziman N, Coleman RR, Starr PA, et al. Pregnancy in a series of dystonia patients treated with deep brain stimulation: outcomes and management recommendations. Stereotact Funct Neurosurg 2016;94(1):60–5.

[70] Bóné B, Kovács N, Balás I, et al. Pregnancy and deep brain stimulation therapy for epilepsy. Epileptic Disord 2021;23(4):633–8.

Advances in Psychiatry and Behavioral Health 2 (2022) 231–239

ADVANCES IN PSYCHIATRY AND BEHAVIORAL HEALTH

The Interface Between Psychiatry and Palliative Medicine

Avani Prabhakar, MD[a,*], Lisa MacLean, MD[b]

[a]Section of Palliative Medicine, Division of General Internal Medicine, Department of Medicine, Johns Hopkins University School of Medicine, 600 North Wolfe Street, Blalock 359, Baltimore, MD 21287, USA; [b]Henry Ford Health System, One Ford Place, 1C, Detroit, MI 48202, USA

KEYWORDS

• Palliative medicine • Psychiatry • Curriculum • Palliative psychiatry

KEY POINTS

- Palliative medicine requires addressing total pain recognizing the whole patient and attending to physical, psychological, spiritual, or social needs.
- The availability of expertise from mental health professionals and a recognized pathway for referral is important within palliative medicine.
- Palliative medicine clinicians would benefit from training in psychiatry and vice versa; psychiatry clinicians would benefit from training in palliative medicine.
- Consultation-liaison psychiatrists should be part of the medical team caring for patients with severe persistent mental illness who are with terminal illness.

INTRODUCTION

With modern medicine, diagnoses that caused death in days to weeks have now become chronic diseases, potentially curable, and patients are living longer. Sadly, despite this lengthening of life, the medical, psychological, spiritual, and social needs during the illness journey are unmet by health care systems, which can negatively affect the patient's and families' quality of life. Palliative care, as defined by the center for advanced palliative care [1], is "specialized medical care for people living with a serious illness. This type of care is focused on providing relief from the symptoms and stress of the illness. The goal is to improve quality of life for both the patient and the family. Palliative care is provided by a specially trained team of doctors, nurses, and other specialists who work together with a patient's other doctors to provide an extra layer of support. Palliative care is based on the needs of the patient, not on the patient's prognosis. It is appropriate at any age and at any stage in a serious illness, and it can be provided along with curative treatment" (Figs. 1 and 2).

The literature supports that there is considerable suffering that occurs for many patients in their last days to months of life due to frequent hospitalizations and extensive medical utilization [2,3]. For many, there is considerable pain. The concept of total pain and the importance of attending to psycho-social-existential domains of serious illness is key to addressing the whole patient in palliative care [4].

Total pain is a common, multidimensional symptom that compromises quality of life for many patients with serious illness. Understanding the concept of total pain and its dimensions is critical for clinicians caring for patients facing a serious illness. Treatable suffering caused by social, psychological, and spiritual components may get missed or overmedicated if the focus is solely on pharmacologically or procedurally treating physical pain (Fig. 3).

*Corresponding author, *E-mail address:* apatel26@jhmi.edu

https://doi.org/10.1016/j.ypsc.2022.03.007

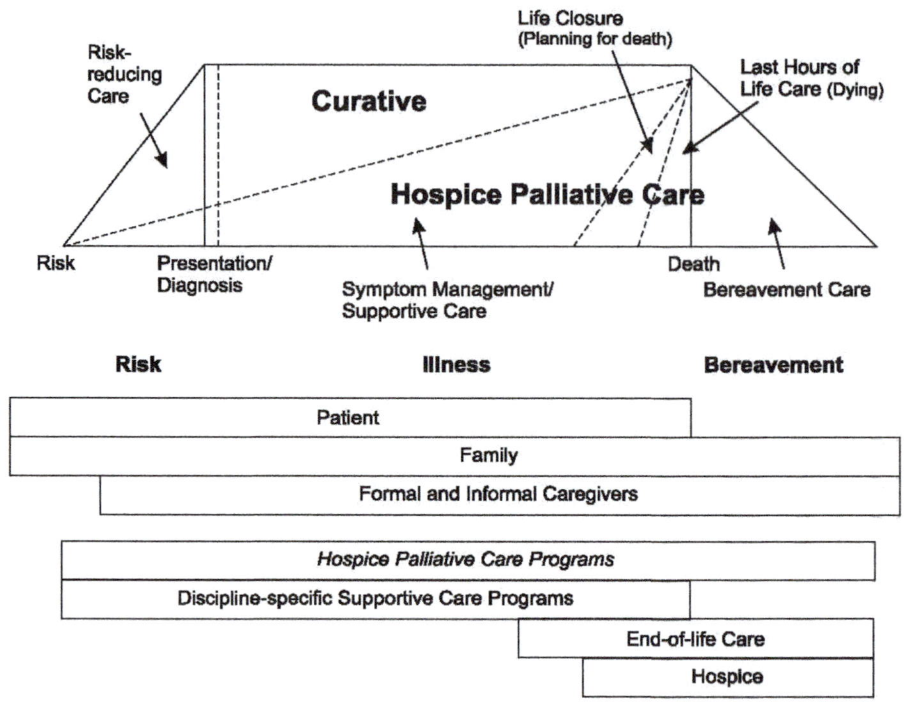

FIG. 1 Continuum of curative modalities and palliative care. (*From* Festic E, Grewal R, Rabatin JT, Divertie GD, Shannon RP, Johnson MM. End-of-life care in the intensive care unit: the perceived barriers, supports, and changes needed. Acta Medica Academica 2010;39:150-8; with permission.)

Although 90% of Americans prefer to die at home, 60% to 80% die in institutional settings [5–7]. Waiting for referral for palliative care when a patient's disease can no longer be cured adds to the burden and suffering of the patient. Sadly, despite significant effort by palliative medicine to recognize this and to minimize overall suffering, the organ that is most often negatively affected is the brain, specifically the mind; this has been recognized by the National Institutes of Health who describe palliative care as a complex interdependence between the physical, social, psychological, and existential/spiritual needs of patients and their families [8]. Some would say, palliative medicine cannot be delivered without a focus on these factors and an understanding of how they affect the mind. And thus, advocating for and focusing attention on the mitigation and management of the psychological factors that affect patients is critical. It is the goal of the palliative care medicine specialist to help guide the patient through the last article of their life. There

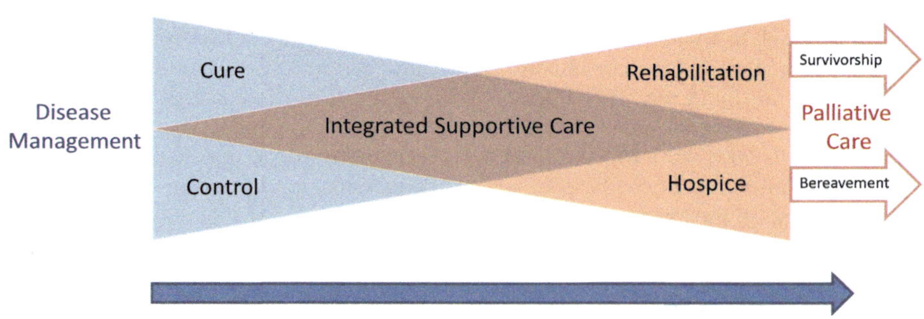

FIG. 2 Palliative care–enhanced care model. (*From* Hawley PH. The bow tie model of 21st century palliative care. J Pain Symptom Manage 2014;47:e2-5; with permission.)

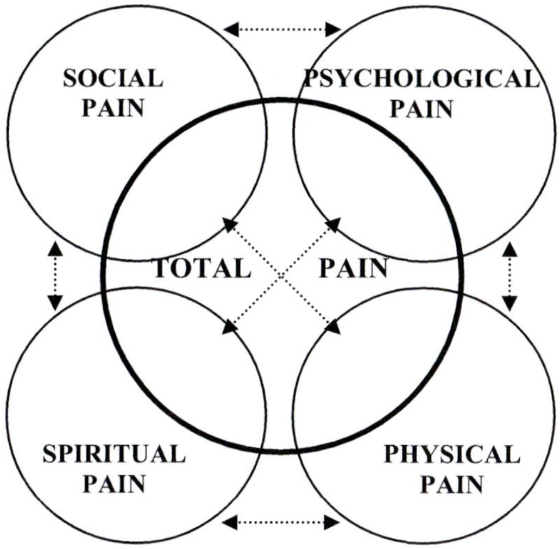

FIG. 3 Total pain diagram. (*From* Mehta A, Chan LS. Understanding of the concept of "total pain": a prerequisite for pain control. J Hosp Palliat Nurs 2008;10:26-32; with permission.)

can be no greater role than this in medicine. Thus, addressing this psychological impact is vital to providing the best care possible. In addition, knowing where to refer the patient if the palliative care specialist is not able to address these psychological needs is essential.

All physicians regardless of specialty should be able to provide basic palliative care including talking with patients and their families about their terminal illness, answering questions, inquiring about goals of care, and striving to alleviate suffering. These basic goals mean holistically attending to the whole person and their family, working to understand the experience of the illness, and prioritizing symptom relief and quality care. Psychiatrist clinicians are uniquely positioned to go beyond these basic goals and build further on these skills, with appropriate training focused on knowledge, skills, and attitudes caring for seriously ill patients.

The literature supports that understanding psychiatry is an integral part of the practice of palliative medicine [9]. "Psychiatry is a branch of medicine focused on the diagnosis, treatment and prevention of mental, emotional and behavioral disorders" [10]. In years past, palliative care seldom involved psychiatrists. The reasons for this are unclear but could be due to a variety of reasons including not feeling that psychiatrists could offer much benefit or feeling that palliative medicine specialists can adequately address the psychological needs of patients [9]. Regardless of the reasons, there has been a growing interest in expanding the interface between psychiatry and palliative medicine from both sides. In addition, there has been agreement that both specialties need to learn from the other and work collaboratively to provide support, training, and advocacy. This article aims to explore the interface of palliative medicine and psychiatry, potential training opportunities, palliative psychiatry, and finally, the suggestion that CL psychiatry might be one way to address the specialized needs of the terminally ill patient with severe mental illness.

THE LINKS BETWEEN PALLIATIVE MEDICINE AND PSYCHIATRY

Psychiatry and palliative care share common ground in the biopsychosocial model and include teams of clinicians: multidisciplinary in psychiatry and interdisciplinary in palliative medicine [11]. Palliative care expands on the biopsychosocial model to include existential elements with a clear mention of care for patient and *the family* (Box 1, Table 1).

Balon and colleagues [12] note that psychiatry itself is a form of palliative care because psychiatric treatments are frequently focused on improving quality of life and many are not curative. The use of basic skills such as thorough and thoughtful communication around diagnosis, prognosis, symptom assessment and management, assessment of caregiver need, and referral for additional medical services are core to these specialties. There is open dialogue about the patient's distress and how best to manage it. Key behaviors such as a caring attitude, empathy, and optimism are useful in managing patients within each specialty. A key challenge for both is maintaining the therapeutic alliance, building trust, and showing a calm composed demeanor even in the face of extreme suffering. In each, the clinician must be person-centered and prioritize the patient's care agenda, striving to understand the patient's goals of care. The primary focus is not only on the physical pain but also on the emotional, spiritual, social, and experiential pain and suffering.

Although there have been significant strides in the development of the intersection between palliative medicine and psychiatry, there is still work to be done. Indeed, there is the continued need for work around ethical issues that arise within both fields–like the withdrawal of medical care in the presence of depression or other significant mental health issues [13,14]. There are also multiple opportunities to further build on the development of clinical care strategies, ethical practice models, and training opportunities.

BOX 1
Common elements of palliative medicine and psychiatry skill sets as relevant to interphase between palliative care and psychiatry

Both palliative medicine and psychiatry share following common elements as part of their specialty skill sets

- Engage in deliberate practice of therapeutic presence
- Bring calm presence to bear witness to patient's illness narrative
- Focus on communication, specifically listening as a key aspect of their practice
- Discuss with patients living with vulnerability
- Explore nuances of each human being's view on what makes life worth living
- Explores what sustains a person's sense of meaning and purpose

No doubt, each field is critically important to the other, and both fields share many common challenges, attitudes, and skills. Having knowledge about each of the fields will not only build on those challenges, attitudes, and skills but help the clinician be stronger. This article discusses where psychiatry and palliative medicine can benefit from crossing the bridge to integrate both fields' approaches to care for seriously ill patients.

TEACHING PALLIATIVE CARE TO PSYCHIATRY CLINICIANS

Unfortunately, historically, the number of psychiatrists entering palliative medicine has been low. Given the aging of the population and increasing clinical needs, the number of psychiatrists with palliative medicine board certification is woefully inadequate. Currently, there are not enough palliative medicine specialists with psychiatry training nor are there enough psychiatrists with palliative medicine training to meet our aging population. The option to rotate in palliative medicine might be an elective option at some academic centers but is rarely required. For trainees without any formal training in palliative care rotation, there is little opportunity to adopt a palliative care mindset into the thoughts or practice patterns of the general psychiatrist.

TABLE 1
Model and focus of care in palliative medicine and psychiatry

	Palliative medicine	Psychiatry
Model	Bio-psycho-social -existential	Bio-psycho-social
Focus of care	Patient and family	Patient

Results of a study performed at San Diego Hospice indicate that training opportunities in palliative care are lacking for psychiatry residents in the United States although residents report strong interest in this area. This study also found that psychiatry residents benefit as much as other disciplines from receiving palliative care training. Therefore, the need to offer such training within psychiatry residencies is highlighted and programs should welcome psychiatrists into palliative care [15]. The benefits of palliative care go beyond the scope of this article. However, there is a strong body of literature that supports that palliative care improves quality of care, reduces costs, provides good stewardship of resources, and improves patient survival [16–18]. Additional training in palliative medicine will help the clinician to grow and develop while improving patient care.

With the recognition of the limited number of specialty trained palliative care providers, a care model that emphasizes primary palliative care is essential. These are skills that all clinicians, especially psychiatrists, should have when caring for seriously ill patients [19]. Teaching psychiatrists about the palliative medicine aspects of care will only strengthen their ability to care for seriously ill patients and their families, including the dying. Further understanding the physical aspects of dying, how to relieve pain, manage fatigue, and eating issues will only enhance the psychiatrist's skill set and help them to be more fully prepared to manage and assist the dying patient. The key is providing a holistic approach that sensitively considers issues such as loss, grief, death, and dying. The explicit application of palliative care principles to psychiatric illnesses has the potential to improve quality of care, person-centeredness, and autonomy for these patients [11]. A representative set of skills for primary palliative care for all psychiatrists should include the items listed in Box 2 [19].

BOX 2
Skill set for all clinicians caring for seriously ill patients

- Basic management of pain and symptoms
- Basic discussions about
  - Prognosis
  - Goals of treatment
  - Suffering
  - Code status

The authors of this article note that psychiatry clinicians are inherently trained in some aspects of specialty palliative care by nature of their psychiatry training, which include the following:

- Management of more complex depression, anxiety, grief, and existential distress
- Assistance with conflict resolution regarding goals or methods of treatment
  - Within families
  - Between staff and families
  - Among treatment teams

Psychiatry clinicians should collaborate with pain, palliative medicine, and ethics consultants when managing following elements of palliative medicine:

- Management of refractory pain and other symptoms
- Assistance in addressing cases of near futility

Residency programs nationally should consider adding palliative medicine as a required rotation for all general psychiatry trainees so that psychiatrists are better prepared to manage all aspects of seriously ill and dying patients. In addition to providing care, psychiatry should participate in palliative medicine education, research, and advocacy, which will significantly benefit their patients, families, and health care systems worldwide.

TEACHING PSYCHIATRY TO PALLIATIVE MEDICINE SPECIALISTS

Psychiatrists bring a unique skill set to the treatment of the terminally ill patient and their skill set can only add to palliative medicine. They are especially qualified to provide dignity therapies and a variety of supportive and cognitive therapies to the dying that ease distress. Unfortunately, the severely anxious, profoundly depressed, and the delirious pose significant management uncertainty for any physician. And yet, these are everyday phenomena for the dying and common symptoms that any psychiatrist can manage. This knowledge and skills would be particularly beneficial for the palliative medicine specialist.

No doubt, there is need for educating palliative care clinicians in psychiatry. Early recognition of psychiatric disease and subsequent psychological distress can reduce the patients' overall distress and may improve the patient's physical illness. Targeted education of the palliative medical and nursing staff may help improve the rate of recognition of these disorders. Growing evidence indicates that psychosocial and psychiatric issues in patients with advanced life-threatening illness are prevalent, often unacknowledged, unassessed, undiagnosed, and undertreated across all health care settings and disciplines [20]. Although many palliative care experts have learned to manage numerous psychiatric issues, most are not experts at assessing, diagnosing, and treating complex situations.

Depression is the most studied mental disorder in seriously ill patients, commonly seen with advanced cancer, frequently untreated, associated with somatic symptoms, and it is known that patients can benefit from treatment of depression even in the last weeks of life [21–24]. Depression is more common in patients with advanced cancer than the general population [25]. Approximately 25% of palliative care patients have depression but many frequently go unrecognized and untreated [23]. One barrier may be that many doctors attribute the somatic symptoms of depression such as fatigue, poor appetite, weight loss, and insomnia to the cancer illness. In addition, diagnostic skills can be improved by recognizing that symptoms such as feelings of worthlessness, helplessness, and hopelessness, excessive or inappropriate guilt, and thoughts of self-harm are helpful in identifying a depression diagnosis in a terminally ill patient [21,26]. Sadly, depression screening tools are not used routinely [22]. Evidence suggests that patients identified as depressed even within the last 4 to 6 weeks of life may still benefit from treatment [23].

Thus, screening for mental illness, and depression in particular, is key to providing comprehensive palliative care. In addition, another recognized psychological issue in the intersection between palliative care and psychiatry is demoralization around end-of-life decision-making [13,14]. There is also the advanced symptom management that requires specialty level psychiatry education to co-manage with specialty level palliative care providers and anesthesia teams to support primary treatment team, such as ketamine for depression [27], and collaboration in careful attention to addressing total pain [4]. Including psychiatry education for palliative care specialists can advance their skills to recognize and meet the recognized gap of underrecognized depression, total pain, and end-of-life decision-making in seriously ill patients [28].

In addition, other psychiatric syndromes, such as anxiety and delirium, are also common in palliative care settings and frequently underrecognized or underappreciated and thus contribute a substantial burden of suffering for patients and families. There has been lessor work on the use of palliative medicine in the severely mentally ill. Learning more about all of these psychiatric disorders and incorporating diagnostic tools and treatment strategies will strengthen the skills of the palliative medicine specialist. This focused knowledge will help them to confidently manage these comorbid diseases, especially in settings where there is a shortage of mental health professionals to aid in the treatment of the dying patient.

AN EMERGING DISCIPLINE: PALLIATIVE CARE PSYCHIATRY

Lack of understanding of psychiatric illness in terminally ill patients has been a barrier for care [12]. From this, the discipline of palliative care psychiatry has emerged [9,32,29. This emerging discipline brings expertise in understanding the psychosocial dimensions of the human experience in the care of the seriously ill and their families. In this field, psychiatrists complete a fellowship in palliative medicine. Unfortunately, the lack of palliative care training opportunities for psychiatrists represents a large obstacle for the introduction of palliative psychiatry as one approach to the treatment of the severely mentally ill. Indeed, in the past, some have questioned the role of psychiatrists in palliative medicine and recommend that palliative medicine trainees just learn about psychiatry in order to fill this gap [9]. This approach is questionable, and it is recommended that psychiatrists, especially those whose work focuses on the interface between medicine and psychiatry (eg, CL work or psycho-oncology) have much to contribute to palliative care [29].

Psychiatrists certainly bring a unique skill set to the care of the seriously ill and dying patient. In terms of end-of-life care, just as with other psychiatric illnesses, a combination of psychotherapy and psychopharmacology is usually the best therapeutic intervention. Supportive psychotherapy by a skilled psychiatrist can provide a safe setting that encourages patients and families to share issues that may be causing suffering. Patients with limited life expectancy need therapies that act quickly. Psychiatrists have the knowledge and experience to use medications in an atypical, off-label way that may benefit these patients, such as stimulants for the rapid relief of depression [30] and first-generation antipsychotics for delirium [10,31]. Psychiatrists can also recommend other strategies such as modifying the environment, teaching family and staff helpful behaviors, providing ongoing support, and recommending other appropriate medications [10].

People with serious mental illness at the end of their lives are a unique and vulnerable population. Palliative medicine physicians need to be careful of diagnostic overshadowing where they attribute physical symptoms to the mental illness, resulting in delayed diagnosis and treatment. The ongoing challenge is to effectively identify and manage patients with serious mental illness and concomitant terminal diagnosis across diverse care settings so that this population has at least equivalent physical health outcomes and quality of life as patients without serious mental illnesses. Palliative medicine is often consulted when the goals of care shift to focus more on comfort and quality than cure. A psychiatrist can help to distinguish between grieving, a normal adjustment, and clinically significant depression.

Psychological issues can affect a person's sense of well-being and impair their ability to realize their full potential. A psychiatrist can help patients to explore issues around meaning and life course, intimacy in relationships, and concerns about treatment. Good management of these psychosocial and psychiatric issues often enables improved management and outcomes of the primary illness. Psychiatry can also be helpful in supporting families and helping them to process and manage their grief. Families often need help facing the loss, coping with their emotions, transitioning their roles and responsibilities, and rebuilding their lives. Helping patients and families maintain their dignity and providing comfort during this stressful period may help to prevent a prolonged grief response later. Death with dignity is something all people desire regardless of whether they have mental illness. Working with mentally ill patients at the end of life can be challenging and rewarding. Palliative psychiatry is a comprehensive way to approach these patients.

ONE POTENTIAL SOLUTION: ROLE OF THE CONSULTATION-LIAISON PSYCHIATRIST IN END-OF-LIFE CARE

Psychiatry clearly has a role to be an integral part of the palliative medicine team, or at least to be regularly involved in consulting roles, given the prevalence of anxiety, mood disorders, and delirium and the complex dynamic of individual and family issues in palliative care[32], this is especially true for patients suffering from severe persistent mental illness (SPMI). Integrating psychiatrists into interdisciplinary palliative care teams will lead to better results for patients and their families [28]. Overall, collaboration between the fields of psychiatry and palliative care has grown significantly in most developed countries over the last 2 decades [33], but there is still room for more growth.

Palliative care for physical illness in mental health patients is critical, given the multiple comorbidities and higher than average mortality rates of patients with SPMI [34]. Patients with SPMI are at risk for either therapeutic neglect or overly aggressive care. Approximately 4.5% of the population lives with SPMI [35]. Individuals with SPMI die approximately 15 to 25 years earlier than those without mental illness and have an all-cause mortality 3.7 times higher than that of the general population [36]. The high burden of SPMI suggests a need for a tailored palliative and end-of-life care.

CL psychiatrists are well positioned to fill this gap and improve the quality of end-of-life care for individuals with SPMI [37]. Quality of life can often be improved and suicide risk reduced when palliative support and attention take places in addition to curative or disorder-specific treatments; this can be especially important for people struggling with SPMI such as treatment refractory depression, severe schizophrenia, and severe anorexia. Indeed, individuals with SPMI have a heavy burden of serious medical illness and experience disparities in availability and kinds of end-of-life care. These barriers are complex and include patient factors such as problems with poor insight, underlying psychiatric symptoms, poor health literacy, and neurobiological differences in pain and symptom response [38]. In addition, health care factors such as health care providers lack of comfort caring for the SPMI or stigma about mentally ill patients can also contribute to poor quality care. Finally, sociocultural factors such as stable housing, poverty, and social supports can add to the burden [38].

CL psychiatrists are well suited to serve as champions for patients with SPMI who need palliative care. They have expertise in managing patients with complex comorbid medical and psychiatric issues clinically. They also have a system level appreciation of the care of such patients and the importance of collaboration with specialty palliative care providers [39]. In particular, CL psychiatrists can help medical providers reframe their assumptions about the care of mentally ill patients, address the advance care planning gap, serve as advocates to involve long-term mental health providers in the end-of-life care, assist patients in assessing their social needs, ensure that psychiatric drug regimens are maintained, serve as advocates for mental care, and address patient suffering [40].

CL psychiatrists are needed to be part of that multidisciplinary team and can help team members to feel better prepared to work with challenging patients and alleviate their negative responses to them. Setting boundaries can be helpful in minimizing disruptive behaviors and reducing staff burnout. CL psychiatrists, when available, add significant benefit to the health care team especially when the patient is struggling with SPMI.

SUMMARY

Palliative care is not just for patients after all curative interventions have been tried. Palliative care's focus is on the quality of life of patients and families and the mitigation of suffering. Palliative care is unevenly available, and there is an insufficient number of trained subspecialists to meet the need [41]. There is value in close engagement of psychiatrists with palliative care teams. There is a clear need for more effective interventions that quickly mitigate depression, address total pain, reduce anxiety, prevent delirium, and minimize agitation. We need to continue to develop learning opportunities for both sides to show that we recognize the value that each can bring to the others. Caring for patients with psychiatric disorders at the end of life is complex, given the nature of psychiatric symptoms and how they affect interactions between the provider, the patient, and their family. When possible, a CL psychiatrist or a palliative care psychiatrist would be a valuable contributor to any health care team.

CLINICS CARE POINTS

- Patients receiving palliative care often have depression that frequently goes undiagnosed.
- Screening for mental illness is key to providing comprehensive palliative care.
- Demoralization around end-of-life decision-making needs to be recognized and appropriately addressed.
- Anxiety and delirium contribute to significant suffering for patients and families receiving palliative care.

DISCLOSURE

The authors have nothing to disclose.

REFERENCES

[1] Center to advance palliative care. About palliative care. 2021. Available at: https://www.capc.org/about/palliative-care/. Accessed December 13, 2021.

[2] Lubitz J, Prihoda R. The use and costs of Medicare services in the last 2 years of life. Health Care Financ Rev 1984;5:117–31.

[3] Lynn J, Harrell F Jr, Cohn F, et al. Prognoses of seriously ill hospitalized patients on the days before death: implications for patient care and public policy. New Horiz 1997;5:56–61.

[4] Prabhakar A, Smith TJ. Total Pain #417. J Palliat Med 2021;24:1100–1.

[5] Hogan C, Ginsburg PB, Gabel JR. Tracking health care costs: inflation returns. Health Aff (Millwood) 2000;19: 217–23.

[6] Lunney JR, Lynn J, Hogan C. Profiles of older medicare decedents. J Am Geriatr Soc 2002;50:1108–12.

[7] Seidlitz L, Duberstein PR, Cox C, et al. Attitudes of older people toward suicide and assisted suicide: an analysis of Gallup Poll findings. J Am Geriatr Soc 1995;43:993–8.

[8] National Institute on Aging. What are palliative care and hospice care?. 2021. Available at: https://www.nia.nih.gov/health/what-are-palliative-care-and-hospice-care. Accessed December 16, 2021.

[9] Macleod AD. Palliative medicine and psychiatry. J Palliat Med 2013;16:340–1.

[10] American Psychiatric Association. What is psychiatry?. 2021. Available at: https://www.psychiatry.org/patients-families/what-is-psychiatry-menu. Accessed December 13, 2021.

[11] Trachsel M, Irwin SA, Biller-Andorno N, et al. Palliative psychiatry for severe persistent mental illness as a new approach to psychiatry? Definition, scope, benefits, and risks. BMC Psychiatry 2016;16:260.

[12] Balon R, Motlova LB, Beresin EV, et al. A case for increased medical student and psychiatric resident education in palliative care. Acad Psychiatry 2016;40: 203–6.

[13] Kissane DW. The contribution of demoralization to end of life decisionmaking. Hastings Cent Rep 2004;34: 21–31.

[14] Kissane DW. Demoralization: a life-preserving diagnosis to make for the severely medically ill. J Palliat Care 2014; 30:255–8.

[15] Irwin SA, Montross LP, Bhat RG, et al. Psychiatry resident education in palliative care: opportunities, desired training, and outcomes of a targeted educational intervention. Psychosomatics 2011;52:530–6.

[16] Kelley AS, Deb P, Du Q, et al. Hospice enrollment saves money for Medicare and improves care quality across a number of different lengths-of-stay. Health Aff (Millwood) 2013;32:552–61.

[17] Temel JS, Greer JA, Muzikansky A, et al. Early palliative care for patients with metastatic non-small-cell lung cancer. N Engl J Med 2010;363:733–42.

[18] Yennurajalingam S, Urbauer DL, Casper KL, et al. Impact of a palliative care consultation team on cancer-related symptoms in advanced cancer patients referred to an outpatient supportive care clinic. J Pain Symptom Manage 2011;41:49–56.

[19] Quill TE, Abernethy AP. Generalist plus specialist palliative care–creating a more sustainable model. N Engl J Med 2013;368:1173–5.

[20] Irwin SA, Rao S, Bower K, et al. Psychiatric issues in palliative care: recognition of depression in patients enrolled in hospice care. J Palliat Med 2008;11:158–63.

[21] Casey PR. Depression in the dying - disorder or distress? Prog Palliat Care 1994;2:1–3.

[22] Lawrie I, Lloyd-Williams M, Taylor F. How do palliative medicine physicians assess and manage depression. Palliat Med 2004;18:234–8.

[23] Maguire P. Improving the detection of psychiatric problems in cancer patients. Soc Sci Med 1985;20: 819–23.

[24] Wasteson E, Brenne E, Higginson IJ, et al. Depression assessment and classification in palliative cancer patients: a systematic literature review. Palliat Med 2009; 23:739–53.

[25] Block SD. Assessing and managing depression in the terminally ill patient. ACP-ASIM end-of-life care consensus panel. american college of physicians - american society of internal medicine. Ann Intern Med 2000;132:209–18.

[26] Endicott J. Measurement of depression in patients with cancer. Cancer 1984;53:2243–9.

[27] Iglewicz A, Morrison K, Nelesen RA, et al. Ketamine for the treatment of depression in patients receiving hospice care: a retrospective medical record review of thirty-one cases. Psychosomatics 2015;56:329–37.

[28] Irwin SA, Ferris FD. The opportunity for psychiatry in palliative care. Can J Psychiatry 2008;53:713–24.

[29] Strouse T. Palliative medicine and psychiatry: a reply. J Palliat Med 2013;16:1166–7.

[30] Homsi J, Nelson KA, Sarhill N, et al. A phase II study of methylphenidate for depression in advanced cancer. Am J Hosp Palliat Care 2001;18:403–7.

[31] Breitbart W, Tremblay A, Gibson C. An open trial of olanzapine for the treatment of delirium in hospitalized cancer patients. Psychosomatics 2002;43:175–82.

[32] Fairman N, Irwin SA. Palliative care psychiatry: update on an emerging dimension of psychiatric practice. Curr Psychiatry Rep 2013;15:374.

[33] Meier DE, Beresford L. Growing the interface between palliative medicine and psychiatry. J Palliat Med 2010; 13:803–6.

[34] Thornicroft G. Physical health disparities and mental illness: the scandal of premature mortality. Br J Psychiatry 2011;199:441–2.

[35] National Institute of Mental Health. Mental illness. 2021. Available at: https://www.nimh.nih.gov/health/statistics/mental-illness. Accessed December 13, 2021.

[36] Olfson M, Gerhard T, Huang C, et al. Premature mortality among adults with schizophrenia in the United States. JAMA Psychiatry 2015;72:1172–81.

[37] Shalev D, Docherty M, Spaeth-Rublee B, et al. Bridging the behavioral health gap in serious illness care: challenges and strategies for workforce development. Am J Geriatr Psychiatry 2020;28:448–62.

[38] Terpstra TL, Williamson S. Palliative care for terminally ill individuals with borderline personality disorder. J Psychosoc Nurs Ment Health Serv 2019;57:24–31.

[39] Shalev D, Nash SS, Levenson JA, et al. Palliative care training for consultation-liaison psychiatry fellows: a national survey project. Psychosomatics 2020;61:336–42.

[40] Shalev D, Fields L, Shapiro PA. End-of-life care in individuals with serious mental illness. Psychosomatics 2020;61:428–35.

[41] Morrison RS, Meier DE. Clinical practice. Palliative care. N Engl J Med 2004;350:2582–90.

Advances in Psychiatry and Behavioral Health 2 (2022) 241–251

ADVANCES IN PSYCHIATRY AND BEHAVIORAL HEALTH

Introduction to Dialectical Behavior Therapy for Psychiatrists and Psychiatry Residents

Andrea L.B. Gottlieb, PhD[a,*], Christopher L. Klinger, LCSW-C[b], Daniela Sampaio, MD[a,c]

[a]Sheppard Pratt, 6501 North Charles Street, Baltimore, MD 21204, USA; [b]Dialectical Behavior Therapy Program, Sheppard Pratt, 6501 North Charles Street, Baltimore, MD 21204, USA; [c]Psychiatry Residency Program, University of Maryland, 22 South Greene Street, Baltimore, MD 21201, USA

KEYWORDS

• Dialectical behavior therapy • Suicide • Behavioral therapy • Psychiatry training

KEY POINTS

- Dialectical behavior therapy (DBT) principles and strategies can be learned during residency training.
- Psychiatrists' awareness of comprehensive DBT is of benefit to both the provider and the patient.
- Some DBT principles can be applied to non-DBT treatments flexibly.

INTRODUCTION

Psychotherapy training is an integral part of psychiatry residency. Exposure to various modalities of psychotherapy not only constitutes a well-rounded experience but also enables psychiatry trainees to better address patient's needs. Dialectical behavior therapy (DBT) is a treatment commonly used in psychotherapy for people with complex psychiatric presentations, as it treats a core problem of emotion dysregulation. Some examples of these presentations include borderline personality disorder (BPD), suicide and self-harm symptoms, trauma disorders, and presentations with multiple comorbidities, to name a few. BPD, arguably the most common diagnosis associated with the application of DBT, is seen in about 15% to 28% psychiatric outpatients [1]. Nonsuicidal self-injury (NSSI) has a lifetime prevalence of about 6% [2] meaning that, in the United States alone, about 20 million persons will engage in this behavior at some point of their lives. With the expansion of availability and access to DBT programs as well as growing evidence supporting the benefits of DBT for specific populations [3–5], there is a growing need for psychiatry residents to learn about this comprehensive and evidence-based treatment.

WHAT IS DIALECTICAL BEHAVIOR THERAPY?

DBT was originally created by Marsha Linehan, PhD to treat chronic suicidality and individuals with BPD [6]. Therefore, it was designed to manage patients with a history of frequent suicidal thoughts and behaviors, nonsuicidal self-injury, and frequent hospitalizations [5]. DBT is classified as a type of cognitive behavioral therapy and brings together acceptance and change through dialectics, a term to describe a synthesis of opposites. In modern descriptions, one of the main goals of treatment involves improvement in chronic emotion dysregulation. However, DBT has a comprehensive approach that involves integration of skills in one's life and focuses on 4 modules—core mindfulness, distress tolerance, emotion regulation, and

*Corresponding author, *E-mail address:* andreagottliebphd@gmail.com

https://doi.org/10.1016/j.ypsc.2022.03.008
2667-3827/22/

ABBREVIATIONS

DBT	Dialectical Behvaior Therapy
BPD	Borderline Personality Disorder
NSSI	Nonsuicidal Self-Injury

interpersonal effectiveness. Each of these skills modules focuses on a specific goal.

DIALECTICAL BEHAVIOR THERAPY IS A SET OF FLEXIBLE PRINCIPLES

DBT is evidence based and follows an overall structure. However, DBT is not a set of procedures guiding the exact nature and path of each patient's DBT treatment. Some describe DBT as being similar to kelp in the ocean with strong and stable foundation holding together many flexible and flowing outgrowths. Although DBT is initially taught to clinicians through books and trainings, there is no specific outline, session-by-session, as other manualized treatments. For the individual therapy, a therapist uses the principles of DBT to determine the treatment course for each therapist-patient pair. Therefore, individual DBT therapy is highly malleable and individualized. In addition, the training manuals provide information about strategies for individual therapy sessions and material for teaching and practicing concepts and skills. Therefore, even the group therapy mode of DBT is a fluid learning experience.

SUMMARY OF EFFICACY AND EFFECTIVENESS OF DIALECTICAL BEHAVIOR THERAPY

Robust evidence shows that DBT is effective in treating various complex psychiatric problems. In addition to a diagnosis of BPD [3,4], DBT shows effectiveness in treating symptoms of bipolar affective disorder, major depressive disorder, and anxiety disorders [7,8]. Further, there is substantial support for the use of DBT to treat individuals with symptoms such as suicidal and parasuicidal behaviors, binge eating behaviors, and substance use disorders, particularly when these behaviors are inadvertently recruited to manage difficult emotions [9–11]. In general, research has supported that standard DBT is effective for individuals experiencing chronic emotion dysregulation and complex-difficult to treat mental health problems. DBT leads to symptom reduction [12,13] and decrease the need for a higher level of psychiatric care such as hospitalizations and emergency room visits [3].

BENEFITS OF TRAINING PSYCHIATRISTS IN DIALECTICAL BEHAVIOR THERAPY

Prevalent psychiatric problems such as suicidal behavior, NSSI, BPD, and posttraumatic stress disorder (PTSD) are linked to substantial subjective distress and interpersonal difficulties, and proper management by psychiatrists is critical in reducing the burden associated with these conditions. Patients with emotional dysregulation may pose challenges including intense emotions toward the provider, potential feelings of failure and frustration in those providing care, and stigmatization of patients. Fortunately, residency training offers a unique opportunity to expand and improve a therapeutic armamentarium of psychiatry trainees.

Teaching DBT to residents and psychiatrists is not only needed but also feasible and welcomed by the stakeholders. Several previous studies of psychiatric residents who underwent training in DBT demonstrate that they go on to incorporate the learned skills in clinical settings and noted that the training improved their confidence in managing patients with BPD and NSSI, while decreasing judgmental attitudes toward persons with BPD [14,15]. Moreover, psychiatry residents and psychiatrists have identified the management of individuals with BPD and suicidal behavior as areas where they need further training [16,17]. DBT education can help fill these training gaps. Therefore, symptom-focused DBT strategies can improve psychiatrists' ability to deal with a wide variety of patients including those with affective disorders, anxiety disorders, substance use disorders, impulse control disorders, trauma-related disorders, and even in patients with subsyndromal presentations.

DIALECTICAL BEHAVIOR THERAPY MODES

DBT consists of 4 core components (referred to in DBT as "modes"): (1) individual outpatient psychotherapy, (2) skills training group, (3) consultation team meetings for therapists, and (4) telephone consultation for patients. Each of these modes serves a specific and complementary function.

Individual therapy has 2 key functions: first, to address specific needs of the client, assisting them in replacing maladaptive behaviors with more effective responses and second, to increase patient's motivation both to engage in treatment and put learned interventions into practice. DBT skills training focuses on patient's acquisition of DBT skills. The skills training curriculum takes approximately 6 months to deliver [18], and patients in standard DBT are required to attend group for at least the first year of their treatment to learn skills in 4 modules.

Core mindfulness skills aim to increase patient's awareness of their internal and external experience, improving their ability to recognize their affective state, control their attention better, and to live life in an effective manner. Distress tolerance skills increase patients' capacity in tolerating and accepting pain in their lives, helping them to decrease impulsive, harmful behaviors that interfere with their long-term goals. Emotion regulation skills provide tools for patients to identify and validate their emotions and to decrease the intensity and duration of painful emotions without avoiding or escaping. Finally, interpersonal effectiveness skills help patients identify their priorities in specific interpersonal situations and offers a framework to obtain their desired outcomes related to their objectives, relationships, and sense of self-respect [6]. Phone consultation (also known as phone coaching) serves to increase patient's ability to assertively address their needs, generalize skills use between session, and address issues within the therapeutic relationship. Finally, case consultation meetings (also referred to as consultation team or "teams") address therapist burnout by improving therapist's responses to their patient's behaviors and increase the effectiveness of their delivery of DBT. Patients in standard DBT are required to attend weekly individual therapy and skills group, whereas DBT therapists conducting DBT are required to attend weekly consultation team meetings and be available to their patients for phone consultation outside of therapy [6,19].

In addition to these 4 modes, Linehan proposed ancillary treatments, including medication management, case management, and peer-run support groups (eg, 12-step programs) that support patient's treatment and goals. These services do not need to be provided by those with a DBT orientation, and, in the cases of psychopharmacology and inpatient hospitalization, there are specific procedures outlined for wider use [6].

DIALECTICAL BEHAVIOR THERAPY STAGES AND TARGETS

One of the central aims of DBT is to assist patients in structuring and organizing their lives, which, at the start of treatment, are often perceived as chaotic and punctuated by crises due to their chronic emotion dysregulation and associated behaviors. To this end, Linehan conceptualized a hierarchy of 5 treatment stages (Table 1). The 5 stages of DBT each have specific goals, as well as behavioral targets (behaviors to either increase or decrease) to achieve that overall goal of that stage. Target behaviors are also organized hierarchically and are categorized into 3 major classes: life-threatening behaviors, therapy-interfering behaviors, and quality-of-life–interfering behaviors. The most serious behaviors are targeted in stage 1 of DBT, particularly life-threatening behaviors (eg, suicidality, NSSI, and so forth and associated ideations/beliefs) and therapy-interfering behaviors (eg, nonattendance, noncollaborative behaviors, and so forth).

The first 2 stages of DBT are the only explicitly linear stages in DBT, as patients must be oriented and commit to DBT before beginning treatment. The pretreatment stage focuses on 2 main goals: (1) educating the patient about DBT principles and practices and (2) establishing a shared commitment between therapist and patient to treatment.

Part of building a commitment to DBT includes a discussion of the individual's life worth living goals (LWLGs), which is a combination of achievable goals, interpersonal connections, and actions that align with core values. This list of goals is tangible, specific, and spans multiple areas of life, acting to anchor treatment in several ways (Box 1). First, discussing this early in treatment helps build rapport through conversation about the patient's interests and wishes. Second, the therapist can align treatment goals and LWLGs to increase motivation for DBT. Last, knowing LWLGs aids the therapist in building a commitment—and recommitment over time—to engage in treatment and coping with difficult life situations and severe symptoms.

Following the pretreatment stage, most patients then move into stage 1 of DBT treatment, learning to control maladaptive behaviors that often offer temporary respite from their painful thoughts and emotions or are otherwise reinforced by their environments. Establishing this behavioral control in the presence of painful emotional cues is integral to moving onto stage 2.

Stage 2 focuses on reduction of emotional suffering through, for example, exposure and acceptance-based strategies. PTSD is commonly treated in stage 2 through evidence-based PTSD treatments [20–22].

Stage 3 and 4 of DBT are the least well defined of the DBT stages, without a specific curriculum or hierarchy of targets (indeed, stage 4 is not mentioned in Linehan's DBT manual). Generally, stage 3 involves establishing a sense of self-respect through achieving a patient's goals (often through problem solving and managing quality-of-life–interfering behaviors), whereas stage 4 focuses on cultivating behaviors that facilitate an increased personal and spiritual connection in their lives [19].

TABLE 1
Stages of dialectical behavior therapy

Stage	Goal
Pretreatment	Orienting patient to DBT and obtaining commitment to treatment
Stage 1	Establish control over life-threatening, therapy-interfering behaviors and significant life-interfering behaviors by increasing behavioral control through DBT skills
Stage 2	Decrease emotional suffering in the face of (though not limited to) avoidance, dissociative symptoms, guilt, shame, and self-invalidation
Stage 3	Increasing self-respect and achieving individual goals
Stage 4	Increasing fulfilment through expanding awareness and increasing sense of freedom

Adapted from Linehan MM. Cognitive-Behavioral Treatment of Borderline Personality Disorder. New York, NY: The Guilford Press; 1993; with permission.

COMPREHENSIVE DIALECTICAL BEHAVIOR THERAPY VERSUS DIALECTICAL BEHAVIOR THERAPY–INFORMED TREATMENT

Fidelity to the DBT model requires all 4 modes of treatment. This structure, often referred to as comprehensive DBT, has significant backing as an evidence-based intervention in both research and community settings for individuals with BPD [23–25]. Despite this documented efficacy, legitimate concerns exist regarding comprehensive DBT implementation in community settings. Some of the main barriers include insufficient training and supervision of clinicians to ensure adherence to the model, lack of adequate reimbursement for certain modes of DBT (particularly multihour skills groups and phone consultation for patients), and challenges related to staff retention due to work with potentially difficult-to-treat patients [26,27].

Recognizing these challenges, some practitioners have simplified the DBT curriculum, focusing exclusively on DBT skills training, to provide the core curriculum of skills in the most cost-effective manner possible. Although this modification does not provide the individualize application of skills found in comprehensive DBT, DBT skills training as a standalone treatment has shown modest efficacy in improving mental health symptoms, particularly depressive symptoms, in a community setting [28]. An additional category, commonly referred to as DBT-informed treatment, is a term used to describe a variety of services that may include DBT groups that do not strictly follow the manuals format, DBT skills training integrating into other individual psychotherapy, or other combination of only some components of comprehensive DBT.

Although DBT was initially conceptualized as an outpatient treatment, it has been modified for more intensive treatment settings including intensive outpatient, partial hospitalization, and inpatient programs.

BOX 1
Life worth living goals examples

Person 1

- Paint again
- Have time connecting with her children
- Improve relationship with her mother
- Get a promotion at work, to be a supervisor
- Be comfortable getting divorced

Person 2

- Sobriety
- Have my own house
- Fulling career (teacher, manager in sales, nursing school)
- Maintain relationships with family, make new relationships with friends
- Creativity
- Get library back
- Have a person to share things with

DBT-informed treatment has shown effectiveness in decreasing anxiety, depression, and hopelessness in an intensive outpatient program [29] and several partial hospitalization programs [30–32]. Although these studies show promise, it is notable that limited research has been done on the efficacy of DBT in these settings. In addition, DBT modifications have shown efficacy for both adults and adolescent inpatient programs [33–36].

DIALECTICAL BEHAVIOR THERAPY ORIENTATION TO PSYCHIATRIC MANAGEMENT

Role of the psychiatrist in comprehensive dialectical behavior therapy

In comprehensive DBT, the roles of primary therapist and of psychiatrists are separated, even if the therapist is a psychiatrist. The individual therapist is considered the primary mental health provider, being the one actively managing emotional crises and associated target behaviors including suicidal ideation, NSSI, substance use, and medication misuse. The psychiatrist, therefore, adopts an ancillary role to DBT, using evidence-based pharmacotherapy when indicated. Ultimately, one long-term goal when prescribing medications for patients enrolled in DBT is to minimize the use of rescue medication for regulation of emotions and behaviors and encouraging patients to use DBT skills to manage affective states.

Psychiatrists who provide care to patients in comprehensive DBT programs must be aware of the uniqueness of the patients they are assisting and the clinical challenges that they might face:

- Severe and chronic emotion dysregulation may influence patients' symptoms presentation and their response to treatment. For example, a depressed patient with BPD may require a different medication regimen than a depressed patient without BPD. Thus, it is of extreme importance for psychiatrists to be familiar with current research literature on pharmacotherapy for this patient population.
- The prevalence of substance use problems in patients with severe emotion dysregulation and impulse control problems is high. Studies have estimated that nearly two-thirds of patients with BPD will be affected by a substance use disorder in their lifetime [37]. With that in mind, medications with potential for misuse, such as benzodiazepines, should be used cautiously or not at all with DBT patients.
- DBT patients tend to struggle with suicidal ideation, suicide behaviors, and chronic hopelessness. Prescribing strategies must provide patients with an effective treatment without prescribing drugs, or amounts of drugs, that could be potentially harmful if taken at once.

When treating such high-risk patients, providers will likely face situations where a hospitalization might be considered. In DBT, inpatient hospitalizations are avoided, when possible, with brief hospitalizations being reserved only for certain conditions; this is based on the lack of data suggesting that hospitalizations are effective in modifying long-term risk of suicide in this patient population [38,39] and other research suggesting iatrogenic effects of hospitalizations in this population [40,41].

PSYCHIATRY TRAINING MODALITIES

The following training modalities can be offered in increasing complexity to residents with interest in advancing their understanding of DBT. Psychiatry training programs that have an affiliation with a standard, comprehensive DBT program can offer a unique experience that includes full participation on a DBT team when possible. Although it is unlikely most trainees will experience, or even choose, this opportunity, when available it can significantly enrich a trainee's understanding of DBT concepts, as well as a solid foundation in how DBT principles guide the treatment of individuals with BPD, suicidality, chronic emotion dysregulation, and related presenting problems.

Traditional psychiatry residency training

The Accreditation Council for Graduate Medical Education (ACGME) is the institution responsible for accrediting residency and fellowship programs. The ACGME's current requirements for psychotherapy in psychiatry residency curricula is that residents "develop competence in ... applying supportive, psychodynamic, and cognitive behavioral psychotherapies to both brief and long-term practice" and that residents have "exposure to family, couples, group and other individual evidence-based psychotherapies" [42]. Despite the elevated rates of BPD in the inpatient and outpatient settings (reportedly around 20% and 10%, respectively) [43], few psychiatry programs provide training in DBT [15]. Surveys of US psychiatry residency programs have shown that although DBT is the most commonly taught form of intervention for BPD, most programs did not have lectures on DBT for residents, and only the minority of programs had didactics focusing on BPD [15]. For example, one survey found that 36% of the psychiatry residency programs have no lectures on DBT, 32% provide no DBT supervision, and 68% of program directors surveyed believed that residents would benefit from more exposure to DBT in their training [44]. Another survey showed that residents spent "none or less than 1 hour" monthly learning DBT, couples/family/group, and child psychotherapy [45].

Didactic learning

Psychotherapy trainees often learn about therapeutic modalities such as DBT as part of their classroom instruction. Traditional didactic education can offer an overview of DBT concepts, including different DBT principles and skills. Trainees are likely to encounter lectures given by faculty who have a range in DBT learning and knowledge, and didactic education by therapists working in standard DBT settings are ideal to teach these lectures.

The length of time allotted to providing lectures and the desired learning outcome likely guides what specific topics trainees learn, as there are countless hours—even days or weeks—worth of material to teach. Nevertheless, psychiatry trainees wanting to learn psychotherapeutic interventions for emotionally dysregulated patients would benefit from instruction in DBT skills. Moreover, there are numerous DBT principles that may benefit a range of psychiatric presentations, such as validation, dialectics, or behavioral assessment.

Observational learning

When comprehensive DBT is available to a trainee, observational learning can be implemented in a curriculum. Medical training often involves shadowing attendings as they provide treatment to patients. Modeling from type of observational learning after classroom instruction in DBT can provide psychiatrists a lens into the way therapists and/or skills trainers interact with patients.

Practical learning, supervision, and consultation

A more immersive experience, learning about DBT by doing the treatment, becomes available when trainees have an option for a rotation or elective in DBT with a comprehensive DBT team. An ideal DBT elective should include participating in all treatment components: (1) participating in a skills training group as a group co-leader with the opportunity to review homework, teach skills, and help patients as needed; (2) functioning as the primary therapist for several patients in stage 1 DBT; (3) providing skills coaching out of session as needed to these individual patients; and (4) attending a full-fidelity consultation team for the course of their time in the DBT elective.

Individual supervision in DBT is an important part of training, and supervisors act as a consultant and a teacher to trainees. Sessions may include observation of videotaped sessions, discussion of sessions and challenges faced, role play of therapeutic situations, and so forth. The supervision process is similar to the therapeutic one in terms of the application of a dialectical balance, the use of behavioral methods, and the balancing of acceptance and change. In addition to individual supervision, trainees participate in consultation meetings as part of the DBT team. The consultation meetings are an important aspect of the program that takes in consideration the challenges in working with such a difficult patient population. The support and guidance of the consultation team is important to assist therapists and trainees to manage the extreme responses of their patients by providing a dialectical balance.

DIALECTICAL BEHAVIOR THERAPY PRINCIPLES AND STRATEGIES

Biosocial theory

A foundational component of DBT is the biosocial theory, which helps in understanding of how people with pervasive difficulties in regulating emotions come to develop this problem. The theory states that biological underpinnings transact with environmental factors to—over time—lead to and/or perpetuate their emotion dysregulation. Biological susceptibility is often observed as greater emotional sensitivity, high reactivity to emotion cues, and slower return to emotional baseline. On the other hand, environmental factors such as chronic invalidation, poor fit between caregivers and the individual during formative developmental times, a surrounding system that believes one's personal attributes are wrong, and trauma can play a significant role in elevating already poor emotion regulation capabilities.

Case scenario: imagine a young child struggling with their gender identity in a community upholding the importance of traditional gender roles. In addition, this child was born to parents who are treated for generalized anxiety disorder and dysthymia with significant irritability. Whenever this youth attempts to talk to their parents about their feelings, parents encourage them to ignore their worries for now as "you're still a kid, just go play with friends." Over the years, such interactions pair with mutterings about "those gay and transgender people." The child learns through these situations (1) to not share their private experience with others in various forms, (2) that emotions are also not to be shared, (3) that their environment may judge them if they outwardly discuss gender identity curiosities.

Validation

The lives of individuals with high emotion dysregulation, past trauma, and suicidality—many of the problems that people in DBT are faced with—are fraught with much invalidation from the world around them. Therefore, as Linehan has written, "it would be difficult to overestimate the importance of validation in DBT" as a strategy used and taught often [46]. Validation is acknowledging the validity of someone else's inner truths.

In DBT, therapists are constantly searching for what is valid through different levels and contexts (Table 2); patients are taught to validate themselves and others. Validation is provided for thoughts, behaviors, emotions, life limits, symptoms, experiences, and the individual themselves, even when it may be necessary to correct their behavioral response. Past, current, and present context also provide frameworks for understanding how to validate. For example, a lifetime of criticism from caregivers (ie, past context) can affect the way someone interprets critique from a close friend (ie, current context).

It is important to differentiate validation from other related concepts. Although empathy is often felt as validating, empathy toward another's internal emotional experience yet does not require communicating this as validation does. In addition, validation does not connote liking or "being OK with" something. Instead, to validate, one has to acknowledge truths regardless of their opinions or judgments. Finally, DBT teaches to only validate what is valid. One essential way this shows up in treatment is, on the one hand, verbalizing understanding for the presence of suicide urges and what led to the presence of or increase in this symptom while, on the other hand, firmly expressing that suicide is not a solution to life's problems and is, therefore, not valid.

Behavioral assessment and management

Case scenario: a person you've been seeing for months continues to act on binge eating urges after months of "trying to stop." When you talk with her about this behavior, conversation often leads to body image concerns and desire to have control over her life. One day, you realize you need to try a different approach. You think: "What exactly does she mean by a binge?" "How much food does she consume at once?" "How often is this happening?" And then you question your conceptualization as well, "Why is she bingeing if she wishes to be thinner; the body image concerns don't seem to line up with increasing food intake" you realize," and "She keeps saying she wants to stop bingeing, we make a plan for skills to use to stop bingeing, and yet she continues to engage in this behavior."

As a behavioral treatment founded on tenants of radical behaviorism, including the teachings of behaviorist John Watson, B. F. Skinner, Ivan Pavlov, and Albert Badura, DBT heavily relies on thorough assessment of a behavior to treat it and basic principles of behaviorism (eg, reinforcement, shaping, and extinction; Table 3).

The treatment is built by using specific tools to assess behaviors: (1) the diary card is used to track each individual's behaviors and emotions. Made to fit each person's specific treatment goals, they are malleable and editable. Using a diary card helps patient and therapist assess presence of and change in life-threatening behavior urge and actions, behaviors to increase, emotions, and skills use, among other items. (2) A behavior chain analysis (BCA) is used to assess and understand what leads to the presence of a target behavior. BCA is a lengthy semistructured set of questions the therapist and person collaborate to complete. The purpose of the BCA is to determine factors leading to or maintaining the target behavior and to, then, pair skillful solutions with links in the chain. This tool starts with details about the target behavior, moving to possible vulnerabilities and the event prompting the behavior, and then into the specific links (actions, body sensations, cognitions/thoughts, events, and feelings) from the prompting event to the behavior being chained. The chain culminates with prevention planning, skillful solutions, and repairs with others if needed. (3) A missing links analysis helps determine why an expected behavior does not occur (eg, follow through on bringing up an important conversation with family, completing therapy homework). In a missing links analysis, the therapist helps the patient go through a set of questions to elucidate why the behavior did not occur, such as not remembering to do it, willfulness around doing the behavior, not understanding what to do, emotion overload, myths about engaging in the behavior, and so forth.

As previously noted, many patients in DBT endorse chronic suicidal thoughts and urges and, over the course of their treatment, may experience periods of acute

TABLE 2
Levels of validation

Level of validation	Definition	Example
V1: Listening and observing	Being present, with active awareness. Paying attending with eyes and ears open.	Direct eye contact. Nodding head in agreement. Leaning in toward someone while talking.
V2: Accurate reflection	Restating what you've observed and heard. Understanding correctly.	"What I'm hearing is you are embarrassed, feeling shame." "You're overwhelmed by many emotions right now?"
V3: Articulating the unverbalized	What is present that isn't being said	"I wonder if you're also scared right now."
V4: Acknowledging through history	Understanding through past events, learning, or environment, or the person's biology	"You're talking about your friend cancelling plans yesterday. You care a lot about how this friend thinks about you and spending time together. I can see how this is disappointing for you."
V5: Acknowledging using current context	Understanding through the context of what is happening in the present. Imparting that the experience is in line with normative functioning.	"I hear this often from other parents as well. Your teenager's behaviors are new for you and pushing the limits. Of course, you're having to re-think consequences."
V6: Radical genuineness	Being a human interacting with another human. Imparting equality.	Using appropriate self-disclosure. In short, being yourself. "This would anger me as well. I would also have had a hard time holding back from my urges."

suicidality. Fortunately, many of DBT's assessment tools including diary cards and behavior chain analyses allow therapists to track monitor for these urges on a consistent basis. When patients endorse an increase in suicidal thoughts or urges, either in session or during phone coaching, DBT requires the therapist to conduct a thorough risk assessment. For example, the Linehan Risk Assessment and Management Protocol (LRAMP [47,48]), similar to DBT generally, is principle based, prompting the therapist to assess known risk factors for suicidal behavior and based on the assessment, recommends interventions both in session and afterward, to manage risk more effectively [49].

Considerations for out-of-session contact are also highly guided by principles of behaviorism. DBT therapists often consider possible or known reinforcers of behaviors, desire to shape behavior, and the principle of extinction when determining when and how to interact with patients between sessions. Complexities such as both (1) wanting people to learn to remember and use skills at times of high emotion dysregulation (shaping) and (2) knowing that being available immediately every time a person asks for it can reinforce *needing* the therapist to solve problems (continuous reinforcement).

Case scenario: a patient who screams at her partner often, has very high dissociative symptoms, and experiences frequent self-harm urges has been in DBT for 2 months. She has made progress in her self-harm urges with the use of phone coaching, specifically using distress tolerance skills and learning to observe and label her precipitating emotions. One day, a few days before the therapist is about to be out of town, the patient sends a message to the therapist telling her she is scared to lose the therapist and asks "why are you leaving me?" The therapist begins to think about the different guiding behavioral principles in relation to this current situation: (1) this patient has been shaped to use skills to avoid target behaviors; (2) this behavior is not wanted, and therapist does not want to increase

TABLE 3
Important behavioral principles

Term	Definition
Behavior	In DBT, anything that can increase or decrease is a behavior, including actions, thoughts, and emotions
Reinforcer	Something that increases the likelihood that a behavior will recur
Punisher	Something that decreases the likelihood that a behavior will recur
Extinction	The removal of a reinforce to decrease a behavior
Shaping	Taking successive steps toward a desired behavior
Modeling	Learning through observing an example of the behavior
Reinforcement schedules	Patterns of reinforcement based on speed and amount of times the reinforcer is used after a behavior occurs
Continuous reinforcement	Pattern of reinforcement based on using a reinforcer every time the behavior occurs
Intermittent reinforcement	Pattern of reinforcement based on using a reinforcer at random times or frequencies; most likely to maintain a behavior

the likelihood it occurs again; (3) punishing the behavior could have unwanted side effects, such as aversive experiences (thoughts, emotions) in patient.

SUMMARY

The authors have provided an overview of important aspects of DBT that psychiatrists and psychiatry trainees can learn and easily adopt in clinical practice. DBT is a comprehensive treatment that requires training in order to practice competently. The treatment is made up of a set of principles and procedures, such as tools for assessing behavior and the DBT treatment hierarchy. Thorough training in DBT is extensive and time consuming and therefore needs proper planning and investment from training programs. On the other hand, individuals can learn aspects of DBT in order to support patients in this treatment, apply DBT principles and procedure to psychiatry practice with chronically suicidal and emotionally dysregulated patients, and participate fully in an adherent DBT team, toward a fulfilling experience in clinical practice.

CLINICS CARE POINTS

- Residency programs should invest in helping ensure exposure and training in this valuable modality.
- Individual therapy component of DBT helps address patient's motivation to engage in treatment.
- DBT skills training focuses on patient's acquisition of skills to build resilience and address maladaptive behaviors.
- Phone consultations help with improvement in patient's ability to generalize skills use between session and address urgent issues.
- Case consultation meetings help address clinician burnout.

DISCLOSURE

The authors have nothing to disclose.

ACKNOWLEDGMENTS

We want to thank our teachers, trainers, including Shari Manning, PhD, who taught us the kelp metaphor, and mentors. We whole-heartedly thank our patients who put their trust in us. We also want to thank the rest of our outpatient DBT team at Sheppard Pratt, for their many contributions.

REFERENCES

[1] Gunderson JG, Herpertz SC, Skodol AE, et al. Borderline personality disorder. Nat Rev Dis Primers 2018;4(1):1–20.
[2] Klonsky ED. Non-suicidal self-injury in United States adults: prevalence, sociodemographics, topography and functions. Psychol Med 2011;41(9):1981–6.

[3] Linehan MM, Dimeff L, Koerner K, et al. Research on dialectical behavior therapy: summary of the data to date 2014 Available from. http://behavioraltech.org/downloads/research-on-dbt_summary-of-data-to-date.pdf.
[4] Storebø OJ, Stoffers-Winterling JM, Völlm BA, et al. Psychological therapies for people with borderline personality disorder. Cochrane Database Syst Rev 2020;5:CD012955. https://doi.org/10.1002/14651858.CD012955.pub2.
[5] Witt KG, Hetrick SE, Rajaram G, et al. Psychosocial interventions for self-harm in adults. Cochrane Database Syst Rev 2021;4:CD013668. https://doi.org/10.1002/14651858.CD013668.pub2.
[6] Linehan MM. Cognitive-behavioral treatment of borderline personality disorder. New York, NY: The Guilford Press; 1993.
[7] Lynch TR, Morse JQ, Mendelson T, et al. Dialectical behavior therapy for depressed older adults: a randomized pilot study. Am J Geriatr Psychiatry 2003;11(1):33–45.
[8] Neacsiu AD, Eberle JW, Kramer R, et al. Dialectical behavior therapy skills for transdiagnostic emotion dysregulation: a pilot randomized controlled trial. Behav Res Ther 2014; 59:40–51. https://doi.org/10.1016/j.brat.2014.05.005.
[9] Telch CF, Agras WS, Linehan MM. Dialectical behavior therapy for binge eating disorder. J Consult Clin Psychol 2001;69(6):1061–5. https://doi.org/10.1037/0022-006X.69.6.1061.
[10] Dimeff LA, Linehan MM. Dialectical behavior therapy for substance abusers. Addict Sci Clin Pract 2008;4(2): 39–47. https://doi.org/10.1151/ascp084239.
[11] Panos PT, Jackson JW, Hasan O, et al. Meta-Analysis and Systematic Review Assessing the Efficacy of Dialectical Behavior Therapy (DBT). Res Soc Work Pract 2014;24(2): 213–23. https://doi.org/10.1177/1049731513503047.
[12] Stoffers JM, Völlm BA, Rücker G, et al. Psychological therapies for people with borderline personality disorder. Cochrane Database Syst Rev 2012;2012(8):CD005652. https://doi.org/10.1002/14651858.CD005652.pub2.
[13] Linehan MM, Comtois KA, Murray AM, et al. Two-year randomized controlled trial and follow-up of dialectical behavior therapy vs therapy by experts for suicidal behaviors and borderline personality disorder. Arch Gen Psychiatry 2006;63(7):757–66. https://doi.org/10.1001/archpsyc.63.7.757.
[14] Frederick JT, Comtois KA. Practice of dialectical behavior therapy after psychiatry residency. Acad Psychiatry 2006; 30(1):63–8.
[15] Brodsky BS, Cabaniss DL, Arbuckle M, et al. Teaching dialectical behavior therapy to psychiatry residents: the Columbia Psychiatry Residency DBT curriculum. Acad Psychiatry 2017;41(1):10–5.
[16] Melton BB, Coverdale JH. What do we teach psychiatric residents about suicide? A national survey of chief residents. Acad Psychiatry 2009;33(1):47–50.
[17] Bodner E, Cohen-Fridel S, Mashiah M, et al. The attitudes of psychiatric hospital staff toward hospitalization and treatment of patients with borderline personality disorder. BMC psychiatry 2015;15(1):1–12.
[18] Linehan ML. DBT skills training manual. Second Edition. Guilford Press; 2015.
[19] Swenson CR. DBT® principles in action: acceptance, change, and dialectics. Guilford Press; 2016.
[20] Bohus M, Dyer AS, Priebe K, et al. Dialectical Behaviour Therapy for Post-traumatic Stress Disorder after Childhood Sexual Abuse in Patients with and without Borderline Personality Disorder: A Randomised Controlled Trial. Psychother Psychosom 2013;82:221–33.
[21] Harned MS, Korslund KE, Foa EB, et al. Treating PTSD in suicidal and self-injuring women with borderline personality disorder: Development and preliminary evaluation of a Dialectical Behavior Therapy Prolonged Exposure protocol. Behav Res Ther 2012;50:381–6.
[22] Harned MS, Korslund KE, Linehan MM. A pilot randomized controlled trial of Dialectical Behavior Therapy with and without the Dialectical Behavior Therapy Prolonged Exposure protocol for suicidal and self-injuring women with borderline personality disorder and PTSD. Behav Res Ther 2014;55:7–17.
[23] Linehan MM, Armstrong HE, Suarez A, et al. Cognitive-Behavioral Treatment of Chronically Parasuicidal Borderline Patients. Arch Gen Psychiatry 1991;48(12):1060–4. https://doi.org/10.1001/archpsyc.1991.01810360024003.
[24] Koons CR, Robins CJ, Tweed JL, et al. Efficacy of dialectical behavior therapy in women veterans with borderline personality disorder. Behav Ther 2001;32: 371–90.
[25] Verheul R, Van Den Bosch LM, Koeter MW, et al. Dialectical behaviour therapy for women with borderline personality disorder: 12-month, randomized clinical trial in The Nether- lands. Br J Psychiatry 2003;182:135–40.
[26] JU Blackford, Love R. Dialectical behavior therapy group skills training in a community mental health setting: a pilot study. Int J Group Psychother 2011;61(4):645–57. https://doi.org/10.1521/ijgp.2011.61.4.645.
[27] Valentine SE, Bankoff SM, Poulin RM, et al. The use of dialectical behavior therapy skills training as stand-alone treatment: a systematic review of the treatment outcome literature. J Clin Psychol 2015;71(1):1–20. https://doi.org/10.1002/jclp.22114.
[28] Harley R, Sprich S, Safren S, et al. Adaptation of dialectical behavior therapy skills training group for treatment-resistant depression. J nervous Ment Dis 2008;196(2):136–43.
[29] Ritschel LA, Cheavens JS, Nelson J. Dialectical behavior therapy in an intensive outpatient program with a mixed-diagnostic sample. J Clin Psychol 2012;68(3): 221–35. https://doi.org/10.1002/jclp.20863.
[30] Lenz AS, Del Conte G. Efficacy of dialectical behavior therapy for adolescents in a partial hospitalization program. J Couns Dev 2018;96(1):15–26. https://doi.org/10.1002/jcad.12174.
[31] Lothes JE II, Mochrie KD, Quickel EJ, et al. Evaluation of a dialectical behavior therapy-informed partial hospital program: outcome data and exploratory analyses. Research in Psychotherapy: Psychopathology, Process

and Outcome 2016;19(2). https://doi.org/10.4081/ripppo.2016.219.

[32] Mochrie KD, Lothes Ii J, Guender E, et al. DBT-informed treatment in a partial hospital and intensive outpatient program: the role of step-down care. Res Psychother 2020;23(2):461. https://doi.org/10.4081/ripppo.2020.461.

[33] Bohus M, Haaf B, Simms T, et al. Effectiveness of inpatient dialectical behavioral therapy for borderline personality disorder: a controlled trial. Behav Res Ther 2004;42(5):487–99. https://doi.org/10.1016/s0005-7967(03)00174.

[34] Katz LY, Cox BJ, Gunasekara S, et al. Feasibility of dialectical behavior therapy for suicidal adolescent inpatients. J Am Acad Child Adolesc Psychiatry 2004;43:276–82. Available at: http://www.ncbi.nlm.nih.gov/pubmed/15076260.

[35] McDonell MG, Tarantino J, Dubose AP, et al. A pilot evaluation of Dialectical behavioural therapy in adolescent long-term inpatient care. Child Adolesc Ment Health 2010;15:193–6.

[36] Tebbett-Mock AA, Saito E, McGee M, et al. Efficacy of Dialectical Behavior Therapy Versus Treatment as Usual for Acute-Care Inpatient Adolescents. J Am Acad Child Adolesc Psychiatry 2019. https://doi.org/10.1016/j.jaac.2019.01.020.

[37] Sansone RA, Sansone LA. Substance use disorders and borderline personality: common bedfellows. Innov Clin Neurosci 2011;8(9):10–3.

[38] Goodman M, Roiff T, Oakes AH, et al. Suicidal risk and management in borderline personality disorder. Curr Psychiatry Rep 2012;14(1):79–85. https://doi.org/10.1007/s11920-011-0249-4.

[39] Paris J. Suicidality in Borderline Personality Disorder. Medicina (Kaunas) 2019;55(6):223. https://doi.org/10.3390/medicina55060223.

[40] Coyle TN, Shaver JA, Linehan MM. On the potential for iatrogenic effects of psychiatric crisis services: The example of dialectical behavior therapy for adult women with borderline personality disorder. J Consult Clin Psychol 2018;86(2):116–24. https://doi.org/10.1037/ccp0000275.

[41] Ward-Ciesielski E, Rizvi S. The potential iatrogenic effects of psychiatric hospitalization for suicidal behavior: A critical review and recommendations for research. Clin Psychol Sci Pract 2020;28. https://doi.org/10.1111/cpsp.12332.

[42] ACGME Program Requirements for Graduate Medical Education in Psychiatry. Available at: https://www.acgme.org/Portals/0/PFAssets/ProgramRequirements/400_Psychiatry_2021.pdf?ver=2021-06-15-161510-003.

[43] Sansone RA, Kay J, Anderson JL. Resident didactic education in borderline personality disorder: is it sufficient? Acad Psychiatr 2013;37(4):287–8.

[44] Sharma B, Dunlop BW, Ninan PT, et al. Use of dialectical behavior behavior therapy in borderline personality disorder: a view from residency. Acad Psychiatr 2007;31(3):218–24.

[45] Kovach JG, Dubin WR, Combs CJ. Psychotherapy Training: Residents' perceptions and experiences. Acad Psychiatry 2015;39(5):567–74. https://doi.org/10.1007/s40596-014-0187-7.

[46] Linehan MM. Validaton and psychotherapy. In: Bohart A, Greenberg L, editors. Empathy Reconsidered new Directions in psychotherapy. Washington DC: American Psychological Association; 1997. p. 353–92.

[47] Linehan MM. University of Washington Risk Assessment Action Protocol: UWRAMP. University of WA, Unpublished Work. 2009.

[48] Linehan MM, Comtois KA, Ward-Ciesielski EF. Assessing and managing risk with suicidal individuals. Cogn Behav Pract 2012;19(2):218–32.

[49] Carmel A, Templeton E, Sorenson SM, et al. Using the Linehan Risk Assessment and Management Protocol With a Chronically Suicidal Patient: A Case Report. Cogn Behav Pract 2018. https://doi.org/10.1016/j.cbpr.

Advances in Psychiatry and Behavioral Health 2 (2022) 253–266

ADVANCES IN PSYCHIATRY AND BEHAVIORAL HEALTH

Recent Advances in Psychopharmacology

Alexander J. Poznanski, MD*, Esther Akinyemi, MD

Department of Behavioral Health, Henry Ford Health, One Ford Place, 1COO, Detroit, MI 48202, USA

KEYWORDS

• Aducanumab • Hypnotics • ADHD • Bremelanotide • Brexanolone • Esketamine • New antipsychotics

KEY POINTS

- Our understanding of psychiatric disorders and underlying causative mechanisms has improved considerably.
- New medications with novel mechanisms of action are being explored for the treatment of psychiatric disorders.
- Older medications are being explored for alternative indications, including their use in combination with other medications and alternative formulations.
- We have an ongoing need to expand our understanding of psychopathology to develop safer and more effective psychopharmacological treatment options.

INTRODUCTION

Our understanding of psychiatric disorders has increased over the last 2 decades, and this has helped spearhead development of new psychotropic medications. In the past 5 years, several medications have been developed that treat psychiatric illnesses while minimizing the burden often associated with side effects. New medications have been approved for a variety of psychiatric indications, including attention-deficit hyperactivity disorder (ADHD), mood disorders, movement disorders, neurocognitive disorders, psychotic disorders, sexual disorders, and sleep disorders.

For ADHD, the primary treatment has been the use of stimulants; however, other mechanisms of action are being explored, and a medication that modulates both serotonin and norepinephrine to target inattention symptoms has been developed. For depression, new medications include esketamine and brexanolone, both of which help alleviate depressive symptoms through mechanisms of action that do not target traditional monoamine systems. For bipolar disorders and psychotic disorders, D2 dopamine receptor blockade remains a major therapeutic mechanism of action driving drug development, with some medications used in combination with others, such as agents targeting opioid receptors, to enhance their effect. Tardive dyskinesia is a significant side effect of D2 blockade, and has historically been difficult to treat; however, we now have new medications to address tardive dyskinesia symptoms, which work by inhibiting vesicular monoamine transporter (VMAT) 2.

Treatment of neurocognitive disorders remains a challenge, with few breakthroughs in the identification of disease-modifying agents until the recent development of a human monoclonal antibody that targets amyloid. For sexual disorders, minimal treatment options for the most common sexual disorders in women are available, which is in contrast to the many medications that have been developed for sexual disorders in men. New medications have been developed to address this disparity including bremelanotide. Finally, medications have been developed for treating excessive daytime sleepiness and for insomnia. Pitolisant was developed to address excessive daytime sleepiness, and this drug

*Corresponding author, *E-mail addresses:* apoznan1@hfhs.org; eakinye2@hfhs.org

https://doi.org/10.1016/j.ypsc.2022.03.009
2667-3827/22/

works through a novel mechanism of action as an antagonist and inverse agonist of the histamine-3 receptor.

Clinicians must remain vigilant in maintaining an up-to-date understanding of the many new psychotropic medications that have been approved and that are in the development pipeline. In this review, we will discuss the new psychiatric medications that have been approved by the United States Food and Drug Administration (FDA) over the last 5 years (Table 1). In particular, we highlight the medications that have novel mechanisms of action and postulate future directions in the pharmacologic treatment of psychiatric illness.

ADUCANUMAB

Aducanumab is a human monoclonal antibody that targets aggregated forms of beta-amyloid in the brain to prevent build-up. It is approved for treating mild cognitive impairment and mild dementia. Aducanumab is given by monthly infusions of 10 mg/kg [1]. Treating patients with aducanumab requires magnetic resonance imaging at baseline, 7 months, and 12 months to monitor for amyloid-related imaging abnormalities. Dangerous side effects of aducanumab therapy include brain hemorrhage, brain edema, and falls. Headaches with confusion and vomiting should raise concern for serious side effects. Other side effects include delirium and diarrhea [2].

Clinical Trials

Aducanumab was studied in the PRIME, EMERGE, and ENGAGE studies. The PRIME study found that aducanumab reduced amyloid plaques in patients with Alzheimer's disease [3]. EMERGE and ENGAGE were 18-month randomized, double-blinded, placebo-controlled studies that compared low-dose, high-dose, and placebo groups. The primary endpoint was a change in clinical dementia rating scores. The EMERGE study showed statistically significant changes in the primary and secondary outcomes compared with placebo in the high-dose group, a reduction in the amyloid deposition as seen by positron emission tomography imaging, and a reduction of tau protein in cerebrospinal fluid. The low-dose group was not significantly different from the placebo group [2]. The ENGAGE study did not show a statistical difference for any of the endpoints. Secondary analysis, however, showed results congruent with the EMERGE study [2]. Aducanumab was approved by the FDA after an initial termination of one study for reasons of futility, leading to the board voting against its approval, which was overturned. This raised some controversy surrounding its approval [4].

BREMELANOTIDE

Bremelanotide is a melanocortin receptor agonist with high affinity for melanocortin type 4, which is a novel mechanism of action. It is approved for acquired hypoactive sexual desire disorders in premenopausal women [5]. It is an on-demand subcutaneous medication given 45 minutes before sexual activity at a dose of 1.75 mg. The half-life is 2.7 hours, and it is metabolized by hydrolysis and excreted mostly in urine. Bremelanotide can be used safely with alcohol [5]. However, bremelanotide can slow absorption and decrease the availability of some medications. The most common side effects of bremelanotide are nausea, injection site reactions, flushing, and headaches [5].

Clinical Trials

Bremelanotide was studied in 2 phase III (RECONNECT) studies. These were 24-week double-blind, randomized, placebo-controlled studies in women 18 years and older who were in stable relationships. The women using bremelanotide in the 2 studies had a significant increase in sexual desire. Satisfaction with desire and arousal was significantly improved in the first study but not in the second study. The bremelanotide group in both studies also showed a decrease on the female sexual distress scale, which was sustained in participants who remained on the medication after the study period [5].

BREXANOLONE

Brexanolone is an allosteric modulator of synaptic and extrasynaptic GABA-A receptors [6]. It mediates the tonic inhibition of GABA receptors, unlike benzodiazepines which mediate phasic inhibition [7]. It is approved to treat postpartum depression in adults [8]. Brexanolone is administered via intravenous infusion lasting 60 hours with a default stepwise infusion rate schedule. It produces rapid antidepressant effects, which may last up to 30 days postinfusion [9]. Brexanolone binds strongly to plasma proteins, with a half-life of 9 hours. It is not known to undergo cytochrome P450 (CYP) metabolism and is associated with minimal QTc prolongation. Most common adverse events include loss of consciousness, excessive sedation, dry mouth, and hot flashes [8]. A risk evaluation and mitigation strategy (REMS) program is required for its

TABLE 1
New Psychopharmacologic Agents in the Last Five Years

Number	Generic Name	Trade Name	Indication	Year of Approval
204370	Cariprazine	Vraylar	Schizophrenia, Bipolar disorder (manic/ mixed/depressive episode) in adults	2015 2019[a]
207318	Pimavanserin	Nuplazid	Parkinson's disease psychosis	2016
208082	Deutetrabenazine	Austedo	Huntington's disease Chorea	2017
209241	Valbenazine	Ingrezza	Tardive Dyskinesia in adults	2017
209229	Lofexidine hydrochloride	Lucemyra	Opioid withdrawal in adults	2018
211371	Brexanolone	Zulresso	Postpartum depression in adults	2019
211230	Solriamfetol	Sunosi	Excessive daytime sleepiness in narcolepsy and obstructive sleep apnea	2019
210557	Bremelanotide	Vyleesi	Hypoactive sexual desire disorder in women	2019
211150	Pitolisant	Wakix	Excessive daytime sleepiness in narcolepsy	2019
209500	Lumateperone tosylate	Caplyta	Schizophrenia, Bipolar disorder (depressive episode) in adults	2019 2021[a]
212028	Lemborexant	Dayvigo	Insomnia in adults	2019
211243	Esketamine	Spravato	Adjunct for treatment-resistant depression and depression with acute suicidal ideation/behavior in adults	2019 2020[a]
212994	Serdexmethylphenidate/ dexmethylphenidate	Azstarys	Attention-deficit hyperactivity disorder in children 6 years + and adults	2019
211964	Viloxazine	Qelbree	Attention-deficit hyperactivity disorder in children ages 6-17	2021
213378	Olanzapine/samidorphan	Lybalvi	Schizophrenia, Bipolar disorder (manic/ mixed episodes and maintenance) in adults	2021
761178	Aducanumab	Aduhelm	Mild cognitive impairment, Mild Alzheimer's disease	2021
214985	Daridorexant	Quviviq	Insomnia in adults	2022

[a] New indication approved.

administration [9]. Patients require continuous pulse oximetry monitoring and must be accompanied at all times while interacting with their children during the infusion [8].

Clinical Trials

Brexanolone was evaluated in 2 double-blind, randomized, placebo-controlled phase 3 studies. In one study, participants diagnosed with postpartum depression were assigned within 6 months of postpartum to receive brexanolone 90 μg/kg/h, brexanolone 60 μg/kg/h, or placebo. In the second study, participants received either brexanolone 90 μg or placebo. The primary endpoint for both studies was a change in Hamilton Depression Rating Scale score from baseline at 60 hours. Patients in all brexanolone groups demonstrated significant improvement in depressive symptoms that persisted at day 30. Laboratory parameters, vital signs, and electrocardiogram results were similar between groups [10].

CARIPRAZINE

Cariprazine is a partial agonist at the D2, D3, and 5-HT1A receptors and an antagonist at 5-HT2A, 5-HT2B, 5-HT2C, 5-HT7, H1, and alpha1a receptors [11,12]. In addition to schizophrenia and manic/mixed episodes, cariprazine has been recently approved to treat depressive episodes in adults with bipolar disorder [12]. Cariprazine has a higher affinity for the D3 receptor than other antipsychotics, and this enhanced agonist activity may provide benefits to cognition, alertness, and depressive symptoms [11,13]. The recommended starting dose for cariprazine is 1.5 mg daily, with a recommended therapeutic dose of 1.5 to 3 mg daily [12]. Most common side effects include extrapyramidal symptoms, akathisia, dyspepsia, nausea, vomiting, and somnolence. Cariprazine has minimal QTc effects. It is primarily metabolized by CYP3A4 and less so by CYP2D6 [12]. The half-life of one of its metabolites, didesmethyl cariprazine, is considerably longer than cariprazine, which can prolong elimination [14].

Clinical Trials

Cariprazine's efficacy for bipolar depression was demonstrated in a double-blind, placebo-controlled phase 2 study. Patients with bipolar I disorder with a current depressive episode were randomized to receive cariprazine 0.75 mg, 1.5 mg, 3 mg, or placebo daily. The primary endpoint was a change in baseline Montgomery-Asberg Depression Rating Scale (MADRS) score at 6 weeks. Patients in cariprazine 1.5 mg and 3 mg groups showed improvement compared with the placebo group, but only the 1.5 mg daily treatment had statistically significant results. The 1.5 mg group had significantly higher rates of response and remission compared with the placebo group, while the 3.0 mg group only had significantly higher response rates. Laboratory parameters were similar between cariprazine and placebo groups. Weight gain was higher in patients in the cariprazine group, and no clinically significant electrocardiogram changes were noted. Suicidal ideation was lower in the 1.5 mg group, and treatment-emergent mania was similar among groups [15].

DARIDOREXANT AND LEMBOREXANT

Daridorexant and lemborexant are dual orexin receptor antagonists (DORAs) like suvorexant. They act as competitive antagonists at both orexin receptors. These medications are approved for both sleep-onset and sleep maintenance insomnia.

Daridorexant is noted to have a limited risk of physical dependence. It promotes natural and surmountable sleep while preserving memory and cognition, and also improves daytime functioning [16]. The recommended dose is 25 to 50 mg nightly, with a half-life of 8 hours. It is metabolized primarily by CYP3A4 and excreted primarily in feces [17]. Nasopharyngitis and headache were the most common adverse events [18].

Lemborexant has also demonstrated efficacy for the treatment of patients with insomnia in dementia [19]. The recommended dose is 5 to 10 mg nightly, and the half-life is between 17 and 19 hours [19]. It is metabolized by CYP3A4 and 3A5 to inactive metabolites and excreted primarily in feces [20]. The most common side effects of lemborexant were somnolence, headaches, and influenza [21].

Note that DORAs are contraindicated for patients with narcolepsy. Physicians should warn patients about potential dangers of driving the day after use of a DORA to avoid medico-legal consequences for both patients and physicians [22].

Clinical Trials

Daridorexant was evaluated in 2 randomized, double-blind, placebo-controlled, phase 3 trials. Adults with insomnia disorder were randomly assigned to receive daridorexant 50 mg, 25 mg, or placebo (study 1) or daridorexant 25 mg, 10 mg, or placebo (study 2) for 3 months. The primary endpoints were a change from baseline in wake time after sleep onset (WASO) and latency to persistent sleep. WASO was improved in both studies for all treatment groups except the 10 mg group. In study 1, latency to persistent sleep and self-reported total sleep time was significantly improved in the treatment groups. The Insomnia Daytime Symptoms and Impact Questionnaire sleepiness domain scores improved in the 50 mg group but not in the 25 mg group. In study 2, the 25 mg group had significant improvement in self-reported total sleep time, but not in Insomnia Daytime Symptoms and Impact Questionnaire sleepiness domain scores [18].

Lemborexant was evaluated in the SUNRISE 1 and 2 studies. SUNRISE 1 found that lemborexant was effective in improving objective measures of sleep compared with placebo and zolpidem [23]. SUNRISE 2, which was a 12-month multicenter, randomized, double-blind, placebo-controlled study, showed that lemborexant improved subjective measures of sleep, with statistically significant reductions in WASO scores [21]. Lemborexant was generally well tolerated compared with placebo and zolpidem [21,24].

DEUTETRABENAZINE AND VALBENAZINE

These medications are VMAT-2 inhibitors thus increasing cytosolic dopamine levels, decreasing synaptic dopamine release and postsynaptic receptor stimulation, and thereby decreasing dyskinesia [25].

Valbenazine is the purified prodrug of the (+)-alpha-isomer of tetrabenazine, the most selective enantiomer for VMAT-2 [26] [94]. Valbenazine is the first medication approved for the treatment of adults with tardive dyskinesia [27]. Valbenazine is administered in doses of 40 to 80 mg orally once daily and has a rapid onset of action within 2 weeks. It is metabolized into 2 metabolites mainly by CYP3A4 and CYP2D6. The half-life is about 20 hours, and it is eliminated primarily in urine [28].

Deutetrabenazine, in addition to tardive dyskinesia, is also approved to treat Huntington's disease-associated chorea in adults. The initial dose is 6 mg daily, with a maximum dose of 24 mg twice daily. It is metabolized by CYP2D6. Deutetrabenazine is contraindicated in patients with hepatic impairment, suicidal ideation, untreated or ineffectively treated depression, and in patients taking reserpine, monoamine oxidase inhibitors (MAOIs), or tetrabenazine. Deutetrabenazine can be safely taken within the setting of impaired renal function [29]. These 2 medications should be avoided in patients with congenital prolonged QTc syndrome and in pregnant and breastfeeding patients [29].

Clinical Trials

Valbenazine was studied in a 6-week double-blind, placebo-controlled, randomized study (KINECT 3). The doses given were 40 mg and 80 mg of valbenazine versus placebo. Effectiveness was measured by the Abnormal Involuntary Movement Scale (AIMS). The results showed a decrease in AIMS score with both dosages compared with placebo, with a larger decrease in the 80 mg group. The most common adverse effects were somnolence, akathisia, and dry mouth. Other side effects were fatigue and headaches [30].

Deutetrabenazine was studied in a 12-week, phase 3, placebo-controlled trial, with an initial open-label arm and a long-term maintenance phase. Efficacy was assessed by changes in the AIMS scores. The results showed a gradual reduction in the AIMS score starting at week 2 [31,32].

ESKETAMINE

Esketamine is a nonselective, noncompetitive antagonist at the N-methyl-D-aspartate (NMDA) receptor [33]. It acts on GABA interneurons to increase glutamatergic neuron activity and may exert its effect via alpha-amino-3-hydroxy-5-methyl-4-isoxazolepropionic acid (AMPA) receptor activation to promote neurotrophic signaling via enhanced brain-derived neurotrophic factor production and stimulation of tropomyosin receptor kinase B [34]. Other potential molecular targets of esketamine include nicotinic, muscarinic, 5HT-3, and D-serine receptor antagonism; cholinesterase inhibition; sigma1/2 and GABA-A receptor agonism; serotonin, norepinephrine, and dopamine reuptake inhibition; and opioid receptor activity. Modulation of many of these receptors can lead to antidepressant or procognitive effects, with some having anxiolytic and euphoric effects [35]. Esketamine is approved for the adjunctive treatment of treatment-resistant depression and depressive symptoms in major depressive disorder with acute suicidal ideation and behavior in adults. It is primarily metabolized via CYP2B6 and 3A4, with some metabolism via 2C9 and 2C19, and its half-life ranges from 7 to 12 hours. Most side effects are transient and include dissociation, dizziness/vertigo, nausea/vomiting, sedation, hypoesthesia, anxiety, euphoria, lethargy, elevated blood pressure, and feeling intoxicated. Esketamine initiation in patients with treatment-resistant depression begins with 56 mg, titrated up to a maximum of 84 mg twice weekly for four weeks, then tapered down. The regimen for the treatment of depressive symptoms in patients with major depressive disorder and acute suicidality is 84 mg twice weekly for 4 weeks, which can be lowered to 56 mg. It is subject to a REMS program and requires administration under physician supervision with subsequent monitoring for at least 2 hours for safety. Patients are advised not to drive before a full night of sleep [33].

Clinical Trials

Esketamine was studied in TRANSFORM-1, 2, and 3, as well as in the SUSTAIN-1 and 2 studies. TRANSFORM-1, 2, and 3 were phase 3, randomized, double-blind, placebo-controlled studies, with TRANSFORM-3 including participants 65 years and older treated with a 28 mg dose in addition to the 56 mg and 84 mg doses used in the other studies. New oral antidepressant medication was given to all participants. The primary endpoint was improvement in MADRS score from baseline at 4 weeks [36–38].

TRANSFORM-1 showed clinically significant improvement in both esketamine groups for all endpoints, and the primary endpoint was statistically significant in the 56 mg group. In TRANSFORM-2, the esketamine group demonstrated significantly improved MADRS scores. In both studies, response and remission rates increased over the treatment period in all groups and suicidal ideation decreased. Dissociative symptoms decreased with repeated dosing and did not appear to affect the response rate. Safety was similar between the treatment groups, and no notable withdrawal symptoms were noted after discontinuation. No evidence of attempted drug abuse or cravings were reported [36,37]. A post hoc analysis of these studies indicated that nonresponse at week 1 did not suggest nonresponse at week 28 [39].

TRANSFORM-3 showed no statistically significant improvement in the esketamine group at 4 weeks. Subgroup analysis did show statistically significant improvement at 4 weeks in patients aged 65 to 74 years and those with depression with onset before age 55. After a second 4-week induction phase, most participants showed improvement in symptoms [38].

SUSTAIN-1 was a phase 3, double-blind randomized withdrawal trial that assessed the long-term effects of esketamine. SUSTAIN-1 evaluated esketamine's ability to prevent relapse of depressive symptoms in patients with remission of treatment-resistant depression and without psychotic features. The study randomized patients in remission to esketamine 56 mg, 84 mg, or placebo for 16 weeks. The primary outcome was time to relapse. Significantly fewer patients from the esketamine group experienced relapse [40,41].

SUSTAIN-2 was an open-label study that evaluated the safety of esketamine in adults and older adults with treatment-resistant depression. Participants initially received intranasal esketamine 28 mg (patients at least 65 years old only) or 56 mg twice weekly for 4 weeks, with maximum titrated dose of 84 mg, plus a new oral antidepressant. Those with adequate response continued into an optimization/maintenance phase, where esketamine was administered every 1 to 2 weeks. Improvements in mean MADRS score during the initiation phase were maintained during the optimization/maintenance phase, with remission seen in most patients. Most improvements in depressive symptoms occurred during the induction phase [40,41].

LOFEXIDINE

Lofexidine is an alpha 2 receptor agonist approved to treat opioid withdrawal symptoms in adults. It reduces norepinephrine and subsequently sympathetic tone, which is a primary mediator of opioid withdrawal [42,43]. Most common side effects from lofexidine include hypotension, bradycardia, dizziness, dry mouth, and somnolence. QTc elevations have been noted in some patients. CYP2D6 is the primary metabolizer of lofexidine, with CYP1A2 and 2C19 also acting on it. The recommended starting and target dose is 0.54 mg every 5 to 6 hours for up to 14 days. It is recommended to taper lofexidine because of the risk of discontinuation syndrome [42].

Clinical Trials

Two clinical trials that evaluated lofexidine randomized participants to receive lofexidine at a total daily dose of 2.16 mg (study 1 only), 2.88 mg, or placebo. The primary outcome was a change in the Short Opiate Withdrawal Scale of Gossop score from the initiation of treatment to 7 days (study 1) or 3 days plus time to discontinuation (study 2). Overall, all lofexidine groups showed statistically significant decreases in Short Opiate Withdrawal Scale of Gossop scores and time to discontinuation was longer in the lofexidine group in study 2. The two doses in study 1 were not significantly different from each other in efficacy [44,45].

LUMATEPERONE TOSYLATE

Lumateperone is a 5-HT2A receptor antagonist with D2 receptor presynaptic partial agonism/postsynaptic antagonism, D1 receptor activity, and serotonin transporter inhibition [46–48]. Its mechanism of action is theorized to involve direct effects on the aforementioned receptors, mesolimbic/mesocortical dopamine phosphoprotein modulation, glutamate GluN2B receptor phosphoprotein modulation, and D1-dependent enhancement of both NMDA and AMPA-mediated circuits via the mTOR signaling pathway [47,48]. It is approved in adults as monotherapy for schizophrenia and as monotherapy or adjunctive therapy with lithium or valproate for depressive episodes in bipolar I/II disorder [46]. This drug's target receptor profile is unique, and it has a much higher affinity for the 5-HT2A receptor than for the D2 receptor [46,47]. Its effect on glutamate transmission may provide procognitive benefits, which may enhance its antidepressant effects [49]. Common side effects of lumateperone include sedation, dry mouth, dizziness, and nausea. Lumateperone is metabolized through CYP3A4, 2C8, and 1A2. Starting and recommended dose is 42 mg daily [46].

Clinical Trials

Lumateperone's efficacy for relieving bipolar depression was evaluated in a phase 3 randomized, double-blind, placebo-controlled clinical trial. Patients with bipolar I or II disorder and a current major depressive episode were randomized to receive either 42 mg of lumateperone or placebo daily, with the primary endpoint being a change in MADRS score at day 43. Lumateperone was significantly superior to placebo, with significantly improved rates of response and remission in the treatment groups. Suicidal ideation was less common with lumateperone use compared with placebo [50].

Lumateperone's efficacy for treating schizophrenia was studied in phase 2 and 3 randomized, double-blind, placebo-controlled clinical trials. In the phase 2 study, patients were randomized to receive lumateperone 42 mg or 84 mg, risperidone 4 mg, or placebo daily. In the phase 3 study, randomized participants received lumateperone 28 mg, 42 mg, or placebo daily. The primary outcome for both studies was a change in Positive and Negative Syndrome Scale (PANSS) score at 4 weeks. In both studies, only lumateperone 42 mg demonstrated greater improvement in the primary endpoint compared with placebo, and was similar to risperidone in the phase 2 study. Participants who received lumateperone in the phase 2 study also had significantly improved psychosocial functioning compared with risperidone. Lumateperone was well tolerated, and side effects were less frequent with lumateperone 42 mg compared with risperidone. Frequency of extrapyramidal symptoms and measures of weight gain were similar between lumateperone and placebo groups. No increase in suicidal ideation was observed in the phase 3 study [51,52].

OLANZAPINE/SAMIDORPHAN

Olanzapine plus samidorphan combines D2 and 5-HT2A antagonism with mu-opioid receptor antagonism. Samidorphan possesses lesser affinity for kappa and delta-opioid receptors, where it functions as a partial agonist [53,54]. It is approved for treating adults with schizophrenia, manic or mixed episodes of bipolar disorder either as monotherapy or adjunctive therapy with lithium or valproate, and for maintenance therapy in bipolar disorder [54]. It is believed that mu-opioid receptor blockade may help to curb food cravings, and therefore weight gain [53]. The starting daily dose for treating bipolar mania is olanzapine 10 to 15 mg, with a recommended maintenance dose of 5 to 20 mg. Starting daily dose for treating schizophrenia is olanzapine 5 to 10 mg, with the recommended treatment dose being 10 to 20 mg. Samidorphan is kept fixed at 10 mg. It is primarily metabolized by CYP1A2 and 3A4, with some involvement of CYP2D6, 3A5, 2C19, and 2C8. Adverse events associated with olanzapine/samidorphan treatment include weight gain, increased appetite, somnolence, dry mouth, and headache [54].

Clinical Trials

Olanzapine/samidorphan therapy was studied in four phase 3 trials: ENLIGHTEN-1, 2, and their extension-EXT studies. ENLIGHTEN-1 and 2 were randomized, double-blind, controlled trials that demonstrated the ability of olanzapine/samidorphan to improve psychotic symptoms similarly to olanzapine alone while reducing weight gain after 6 weeks. Patient metabolic parameters were similar between the olanzapine groups. Extrapyramidal symptoms were comparable between treatment groups and were not significantly different from baseline. No reports of suicidal ideation or changes in suicide risk scores were observed in the olanzapine/samidorphan groups [55,56].

The ENLIGHTEN-1- and 2-EXT studies were 52-week open-label follow-up studies, wherein all participants received olanzapine/samidorphan to evaluate efficacy and adverse events. Rates of psychotic symptoms remained stable or were reduced, and the response rate increased throughout the study period. Weight gain and somnolence were the most common adverse events, and weight gain seemed to stabilize after 6 weeks of samidorphan treatment. Vital sign, electrocardiogram, movement disorder, metabolic, hematologic, and liver function parameters were all stable. Mean prolactin level increased slightly in women and decreased in men in the first extension study, but prolactin decreased in both groups in the second study. Suicidal ideation/behavior was noted, but no completed suicides occurred [57,58].

Clinical studies evaluating the efficacy of olanzapine/samidorphan for treating bipolar disorder are lacking, and approval of this combination treatment for bipolar disorder is based primarily on the above studies and past FDA approval of olanzapine for bipolar disorder [59].

PIMAVANSERIN

Pimavanserin is an inverse agonist/antagonist that has strong affinity for the 5-HT2A receptor, low affinity for the 5-HT2C receptor, and activity at the sigma-1 receptor. It is approved for treating psychosis in patients with Parkinson's disease [60]. Pimavanserin is the first FDA-approved non-D2-acting antipsychotic drug; hence, it should not worsen parkinsonian symptoms [61]. It does not seem to worsen cognition [62], and it may reduce extrapyramidal symptoms and augment efficacy when used adjunctively with other antipsychotic drugs [63]. The recommended starting and target dose for pimavanserin is 34 mg daily. Its half-life is about 57 hours, and it is primarily metabolized by CYP3A4 and 3A5. Most common side effects include peripheral edema and confusion [60].

Clinical Trials

Pimavanserin was evaluated in a phase 3, randomized, double-blind, placebo-controlled trial [64]. Patients with Parkinson's disease-related psychosis, after a 2-week nonpharmacological lead-in phase to limit the placebo response, were randomized to receive pimavanserin 40 mg or placebo daily. The primary outcome was antipsychotic benefit assessed via the Parkinson's disease-adapted Scale for the Assessment of Positive Symptoms (SAPS-PD) [64]. The study showed that pimavanserin was associated with a statistically significant reduction in SAPS-PD scores compared with placebo. Pimavanserin was well tolerated, with no significant safety concerns or worsening of motor function [64].

PITOLISANT

Pitolisant is a histamine (H3) receptor antagonist/inverse agonist, which is a novel mechanism of action. It is approved for treating hypersomnolence in patients with narcolepsy. It releases histamine in the brain, promoting wakefulness and preferentially increasing dopamine in the prefrontal cortex [65]. Pitolisant is the first medication approved for treating hypersomnolence that is not a controlled medication, with abuse potential comparable to placebo [65].

The starting dose for pitolisant is 8.9 mg daily, and the recommended dose is 17.8 to 35.6 mg daily. Its half-life is 7.5 to 24.2 hours [66]. It is metabolized by CYP3A4 and 2D6 and excreted mainly in urine. Lower doses should be used in patients with renal or mild hepatic impairment, and pitolisant should be avoided in patients with end-stage renal disease or severe hepatic impairment [66]. Common adverse effects from pitolisant use include headaches, insomnia, nausea, and anxiety [66,67].

Clinical Trials

Pitolisant was evaluated in 4 main studies: HARMONY 1, HARMONY Ibis, HARMONY CTP, and HARMONY III. The HARMONY 1 and Ibis trials compared pitolisant to placebo and modafinil and showed that pitolisant was superior to placebo but not to modafinil. The HARMONY Ibis trial used lower doses and did not show a consistent improvement in the Epworth Sleepiness Scale score or in reducing cataplexy [67].

The HARMONY CTP trial evaluated pitolisant in patients with cataplexy. The 7-week study evaluated the effectiveness of pitolisant compared with placebo and showed that pitolisant reduced episodes of cataplexy by 75% compared with 38% in the placebo group [68].

The HARMONY III trial studied the long-term efficacy of pitolisant over 12 months and extending to 5 years. After 12 months, pitolisant use was associated with a decrease in Epworth Sleepiness Scale scores, as well as reduction in the frequency of sleep attacks, sleep paralysis, cataplexy, and hallucinations [69].

SERDEXMETHYLPHENIDATE/ DEXMETHYLPHENIDATE

Serdexmethylphenidate/dexmethylphenidate (SDX/d-MPH) is a combined schedule II stimulant medication. It is approved for the treatment of ADHD in both children and adults. Serdexmethylphenidate is a prodrug of dexmethylphenidate [70]. Dexmethylphenidate increases norepinephrine and dopamine release from the presynaptic neuron and prevents their reuptake. The half-lives of these compounds are 5.7 hours and 11.7 hours, respectively. Dexmethylphenidate is metabolized to inactive forms, and excretion is primarily in urine.

Recommended starting dose for all ages is 39.2 mg/7.8 mg daily, with maximum dose of 52.3 mg/10.4 mg daily. Like other stimulants, SDX/d-MPH can interfere with growth in children and must not be given with MAOIs. Common side effects include nausea, indigestion, mood swings, blood pressure increases, poor appetite, dizziness, anxiety, and irritability [70].

Clinical Trials

SDX/d-MPH was studied in a 3-week, open-label study in 6- to 12-year-old children with ADHD. Subjects were initiated with open-label treatment at 39.2 mg/7.8 mg daily of SDX/d-MPH, titrated weekly to an optimal dose, then moved to a double-blind treatment phase during which subjects were randomized to receive their optimal dose or placebo. Efficacy was assessed on day 7. The results showed significant improvement with SDX/d-MPH versus placebo. A significant treatment effect from SDX/d-MPH compared with placebo was observed from 1 to 10 hours postdose [71].

SOLRIAMFETOL

Solriamfetol is a selective dopamine and norepinephrine reuptake inhibitor that is FDA-approved for the treatment of excessive daytime sleepiness in patients with narcolepsy and obstructive sleep apnea (OSA) [72]. Starting dose is 37.5 mg daily for OSA and 75 mg daily for narcolepsy, with a maximum dose of 150 mg daily. It has a half-life of 7 hours and is renally excreted. Side effects seem to be dose-dependent and include increased systolic/diastolic blood pressure, insomnia, anxiety, jitteriness, nausea, chest discomfort, headaches, decreased appetite, and nasopharyngitis. Solriamfetol is contraindicated in patients with unstable cardiovascular status [73] and in patients taking MAOIs [74] [92].

Clinical Trials

Solriamfetol was evaluated in the TONES 3 trial [73]. The study evaluated its effectiveness in treating patients with excessive daytime sleepiness due to OSA. The study was a randomized, double-blind, placebo-controlled parallel study. Solriamfetol improved wakefulness at all doses compared with placebo, and the rate of effectiveness was dose-dependent [73].

VILOXAZINE

Viloxazine is a nonstimulant medication approved for the treatment of ADHD in children. It is a serotonin-norepinephrine modulating agent. Viloxazine modulates serotonergic activity via selective 5-HT2B receptor antagonism and 5-HT2C receptor agonism, and it moderately inhibits the norepinephrine transporter by blocking the reuptake of norepinephrine. Viloxazine increases serotonin levels in the prefrontal cortex but not significantly in the nucleus accumbens, suggesting low abuse potential [75,76]. Starting dose is 100 mg daily for patients ages 6-11 and 200 mg daily in ages 12-17. Maximum dose is 400 mg daily. The half-life of regular viloxazine is 2 to 5 hours, with extended release being about 7 hours. It is mostly renally excreted. Common adverse effects include somnolence, insomnia, fatigue, nausea/vomiting, irritability, headache, and decreased appetite. [93] The incidence of somnolence and headache from viloxazine use seemed to be dose-related [77]. Adverse effects may be milder with viloxazine compared with other antidepressant medications [76].

Clinical Trials

Viloxazine extended-release was studied in an 8-week, randomized, double-blind, placebo-controlled, phase 2 study [77]. The results showed significant improvements in ADHD Rating Scale-IV total score in the 200 mg, 300 mg, and 400 mg dose groups versus placebo. Clinical Global Impression-Improvement (CGI-I) scores for the 300 mg group and Clinical Global Impression-Severity (CGI-S) scores for all extended-release viloxazine groups (except the 100 mg group) were also improved significantly compared with placebo.

Another study of viloxazine was a 6-week randomized, double-blind, placebo-controlled trial to assess the efficacy and safety of daily 100 mg and 200 mg doses of extended-release viloxazine for treating 6- to 12-year-old children with ADHD. The primary efficacy endpoint was the change from baseline in ADHD Rating Scale-5 total score [78]. The study showed significant improvements in ADHD Rating Scale-5 total score in both treatment groups at week 1 of treatment, which was maintained through the end of study. Significant improvements were also observed in the CGI-I scale, Conners 3-PS Composite T-score, and WFIRS-P total average score [78].

DISCUSSION

In this review article, we provided an overview of some of the latest FDA-approved medications for treating psychiatric disorders, with a special focus on therapies with novel molecular mechanisms of action. The field of psychiatry continues to evolve with increasing knowledge of the pathophysiology of psychiatric disorders, and this knowledge will continually lead to the development of more medications with novel mechanisms of actions. Many new and old agents are being explored for the treatment of psychiatric disorders, and the need for effective medications with limited side effects is ongoing. For ADHD, developing medications that can effectively treat all ADHD symptoms and that have less abuse potential and greater ease of prescription is important. For treating mood disorders, the long-term effects of newer agents such as esketamine and brexanolone are still unclear, and the dosing structure for repeated administration and frequency of treatment of such agents still needs to be delineated. Additionally, mood stabilizers are often fraught with side effects that make long-term adherence to treatment difficult. Newer agents working outside of the monoaminergic system are under investigation, including glutamatergic agents such as arketamine [79]. Opioid receptor antagonist/partial agonists are also being evaluated, with several under investigation, and this approach is supported by evidence that agonism of certain opioid receptors can produce mood symptoms [80]. Zuranolone, an oral GABA-A modulator similar to brexanolone, has shown benefits for treating depressive symptoms and may present a more practical option for treating postpartum depression and other depressive disorders [81]. Strong associations between depression and inflammation are known, and medications such as minocycline have shown how anti-inflammatory treatments may help treat depressive symptoms [82].

Research into the utility of psychedelic/hallucinogenic drugs for treating psychiatric disorders is also experiencing a resurgence, and studies are underway to assess the benefits of psilocybin, ayahuasca, and LSD [83]. Ideally, the development of medications with faster onset of action, increased response rates, and minimal side effects in the treatment of mood disorders should be prioritized. While approved medications for treating tardive dyskinesia exist, reexamining older generation drugs for efficacy and the ability to bind new targets, such as GABA and glutamate receptors, will also be important [84].

For the treatment of neurocognitive disorders, several medications with novel mechanisms of action are being studied, including medications that target the tau protein, modulate glucose and lipid metabolism, and reduce inflammation. Existing medications are being reexamined for possible use in Alzheimer's disease, including leuprolide, bromocriptine, and levetiracetam [85–87].

For antipsychotic agents, newer pharmacotherapies continue to break out of the confines of older neuroleptic drugs, with non-D2-acting medications receiving significant attention. Some of the targets of these drugs include cannabinoid receptors, with cannabidiol showing some therapeutic benefits. Roluperidone is a 5-HT2A, sigma-2, and alpha-1 antagonist that targets negative and cognitive symptoms. Phosphodiesterase 10A inhibitors target secondary messengers to modulate dopaminergic and glutamatergic pathways via phosphorylation [88]. Trace amino acid receptor 1 agonists target G-protein-coupled receptors that are relatively selective for amino acids and share similarities with dopamine, and they may modulate dopaminergic transmission [89]. D-amino acid oxidase inhibitors degrade D-serine, which modulates NMDA receptor, possibly improving the negative symptoms of schizophrenia. Therefore, agonist agents are being investigated to target these receptors [90]. LuAF-35700 is an experimental molecule with primarily D1 over D2 antagonism and 5-HT2A and 5-HT6 antagonism activity that is in phase 3 trials. It has shown similar efficacy to current antipsychotic drugs for helping patients with treatment-resistant psychosis [53]. LuAF-35700 is one of the several reagents in current studies with a greater emphasis on the modulation of serotonergic action for treating schizophrenia [91].

SUMMARY

The search continues for more efficacious and safer medications to treat patients who have psychiatric disorders. The advancements in drug therapy made in recent years have helped the field make strides toward this end. Future medications will need to separate themselves from the current repertoire in regard to having milder side effect profiles, greater efficacy, and a wider range of targeted symptoms.

CLINICAL CARE POINTS

- Newer medications may provide similar or improved clinical outcomes but must be weighed against the cost and convenience of older medications.
- Novel mechanisms of action for antidepressant medications have resulted in more rapid-acting treatments compared with traditional medications.
- New medications for insomnia have low risk of physical dependence while remaining effective for sleep.
- The vesicular monoamine inhibitors are a new class that offers relief from tardive dyskinesia.
- Pimavanserin offers treatment for symptoms of psychosis in Parkinson's disease without worsening parkinsonian symptoms.
- Pitolisant provides treatment of narcolepsy without significant abuse potential.
- Further study is needed to better elucidate mechanisms of disorders to drive increasingly effective treatments.

DISCLOSURE

The authors have nothing to disclose.

REFERENCES

[1] Dhillon S. Aducanumab: first approval. Drugs 2021;81:1437–43.

[2] Salloway S, Chalkias S, Barkhof F, et al. Amyloid-related imaging abnormalities in 2 phase 3 studies evaluating aducanumab in patients with early Alzheimer disease. JAMA Neurol 2022;79:13–21.

[3] Sevigny J, Chiao P, Bussière T, et al. The antibody aducanumab reduces Aβ plaques in Alzheimer's disease. Nature 2016;537:50–6.

[4] Kuller LH, Lopez OL. ENGAGE and EMERGE: truth and consequences? Alzheimers Dement 2021;17:692–5.

[5] Dhillon S, Keam SJ. Bremelanotide: first approval. Drugs 2019;79:1599–606.

[6] Reddy HM, Poole JS, Maguire GA, et al. New medications for neuropsychiatric disorders. Psychiatr Clin North Am 2020;43:399–413.

[7] Farrant M, Nusser Z. Variations on an inhibitory theme: phasic and tonic activation of $GABA_A$ receptors. Nat Rev Neurosci 2005;6:215–29.

[8] Zulresso. Prescribing information. Sage Therapeutics. 2019. Available at: https://www.accessdata.fda.gov/drugsatfda_docs/label/2019/211371s002lbl.pdf. Accessed March 20, 2022.

[9] Ragguett RM, Tamura JK, McIntyre RS. Keeping up with the clinical advances: depression. CNS Spectr 2019;24: 25–37.

[10] Meltzer-Brody S, Colquhoun H, Riesenberg R, et al. Brexanolone injection in post-partum depression: two multicentre, double-blind, randomised, placebo-controlled, phase 3 trials. Lancet 2018;392:1058–70.

[11] Frankel JS, Schwartz TL. Brexpiprazole and cariprazine: distinguishing two new atypical antipsychotics from the original dopamine stabilizer aripiprazole. Ther Adv Psychopharmacol 2017;7:29–41.

[12] Vraylar. Prescribing information. Allergan. 2019. Available at: https://www.accessdata.fda.gov/drugsatfda_docs/label/2019/204370s006lbl.pdf. Accessed March 20, 2022.

[13] Gross G, Wicke K, Drescher KU. Dopamine D_3 receptor antagonism–still a therapeutic option for the treatment of schizophrenia. Naunyn Schmiedebergs Arch Pharmacol 2013;386:155–66.

[14] Citrome L. Cariprazine: chemistry, pharmacodynamics, pharmacokinetics, and metabolism, clinical efficacy, safety, and tolerability. Expert Opin Drug Metab Toxicol 2013;9:193–206.

[15] Durgam S, Earley W, Lipschitz A, et al. An 8-week randomized, double-blind, placebo-controlled evaluation of the safety and efficacy of cariprazine in patients with bipolar I depression. Am J Psychiatry 2016;173:271–81.

[16] Roch C, Bergamini G, Steiner MA, et al. Nonclinical pharmacology of daridorexant: a new dual orexin receptor antagonist for the treatment of insomnia. Psychopharmacology (Berl) 2021;238:2693–708.

[17] Quviviq. Prescribing information. Idorsia Pharmaceuticals. 2022. Available at: https://www.accessdata.fda.gov/drugsatfda_docs/label/2022/214985s000lbl.pdf. Accessed March 20, 2022.

[18] Mignot E, Mayleben D, Fietze I, et al. Safety and efficacy of daridorexant in patients with insomnia disorder: results from two multicentre, randomized, double-blind, placebo-controlled, phase 3 trials. Lancet Neurol 2022; 21:125–39.

[19] Moline M, Thein S, Bsharat M, et al. Safety and efficacy of lemborexant in patients with irregular sleep-wake rhythm disorder and Alzheimer's disease dementia: results from a phase 2 randomized clinical trial. J Prev Alzheimers Dis 2021;8:7–18.

[20] Dayvigo. Prescribing information. Eisai. Available at: https://www.accessdata.fda.gov/drugsatfda_docs/label/2022/212028s006lbl.pdf, 2022. Accessed April 22, 2022.

[21] Kärppä M, Yardley J, Pinner K, et al. Long-term efficacy and tolerability of lemborexant compared with placebo in adults with insomnia disorder: results from the phase 3 randomized clinical trial SUNRISE 2. Sleep 2020;43: zsaa123.

[22] Earl DC, Van Tyle KM. New pharmacologic agents for insomnia and hypersomnia. Curr Opin Pulm Med 2020;26:629–33.

[23] Moline M, Zammit G, Cheng JY, et al. Comparison of the effect of lemborexant with placebo and zolpidem tartrate extended release on sleep architecture in older adults with insomnia disorder. J Clin Sleep Med 2021;17:1167–74.

[24] Murphy P, Kumar D, Zammit G, et al. Safety of lemborexant versus placebo and zolpidem: effects on auditory awakening threshold, postural stability, and cognitive performance in healthy older participants in the middle of the night and upon morning awakening. J Clin Sleep Med 2020;16:765–73.

[25] German CL, Baladi MG, McFadden LM, et al. Regulation of the dopamine and vesicular monoamine transporters: pharmacological targets and implications for disease. Pharmacol Rev 2015;67:1005–24.

[26] Müller T. Valbenazine granted breakthrough drug status for treating tardive dyskinesia. Expert Opin Investig Drugs 2015;24:737–42.

[27] US Food and Drug Administration. FDA approves first drug to treat tardive dyskinesia. April 11, 2017. Available at: https://www.fda.gov/news-events/press-announcements/fda-approves-first-drug-treat-tardive-dyskinesia. Accessed January 27, 2022.

[28] Witek N, Comella C. Valbenazine in the treatment of tardive dyskinesia. Neurodegener Dis Manag 2019;9: 73–81.

[29] Arya D, Khan T, Margolius AJ, et al. Tardive dyskinesia: treatment update. Curr Neurol Neurosci Rep 2019;19:69.

[30] Hauser RA, Factor SA, Marder SR, et al. KINECT 3: a phase 3 randomized, double-blind, placebo-controlled trial of valbenazine for tardive dyskinesia. Am J Psychiatry 2017;174:476–84.

[31] O'Brien CF, Jimenez R, Hauser RA, et al. NBI-98854, a selective monoamine transport inhibitor for the treatment of tardive dyskinesia: a randomized, double-blind, placebo-controlled study. Mov Disord 2015;30:1681–7.

[32] Khorassani F, Luther K, Talreja O. Valbenazine and deutetrabenazine: vesicular monoamine transporter 2 inhibitors for tardive dyskinesia. Am J Health Syst Pharm 2020;77:167–74.

[33] Spravato. Prescribing information. Janssen Pharmaceuticals. 2020. Available at: https://www.accessdata.fda.gov/drugsatfda_docs/label/2020/211243s004lbl.pdf. Accessed March 20, 2022.

[34] Salahudeen MS, Wright CM, Peterson GM. Esketamine: new hope for the treatment of treatment-resistant depression? A narrative review. Ther Adv Drug Saf 2020;11: 2042098620937899.

[35] McIntyre RS, Rosenblat JD, Nemeroff CB, et al. Synthesizing the evidence for ketamine and esketamine in treatment-resistant depression: an international expert opinion on the available evidence and implementation. Am J Psychiatry 2021;178:383–99.

[36] Fedgchin M, Trivedi M, Daly EJ, et al. Efficacy and safety of fixed-dose esketamine nasal spray combined with a new oral antidepressant in treatment-resistant depression: results of a randomized, double-blind, active-controlled study (TRANSFORM-1). Int J Neuropsychopharmacol 2019;22:616–30.

[37] Popova V, Daly EJ, Trivedi M, et al. Efficacy and safety of flexibly dosed esketamine nasal spray combined with a newly initiated oral antidepressant in treatment-resistant depression: a randomized double-blind active-controlled study. Am J Psychiatry 2019;176:428–38.

[38] Turkoz I, Daly E, Singh J, et al. Treatment response with esketamine nasal spray plus an oral antidepressant in patients with treatment-resistant depression without evidence of early response: a pooled post hoc analysis of the TRANSFORM studies. J Clin Psychiatry 2021;82: 20m13800.

[39] Ochs-Ross R, Daly EJ, Zhang Y, et al. Efficacy and safety of esketamine nasal spray plus an oral antidepressant in elderly patients with treatment-resistant depression-TRANSFORM-3. Am J Geriatr Psychiatry 2020;28:121–41.

[40] Daly EJ, Trivedi MH, Janik A, et al. Efficacy of esketamine nasal spray plus oral antidepressant treatment for relapse prevention in patients with treatment-resistant depression: a randomized clinical trial. JAMA Psychiatry 2019; 76:893–903.

[41] Wajs E, Aluisio L, Holder R, et al. Esketamine nasal spray plus oral antidepressant in patients with treatment-resistant depression: assessment of long-term safety in a phase 3, open-label study (SUSTAIN-2). J Clin Psychiatry 2020;81:19m12891.

[42] Lucemyra. Prescribing information. US WorldMeds. 2018. Available at: https://www.accessdata.fda.gov/drugsatfda_docs/label/2018/209229s000lbl.pdf. Accessed March 20, 2022.

[43] Urits I, Patel A, Zusman R, et al. A comprehensive update of lofexidine for the management of opioid withdrawal symptoms. Psychopharmacol Bull 2020;50:76–96.

[44] Fishman M, Tirado C, Alam D, et al, CLEEN-SLATE Team. Safety and efficacy of lofexidine for medically managed opioid withdrawal: a randomized controlled clinical trial. J Addict Med 2019;13:169–76.

[45] Gorodetzky CW, Walsh SL, Martin PR, et al. A phase III, randomized, multi-center, double blind, placebo controlled study of safety and efficacy of lofexidine for relief of symptoms in individuals undergoing inpatient opioid withdrawal. Drug Alcohol Depend 2017;176: 79–88.

[46] Caplyta. Prescribing information. Intra-Cellular Therapies. 2021. Available at: https://www.accessdata.fda.gov/drugsatfda_docs/label/2021/209500s005s006lbl.pdf. Accessed March 20, 2022.

[47] Davis RE, Correll CU. ITI-007 in the treatment of schizophrenia: from novel pharmacology to clinical outcomes. Expert Rev Neurother 2016;16:601–14.

[48] Vanover K, Dmitrienko A, Glass S, et al. Lumateperone (ITI-007) for the treatment of schizophrenia: placebo-controlled clinical trials and an open-label safety switching study [abstract]. Schizophr Bull 2018;44(Suppl 1): S341.

[49] Corponi F, Fabbri C, Bitter I, et al. Novel antipsychotics specificity profile: a clinically oriented review of lurasidone, brexpiprazole, cariprazine and lumateperone. Eur Neuropsychopharmacol 2019;29: 971–85.

[50] Calabrese JR, Durgam S, Satlin A, et al. Efficacy and safety of lumateperone for major depressive episodes associated with bipolar I or bipolar II disorder: a phase 3 randomized placebo-controlled trial. Am J Psychiatry 2021; 178:1098–106.

[51] Lieberman JA, Davis RE, Correll CU, et al. ITI-007 for the treatment of schizophrenia: a 4-week randomized, double-blind, controlled trial. Biol Psychiatry 2016;79: 952–61.

[52] Correll CU, Davis RE, Weingart M, et al. Efficacy and safety of lumateperone for treatment of schizophrenia: a randomized clinical trial. JAMA Psychiatry 2020;77: 349–58.

[53] Krogmann A, Peters L, von Hardenberg L, et al. Keeping up with the therapeutic advances in schizophrenia: a review of novel and emerging pharmacological entities. CNS Spectr 2019;24:38–69.

[54] Lybalvi. Prescribing information. Alkermes. 2021. Available at: https://www.accessdata.fda.gov/drugsatfda_docs/label/2021/213378s000lbl.pdf. Accessed March 20, 2022.

[55] Potkin SG, Kunovac J, Silverman BL, et al. Efficacy and safety of a combination of olanzapine and samidorphan in adult patients with an acute exacerbation of schizophrenia: outcomes from the randomized, phase 3 ENLIGHTEN-1 study. J Clin Psychiatry 2020;81: 19m12769.

[56] Correll CU, Newcomer JW, Silverman B, et al. Effects of olanzapine combined with samidorphan on weight gain in schizophrenia: a 24-week phase 3 study. Am J Psychiatry 2020;177:1168–78.

[57] Yagoda S, Graham C, Simmons A, et al. Long-term safety and durability of effect with a combination of olanzapine and samidorphan in patients with schizophrenia: results from a 1-year open-label extension study. CNS Spectr 2021;26:383–92.

[58] Kahn RS, Silverman BL, DiPetrillo L, et al. A phase 3, multicenter study to assess the 1-year safety and tolerability of a combination of olanzapine and samidorphan in patients with schizophrenia: Results from the ENLIGHTEN-2 long-term extension. Schizophr Res 2021;232:45–53.

[59] Alkermes. Alkermes announces commercial availability of LYBALVI® for the treatment of schizophrenia and bipolar I disorder. 2021. Available at: https://www.prnewswire.com/news-releases/alkermes-announces-commercial-availability-of-lybalvi-for-the-treatment-of-schizophrenia-and-bipolar-i-disorder-301401658.html. Accessed March 18, 2022.

[60] Nuplazid. Prescribing information. Acadia Pharmaceuticals. 2020. Available at: https://www.accessdata.fda.gov/drugsatfda_docs/label/2020/207318s010lbl.pdf. Accessed March 20, 2022.

[61] Abbas A, Roth BL. Pimavanserin tartrate: a 5-HT2A inverse agonist with potential for treating various neuropsychiatric disorders. Expert Opin Pharmacother 2008;9:3251–9.

[62] Ballard C, Foff EP, Tariot P, et al. Impact of pimavanserin on cognitive measures in patients with neurodegenerative disease (NDD): results from 4 placebo-controlled clinical studies [abstract]. Neurology 2021;96(15 Suppl):2369.

[63] Meltzer HY, Elkis H, Vanover K, et al. Pimavanserin, a selective serotonin (5-HT)2A-inverse agonist, enhances the efficacy and safety of risperidone, 2mg/day, but does not enhance efficacy of haloperidol, 2mg/day: comparison with reference dose risperidone, 6mg/day. Schizophr Res 2012;141:144–52.

[64] Cummings J, Isaacson S, Mills R, et al. Pimavanserin for patients with Parkinson's disease psychosis: a randomised, placebo-controlled phase 3 trial. Lancet 2014;383:533–40.

[65] Guevarra JT, Hiensch R, Varga AW, et al. Pitolisant to treat excessive daytime sleepiness and cataplexy in adults with narcolepsy: rationale and clinical utility. Net Sci Sleep 2020;12:709–19.

[66] Wakix package insert. Summary of product characteristics. Bioprojet Pharma; 2016. Available at: https://www.accessdata.fda.gov/drugsatfda_docs/label/2020/211150_Orig2s000lbl.pdf. Accessed March 20, 2022.

[67] Dauvilliers Y, Bassetti C, Lammers GJ, et al, HARMONY I Study Group. Pitolisant versus placebo or modafinil in patients with narcolepsy: a double-blind, randomised trial. Lancet Neurol 2013;12:1068–75.

[68] Szakacs Z, Dauvilliers Y, Mikhaylov V, et al, HARMONY-CTP Study Group. Safety and efficacy of pitolisant on cataplexy in patients with narcolepsy: a randomised, double-blind, placebo-controlled trial. Lancet Neurol 2017;16:200–7.

[69] Dauvilliers Y, Arnulf I, Szakacs Z, et al, HARMONY III Study Group. Long-term use of pitolisant to treat patients with narcolepsy: Harmony III Study. Sleep 2019;42:zsz174.

[70] Azstarys. Prescribing information. Corium. 2021. Available at: https://www.accessdata.fda.gov/drugsatfda_docs/label/2021/212994s000lbl.pdf. Accessed March 20, 2022.

[71] Kollins SH, Braeckman R, Guenther S, et al. A randomized, controlled laboratory classroom study of serdexmethylphenidate and d-methylphenidate capsules in children with attention-deficit/hyperactivity disorder. J Child Adolesc Psychopharmacol 2021;31:597–609.

[72] Markham A. Solriamfetol: first global approval. Drugs 2019;79:785–90.

[73] Schweitzer PK, Rosenberg R, Zammit GK, et al, TONES Study Investigators. Solriamfetol for excessive sleepiness in obstructive sleep apnea (TONES 3). A randomized controlled trial. Am J Respir Crit Care Med 2019;199:1421–31.

[74] Javaheri S, Javaheri S. Update on persistent excessive daytime sleepiness in OSA. Chest 2020;158:776–86.

[75] Edinoff AN, Akuly HA, Wagner JH, et al. Viloxazine in the treatment of attention deficit hyperactivity disorder. Front Psychiatry 2021;12:789982.

[76] Mathew BM, Nguyen H. Viloxazine. In: StatPearls. Treasure Island. FL: StatPearls Publishing; 2021. Available at: https://www.ncbi.nlm.nih.gov/books/NBK576423/. Accessed January 27, 2022.

[77] Johnson JK, Liranso T, Saylor K, et al. A phase II double-blind, placebo-controlled, efficacy and safety study of SPN-812 (extended-release viloxazine) in children with ADHD. J Atten Disord 2020;24:348–58.

[78] Nasser A, Liranso T, Adewole T, et al. A phase III, randomized, placebo-controlled trial to assess the efficacy and safety of once-daily SPN-812 (viloxazine extended-release) in the treatment of attention-deficit/hyperactivity disorder in school-age children. Clin Ther 2020;42:1452–66.

[79] Leal GC, Bandeira ID, Correia-Melo FS, et al. Intravenous arketamine for treatment-resistant depression: open-label pilot study. Eur Arch Psychiatry Clin Neurosci 2021;271:577–82.

[80] Browne CA, Jacobson ML, Lucki I. Novel targets to treat depression: opioid-based therapeutics. Harv Rev Psychiatry 2020;28:40–59.

[81] Gunduz-Bruce H, Silber C, Kaul I, et al. Trial of SAGE-217 in patients with major depressive disorder. N Engl J Med 2019;381:903–11.

[82] Rosenblat JD, McIntyre RS. Efficacy and tolerability of minocycline for depression: a systematic review and meta-analysis of clinical trials. J Affect Disord 2018;227:219–25.

[83] Sanches M, Quevedo J, Soares JC. New agents and perspectives in the pharmacological treatment of major depressive disorder. Prog Neuropsychopharmacol Biol Psychiatry 2021;106:110157.

[84] Caroff SN. Recent advances in the pharmacology of tardive dyskinesia. Clin Psychopharmacol Neurosci 2020;18:493–506.

[85] Abyadeh M, Gupta V, Gupta V, et al. Comparative analysis of aducanumab, zagotenemab and pioglitazone as targeted treatment strategies for Alzheimer's disease. Aging Dis 2021;12:1964–76.

[86] Bowen RL, Perry G, Xiong C, et al. A clinical study of lupron depot in the treatment of women with Alzheimer's disease: preservation of cognitive function in patients taking an acetylcholinesterase inhibitor and treated with high dose lupron over 48 weeks. J Alzheimers Dis 2015;44:549–60.

[87] Sen A, Akinola M, Tai XY, et al. An Investigation of Levetiracetam in Alzheimer's Disease (ILiAD): a double-blind, placebo-controlled, randomised crossover proof of concept study. Trials 2021;22:508.

[88] Grauer SM, Pulito VL, Navarra RL, et al. Phosphodiesterase 10A inhibitor activity in preclinical models of the positive, cognitive, and negative symptoms of schizophrenia. J Pharmacol Exp Ther 2009;331:574–90.

[89] Schwartz MD, Canales JJ, Zucchi R, et al. Trace amine-associated receptor 1: a multimodal therapeutic target for neuropsychiatric diseases. Expert Opin Ther Targets 2018;22:513–26.

[90] Sacchi S, Rosini E, Pollegioni L, et al. D-amino acid oxidase inhibitors as a novel class of drugs for schizophrenia therapy. Curr Pharm Des 2013;19:2499–511.

[91] Capuzzi E, Caldiroli A, Ciscato V, et al. Experimental serotonergic agents for the treatment of schizophrenia. J Exp Pharmacol 2021;13:49–67.

[92] Sunosi. Prescribing information. Jazz Pharmaceuticals. Available at: https://www.accessdata.fda.gov/drugsatfda_docs/label/2019/211230_Orig1Orig2s000lbl.pdf, 2019. Accessed April 22, 2022

[93] Qelbree. Prescribing information. Supernus Pharmaceuticals. Available at: https://www.accessdata.fda.gov/drugsatfda_docs/label/2021/211964s000lbl.pdf, 2021. Accessed April 22, 2022.

[94] Austedo. Prescribing information. Teva Neuroscience. Available at: https://www.accessdata.fda.gov/drugsatfda_docs/label/2017/208082s000lbl.pdf, 2017. Accessed April 22, 2022.

9780323920155